Artificial Intelligence in Modeling and Simulation

Artificial Intelligence in Modeling and Simulation

Editors

Nuno Fachada
Nuno David

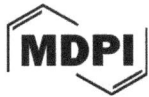

Basel • Beijing • Wuhan • Barcelona • Belgrade • Novi Sad • Cluj • Manchester

Editors
Nuno Fachada
COPELABS
Lusófona University
Lisboa
Portugal

Nuno David
DINÂMIA'CET
Iscte—Instituto Universitário
de Lisboa
Lisboa
Portugal

Editorial Office
MDPI AG
Grosspeteranlage 5
4052 Basel, Switzerland

This is a reprint of articles from the Special Issue published online in the open access journal *Algorithms* (ISSN 1999-4893) (available at: https://www.mdpi.com/journal/algorithms/special_issues/AI_Model_Simu).

For citation purposes, cite each article independently as indicated on the article page online and as indicated below:

Lastname, A.A.; Lastname, B.B. Article Title. *Journal Name* **Year**, *Volume Number*, Page Range.

ISBN 978-3-7258-1517-3 (Hbk)
ISBN 978-3-7258-1518-0 (PDF)
doi.org/10.3390/books978-3-7258-1518-0

Cover image courtesy of Nuno Fachada

© 2024 by the authors. Articles in this book are Open Access and distributed under the Creative Commons Attribution (CC BY) license. The book as a whole is distributed by MDPI under the terms and conditions of the Creative Commons Attribution-NonCommercial-NoDerivs (CC BY-NC-ND) license.

Contents

About the Editors vii

Preface ix

Nuno Fachada and Nuno David
Artificial Intelligence in Modeling and Simulation
Reprinted from: *Algorithms* 2024, 17, 265, doi:10.3390/a17060265 1

Eva Holasova, Radek Fujdiak and Jiri Misurec
Comparative Analysis of Classification Methods and Suitable Datasets for Protocol Recognition in Operational Technologies
Reprinted from: *Algorithms* 2024, 17, 208, doi:10.3390/a17050208 5

Mattia Neroni, Massimo Bertolini and Angel A. Juan
A Biased-Randomized Discrete Event Algorithm to Improve the Productivity of Automated Storage and Retrieval Systems in the Steel Industry
Reprinted from: *Algorithms* 2024, 17, 46, doi:10.3390/a17010046 25

Ken Jom Ho, Ender Özcan and Peer-Olaf Siebers
Efficient Multi-Objective Simulation Metamodeling for Researchers
Reprinted from: *Algorithms* 2024, 17, 41, doi:10.3390/a17010041 45

Ștefan Ionescu, Camelia Delcea, Nora Chiriță and Ionuț Nica
Exploring the Use of Artificial Intelligence in Agent-Based Modeling Applications: A Bibliometric Study
Reprinted from: *Algorithms* 2024, 17, 21, doi:10.3390/a17010021 72

Rajiv Paudel and Arika Ligmann-Zielinska
A Largely Unsupervised Domain-Independent Qualitative Data Extraction Approach for Empirical Agent-Based Model Development
Reprinted from: *Algorithms* 2023, 16, 338, doi:10.3390/a16070338 110

Elizabeth Hunter and John. D. Kelleher
Validating and Testing an Agent-Based Model for the Spread of COVID-19 in Ireland
Reprinted from: *Algorithms* 2022, 15, 270, doi:10.3390/a15080270 126

Kara Combs, Adam Moyer and Trevor J. Bihl
Uncertainty in Visual Generative AI
Reprinted from: *Algorithms* 2024, 17, 136, doi:10.3390/a17040136 148

Wenny Hojas-Mazo, Francisco Maciá-Pérez, José Vicente Berná Martínez, Mailyn Moreno-Espino, Iren Lorenzo Fonseca and Juan Pavón
Framework Based on Simulation of Real-World Message Streams to Evaluate Classification Solutions
Reprinted from: *Algorithms* 2024, 17, 47, doi:10.3390/a17010047 168

Md. Monirul Islam, Md. Belal Hossain, Md. Nasim Akhtar, Mohammad Ali Moni and Khondokar Fida Hasan
CNN Based on Transfer Learning Models Using Data Augmentation and Transformation for Detection of Concrete Crack
Reprinted from: *Algorithms* 2022, 15, 287, doi:10.3390/a15080287 183

Olivier Pantalé
Comparing Activation Functions in Machine Learning for Finite Element Simulations in Thermomechanical Forming
Reprinted from: *Algorithms* **2023**, *16*, 537, doi:10.3390/a16120537 . . . . **200**

Angel E. Muñoz-Zavala, Jorge E. Macías-Díaz, Daniel Alba-Cuellar and Antonio Guerrero-Díaz-de-León
A Literature Review on Some Trends in Artificial Neural Networks for Modeling and Simulation with Time Series
Reprinted from: *Algorithms* **2024**, *17*, 76, doi:10.3390/a17020076 . . . . **222**

About the Editors

Nuno Fachada

Dr. Nuno Fachada is an Assistant Professor at Universidade Lusófona-Centro Universitário de Lisboa (UL-CUL) in Lisbon, Portugal, and a researcher at the COPELABS research unit. He teaches Programming, Research Software, and Artificial Intelligence across Undergraduate, Master's, and Doctoral programs.

Dr. Fachada's research interests focus on modeling and simulation, artificial intelligence, research software, and computer science education. He earned his Electrical and Computer Engineering degree from Instituto Superior Técnico (IST) in Lisbon in 2005, followed by a Master's degree in 2008 with a thesis on immune system simulation from the same institute. In 2016, he completed his Ph.D. at IST with a dissertation titled "Agent-Based Modeling on High-Performance Computing Architectures," receiving the highest distinction, "Pass with Distinction and Honour". Following a postdoctoral research position at LaSEEB/ISR, Dr. Fachada joined UL-CUL, where he continues to contribute to his fields of expertise.

Nuno David

Dr. Nuno David is a professor at Iscte-Instituto Universitário de Lisboa (Iscte-IUL). He teaches "Professional Ethics, Computing, and Society" and the Ethics and Privacy module in the "Security, Ethics, and Privacy" course for the Master's in Computer Engineering and the Bachelor's in Data Science programs. He serves as the Data Protection Officer at Iscte-IUL.

Dr. David's research interests include social simulation, agent-based models, computational ethics, privacy, data protection, computer science philosophy, the epistemology of computational social sciences, and the implications of computational and interdisciplinary approaches for theories and methodologies in social sciences.

He holds a Bachelor's degree in Computer Engineering from the University of Coimbra and a Master's and Ph.D. in Computer Science from the University of Lisbon and the University of São Paulo, Brazil.

Preface

This Special Issue on "Artificial Intelligence in Modeling and Simulation" addresses the integration of AI in improving the accuracy and efficiency of simulation models across various domains. The collection, featuring contributions from leading researchers, investigates AI-driven optimization, data processing, and agent-based modeling, often focusing on model validation. Aimed at researchers and practitioners, this issue offers valuable insights into AI applications in modeling and simulation. We acknowledge the contributions of the authors and the efforts of the reviewers and editorial team in bringing this work to completion.

Nuno Fachada and Nuno David
Editors

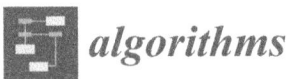 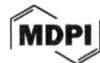

Editorial

Artificial Intelligence in Modeling and Simulation

Nuno Fachada [1],* and Nuno David [2]

1 COPELABS, Lusófona University, 1749-024 Lisboa, Portugal
2 DINÂMIA'CET-Iscte, 1649-026 Lisboa, Portugal; nuno.david@iscte-iul.pt
* Correspondence: nuno.fachada@ulusofona.pt

1. Introduction

Modeling and simulation (M&S) serve as essential tools in various scientific and engineering domains, enabling the representation of complex systems and processes without the constraints of physical experimentation [1]. These tools have evolved significantly with the integration of artificial intelligence (AI), which offers advanced capabilities in essential aspects of M&S such as optimization [2,3], data analysis [4,5], and verification and validation [6]. AI's capacity to enhance M&S is demonstrated in applications ranging from engineering [7] and physics [8,9] to social sciences [10] and biology [11], providing novel approaches to problem-solving and system understanding.

In this Special Issue, entitled "Artificial Intelligence in Modeling and Simulation", we received 18 submissions from researchers worldwide. After a rigorous peer-review process, 11 papers were selected for publication, reflecting the diversity and depth of current research in the combined fields of AI and M&S. These papers encompass a wide range of topics, including the use of AI in developing and optimizing simulation models, AI-driven metamodeling, and the application of AI techniques in various domains such as industrial systems, agent-based modeling (ABM), and public health.

2. Contents

The accepted submissions can be broadly grouped into four main categories: (1) AI techniques for simulation and optimization [2,3], (2) AI in ABM [12], (3) AI for data processing and classification models [13], and (4) Artificial Neural Network (ANN) methods for improved M&S [14]. These are organized as follows:

AI techniques for simulation and optimization

1. Comparative Analysis of Classification Methods and Suitable Datasets for Protocol Recognition in Operational Technologies (2024), by Holasova et al., in *Algorithms* 17:208, https://doi.org/10.3390/a17050208.
2. A Biased-Randomized Discrete Event Algorithm to Improve the Productivity of Automated Storage and Retrieval Systems in the Steel Industry (2024), by Neroni et al., in *Algorithms* 17:46, https://doi.org/10.3390/a17010046.
3. Efficient Multi-Objective Simulation Metamodeling for Researchers (2024), by Ho et al., in *Algorithms* 17:41, https://doi.org/10.3390/a17010041.

AI in ABM

4. Exploring the Use of Artificial Intelligence in Agent-Based Modeling Applications: A Bibliometric Study (2024), by Ionescu et al., in *Algorithms* 17:21, https://doi.org/10.3390/a17010021.
5. A Largely Unsupervised Domain-Independent Qualitative Data Extraction Approach for Empirical Agent-Based Model Development (2023), by Paudel et al., in *Algorithms* 16:338, https://doi.org/10.3390/a16070338.
6. Validating and Testing an Agent-Based Model for the Spread of COVID-19 in Ireland (2022), by Hunter et al., in *Algorithms* 15:270, https://doi.org/10.3390/a15080270.

AI for data processing and classification models

7. Uncertainty in Visual Generative AI (2024), by Combs et al., in *Algorithms* 17:136, https://doi.org/10.3390/a17040136.
8. Framework Based on Simulation of Real-World Message Streams to Evaluate Classification Solutions (2024), by Hojas-Mazo et al., in *Algorithms* 17:47, https://doi.org/10.3390/a17010047.
9. CNN Based on Transfer Learning Models Using Data Augmentation and Transformation for Detection of Concrete Crack (2022), by Islam et al., in *Algorithms* 15:287, https://doi.org/10.3390/a15080287.

ANN methods for improved M&S

10. Comparing Activation Functions in Machine Learning for Finite Element Simulations in Thermomechanical Forming (2023), by Pantalé, in *Algorithms* 16:537, https://doi.org/10.3390/a16120537.
11. A Literature Review on Some Trends in Artificial Neural Networks for Modeling and Simulation with Time Series (2024), by Muñoz-Zavala et al., in *Algorithms* 17:76, https://doi.org/10.3390/a17020076.

These publications are described in detail in the following subsections, one per subject category.

2.1. AI Techniques for Simulation and Optimization

Several papers focus on the integration of AI techniques to enhance simulation and optimization processes.

In *Comparative Analysis of Classification Methods and Suitable Datasets for Protocol Recognition in Operational Technologies*, Holasova et al. analyze different machine learning methods for protocol recognition in operational technology (OT) networks, addressing the unique challenges of OT environments and highlighting the need for relevant datasets.

Neroni et al. present a hybrid approach in *A Biased-Randomized Discrete Event Algorithm to Improve the Productivity of Automated Storage and Retrieval Systems in the Steel Industry*, combining discrete event simulation with biased-randomized heuristics to minimize makespan in automated storage and retrieval systems, showcasing significant improvements over traditional methods.

In *Efficient Multi-Objective Simulation Metamodeling for Researchers*, Ho et al. introduce a methodology for multi-objective optimization using metamodels and heuristics, demonstrating the varying performance of different metamodel–optimizer pairs across several problem scenarios.

2.2. AI in Agent-Based Modeling

The application of AI within ABM is addressed in three studies featured in this Special Issue.

Ionescu et al. provide a bibliometric analysis in *Exploring the Use of Artificial Intelligence in Agent-Based Modeling Applications: A Bibliometric Study*, revealing trends and influential research in the convergence of these fields, with significant growth observed post 2006.

Paudel and Ligmann-Zielinska propose a novel approach in *A Largely Unsupervised Domain-Independent Qualitative Data Extraction Approach for Empirical Agent-Based Model Development*, using natural language processing tools to automate qualitative data extraction for ABM, reducing biases and improving efficiency.

Hunter and Kelleher detail the validation of an ABM in *Validating and Testing an Agent-Based Model for the Spread of COVID-19 in Ireland*, utilizing a scaling factor to manage computational costs while maintaining model accuracy in simulating pandemic dynamics.

2.3. AI for Data Processing and Classification Models

The potential of AI in improving data processing and classification models is demonstrated by three articles included in this Special Issue.

In the first of these articles, *Uncertainty in Visual Generative AI*, Combs et al. address the issue of uncertainty in generative AI models, proposing a pipeline to quantify uncertainty and improve model reliability.

In the following article, *Framework Based on Simulation of Real-World Message Streams to Evaluate Classification Solutions*, Hojas-Mazo et al. develop a simulation-based framework for enhancing the evaluation of message classification solutions under realistic conditions.

In the third article, *CNN Based on Transfer Learning Models Using Data Augmentation and Transformation for Detection of Concrete Crack*, Islam et al. focus on structural health monitoring in leveraging transfer learning and CNNs for accurate and efficient crack detection in concrete structures.

2.4. Artificial Neural Network Architectures and Methodologies for Improved Modeling and Simulation

ANNs are powerful tools for improving model efficiency and validity. The two final papers in this Special Issue address this theme, demonstrating the effectiveness of ANNs in complex simulation scenarios.

Pantalé investigates the impact of different activation functions on prediction accuracy and computational efficiency in *Comparing Activation Functions in Machine Learning for Finite Element (FE) Simulations in Thermomechanical Forming*.

Finally, Muñoz-Zavala et al. review trends in *A Literature Review on Some Trends in Artificial Neural Networks for Modeling and Simulation with Time Series*, summarizing ANN applications in time series prediction and suggesting future research directions.

3. Final Remarks

These papers highlight the substantial progress and varied uses of AI in modeling and simulation, offering useful insights and methods for both researchers and practitioners. The Editors thank all authors, reviewers, and the editorial team in making this Special Issue possible.

Author Contributions: Special Issue Editorial by N.F. and N.D. All authors have read and agreed to the published version of the manuscript.

Funding: This work was funded by Fundação para a Ciência e a Tecnologia under grants CEECINST/00002/2021/CP2788/CT0001 and UIDB/04111/2020.

Acknowledgments: The Editors would like to thank the authors of the submitted manuscripts and the reviewers for their contributions. The Editors would also like to thank the Managing Editor and supporting MDPI staff for their help in publishing this Special Issue.

Conflicts of Interest: The authors declare no conflicts of interest.

Abbreviations

The following abbreviations are used in this manuscript:

ABM	Agent-Based Modeling
AI	Artificial Intelligence
ANN	Artificial Neural Network
FE	Finite Elements
M&S	Modeling and Simulation
OT	Operational Technology

References

1. Law, A.M. *Simulation Modeling and Analysis*, 5th ed.; McGraw-Hill: Columbus, OH, USA, 2015.
2. Bakhtiyari, A.N.; Wang, Z.; Wang, L.; Zheng, H. A review on applications of artificial intelligence in modeling and optimization of laser beam machining. *Opt. Laser Technol.* **2021**, *135*, 106721. https://doi.org/10.1016/j.optlastec.2020.106721.
3. de la Torre, R.; Corlu, C.G.; Faulin, J.; Onggo, B.S.; Juan, A.A. Simulation, optimization, and machine learning in sustainable transportation systems: Models and applications. *Sustainability* **2021**, *13*, 1551. https://doi.org/10.3390/su13031551.

4. Zhu, H. Big data and artificial intelligence modeling for drug discovery. *Annu. Rev. Pharmacol. Toxicol.* **2020**, *60*, 573–589. https://doi.org/10.1146/annurev-pharmtox-010919-023324.
5. Fachada, N.; Lopes, V.V.; Martins, R.C.; Rosa, A.C. Model-independent comparison of simulation output. *Simul. Model. Pract. Theory* **2017**, *72*, 131–149. https://doi.org/10.1016/j.simpat.2016.12.013.
6. David, N.; Fachada, N.; Rosa, A.C. Verifying and Validating Simulations. In *Simulating Social Complexity: A Handbook*; Edmonds, B., Meyer, R., Eds.; Springer International Publishing: Berlin/Heidelberg, Germany, 2017; pp. 173–204. https://doi.org/10.1007/978-3-319-66948-9_9.
7. Wagg, D.; Worden, K.; Barthorpe, R.; Gardner, P. Digital twins: State-of-the-art and future directions for modeling and simulation in engineering dynamics applications. *Asce-Asme J. Risk Uncertain. Eng. Syst. Part B Mech. Eng.* **2020**, *6*, 030901. https://doi.org/10.1115/1.4046739.
8. Willard, J.; Jia, X.; Xu, S.; Steinbach, M.; Kumar, V. Integrating scientific knowledge with machine learning for engineering and environmental systems. *ACM Comput. Surv.* **2022**, *55*, 1–37. https://doi.org/10.1145/3514228.
9. Hennigh, O.; Narasimhan, S.; Nabian, M.A.; Subramaniam, A.; Tangsali, K.; Fang, Z.; Rietmann, M.; Byeon, W.; Choudhry, S. NVIDIA SimNet™: An AI-accelerated multi-physics simulation framework. In *Computational Science—ICCS 2021*; Lecture Notes in Computer Science; Springer: Berlin/Heidelberg, Germany, 2021; Volume 12746, pp. 447–461. https://doi.org/10.1007/978-3-030-77977-1_36.
10. David, N.; Sichman, J.S.; Coelho, H. The Logic of the Method of Agent-Based Simulation in the Social Sciences: Empirical and Intentional Adequacy of Computer Programs. *J. Artif. Soc. Soc. Simul.* **2005**, *8*, 2.
11. Fages, F. Artificial intelligence in biological modelling. In *A Guided Tour of Artificial Intelligence Research: Volume III: Interfaces and Applications of Artificial Intelligence*; Springer: Berlin/Heidelberg, Germany, 2020; pp. 265–302. https://doi.org/10.1007/978-3-030-06170-8_8.
12. Fachada, N.; Lopes, V.V.; Martins, R.C.; Rosa, A.C. Towards a standard model for research in agent-based modeling and simulation. *PeerJ Comput. Sci.* **2015**, *1*, e36. https://doi.org/10.7717/peerj-cs.36.
13. Ghahramani, M.; Qiao, Y.; Zhou, M.C.; O'Hagan, A.; Sweeney, J. AI-based modeling and data-driven evaluation for smart manufacturing processes. *IEEE CAA J. Autom. Sin.* **2020**, *7*, 1026–1037. https://doi.org/10.1109/JAS.2020.1003114.
14. Legaard, C.; Schranz, T.; Schweiger, G.; Drgoňa, J.; Falay, B.; Gomes, C.; Iosifidis, A.; Abkar, M.; Larsen, P. Constructing neural network based models for simulating dynamical systems. *ACM Comput. Surv.* **2023**, *55*, 1–34. https://doi.org/10.1145/3567591.

Disclaimer/Publisher's Note: The statements, opinions and data contained in all publications are solely those of the individual author(s) and contributor(s) and not of MDPI and/or the editor(s). MDPI and/or the editor(s) disclaim responsibility for any injury to people or property resulting from any ideas, methods, instructions or products referred to in the content.

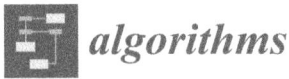

Article

Comparative Analysis of Classification Methods and Suitable Datasets for Protocol Recognition in Operational Technologies

Eva Holasova *, Radek Fujdiak * and Jiri Misurec

Department of Telecommunications, Faculty of Electrical Engineering and Communication, Brno University of Technology, Technicka 12, 616 00 Brno, Czech Republic; misurec@vut.cz
* Correspondence: eva.holasova@vut.cz (E.H.); fujdiak@vut.cz (R.F.)

Abstract: The interconnection of Operational Technology (OT) and Information Technology (IT) has created new opportunities for remote management, data storage in the cloud, real-time data transfer over long distances, or integration between different OT and IT networks. OT networks require increased attention due to the convergence of IT and OT, mainly due to the increased risk of cyber-attacks targeting these networks. This paper focuses on the analysis of different methods and data processing for protocol recognition and traffic classification in the context of OT specifics. Therefore, this paper summarizes the methods used to classify network traffic, analyzes the methods used to recognize and identify the protocol used in the industrial network, and describes machine learning methods to recognize industrial protocols. The output of this work is a comparative analysis of approaches specifically for protocol recognition and traffic classification in OT networks. In addition, publicly available datasets are compared in relation to their applicability for industrial protocol recognition. Research challenges are also identified, highlighting the lack of relevant datasets and defining directions for further research in the area of protocol recognition and classification in OT environments.

Keywords: classification methods; datasets; machine learning; operational technology; protocol classification; protocol recognition; security

Citation: Holasova, E.; Fujdiak, R.; Misurec, J. Comparative Analysis of Classification Methods and Suitable Datasets for Protocol Recognition in Operational Technologies. *Algorithms* 2024, 17, 208. https://doi.org/10.3390/a17050208

Academic Editors: Nuno Fachada and Nuno David

Received: 31 March 2024
Revised: 8 May 2024
Accepted: 9 May 2024
Published: 11 May 2024

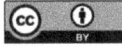

Copyright: © 2024 by the authors. Licensee MDPI, Basel, Switzerland. This article is an open access article distributed under the terms and conditions of the Creative Commons Attribution (CC BY) license (https://creativecommons.org/licenses/by/4.0/).

1. Introduction

Cyber security is now an essential part of industrial networks. As a result of the interconnection of Operational Technology (OT) and Information Technology (IT), new possibilities for remote management, the use of cloud storage, real-time data transfer over long distances, or integration between different OT and IT networks, for example, are emerging. On the other hand, there are new security risks to which OT networks are exposed [1]. OT networks used to be completely isolated from IT networks, so there was not much emphasis on cyber security [2]. For this reason, there is a new emphasis on monitoring and analyzing OT traffic.

Protocol recognition and classification is an important task in security control and can be conducted via data analysis [3]. Knowledge of the protocols used in the network contributes to network optimization and helps to understand how traffic is distributed and what data are present in the network. Based on protocol recognition and data classification, traffic routes can be optimized, the quality of traffic and transmitted data can be improved, and network management strategies can be developed. Based on the automatic inspection of traffic data, redundant messages can be filtered, and the volume of transmitted messages can be reduced, thereby reducing the computational complexity and cost of transmission. In terms of network security, the use of protocol recognition leads to earlier and timely detection of threats, for example, in the case of a Man in the Middle attack. It is also possible to detect and find a virus early. There is a large number of methods that can be used to achieve protocol identification both in IT and OT networks. It is possible to use traditional methods, which include classification based on ports used, or more sophisticated approaches using Artificial Intelligence (AI). Using such approaches, it is possible to perform an in-depth analysis of the monitored data stream (or other data units) and classify not only the protocol used but also, for example, the cipher suite used. Performing classification in OT networks is currently less common, but it provides great potential in terms of security benefits for such networks. It is for this reason that this paper has been created, in order to describe and summarize the different protocol classification methods (especially in OT networks) and also the available datasets.

This paper focuses on the protocol recognition aspects of OT networks. Advanced methods using AI techniques can be used to perform protocol recognition with additional recognition capability. Conventional techniques, such as relying on known ports, may not be fully sufficient and thus more advanced techniques that are able to directly detect/recognize the protocol itself (trained marks of the protocol) need to be employed. Based on the analysis of the current state of the art, it is clear that the recognition of industrial protocols is rather minor, as is the current state of publicly available datasets. Thus, this paper points out this gap (research gap), and for this reason, it performs (i) a summarization of methods for network traffic classification, (ii) a summarization of methods for recognition and identification of the protocol used in the network, (iii) the use of machine learning methods for industrial protocol recognition. Finally, (iv) an analysis of publicly available datasets that can be used for industrial protocol classification was performed. This article takes aim at the scientific question: How can industrial protocol classification be achieved? What publicly available datasets can currently be used specifically for the purpose of classifying these protocols? OT networks require increased attention due to IT and OT convergence, in particular, due to the increased risk of cyber-attacks that may target these networks. Convergence has caused, among other things, a proliferation of attack vectors, making advanced data monitoring necessary and using a software-as-a-service (SaaS) approach. Industrial protocol classification thus enables (i) automatic detection of the protocol used to assess security, including the cipher suite used, (ii) diagnostic data, network monitoring (protocol usage within different sectors, etc.), (iii) automation of audit tools, and (iv) development of protocol adaptive solutions—automatic protocol detection and further actions following this knowledge.

The structure of this paper is as follows: Section 2 describes the specifics of OT networks, the effects of the convergence of IT and OT networks, and, hence, the need to use sophisticated methods to enhance security in the OT industry. Section 3 presents an analysis and comparison of the current state of the art, focusing mainly on the issues of protocol recognition and traffic classification. Furthermore, Section 4 presents various methods for the purpose of traffic analysis. The section presents approaches to protocol classification, recognition and identification, Machine Learning (ML) methods, and metrics used to evaluate models. Section 5 focuses on the available datasets usable for the purpose of traffic classification and the chosen protocol, and a comparison of the most relevant datasets in terms of several parameters is also provided.

2. Operational Technology Networks Specifics

A significant difference between classical IT networks and OT networks is their purpose and related use. OT networks have the main purpose of controlling and monitoring the industrial process, whereas IT networks aim mainly at data transmission (by nature non-critical in comparison with OT networks). Another distinction is the elements and components of the individual networks themselves. IT networks use end stations (laptops, desktop PCs, mobiles, tablets, etc.). Network elements and infrastructure provide data transfer mainly between end-user elements using data stored on servers (located and connected to the Internet). On the other hand, OT networks typically use specific devices with a well-defined purpose to provide/monitor a specific activity within an industrial process. These can be single active/passive elements (actuators and sensors), control PLCs, HMIs (providing visualization of the current process status to the operator), or SCADA/DCS components. Another difference is the data transmitted itself and the typical orientation of the data flow. Within IT, it is mainly the use of data obtained from higher layers (Internet) and its local modification/processing/consumption by the user. OT networks mainly generate data from sensors and perform operations by actuators. Thus, the data occurring in an industrial network mainly contains data acquired from sensors (temperature, pressure, speed—numerical data), and based on these data, actuators (motors, pumps, valves—binary state I/O) are activated/deactivated [4].

Another major difference is the security of individual networks. IT networks are evolving at a very fast pace, the lifetime of equipment within IT networks is typically 3–5 years (servers, workstations, laptops and network components), and the frequency of updates is also very high. Systems and software are regularly updated and upgraded to improve performance, security, and functionality. In terms of basic requirements, the priority is security, i.e., confidentiality of data, followed by data integrity, with availability (CIA triad) coming in third. Thus, it is necessary to transfer the data primarily in a confidential manner (encryption), ensuring their integrity (preserving the content without modification), followed by their availability (slight delays and outages are tolerated to provide more critical services—there is no security risk not to deliver the message immediately). In contrast, OT networks are completely identical in these aspects. Development within OT is slow and gradual, equipment lifetimes are typically 10–20 years (i.e., decades), so the frequency of updates is conducted at large intervals (industrial process is affected—creating downtime and slowing production efficiency). Systems often require long-term stability and reliability, which means that updates or changes are made less frequently to avoid the risk of disrupting critical operations [4].

In terms of basic requirements, the priority is data and service availability, followed by integrity and thirdly confidentiality (AIC triad). It is, therefore, necessary to have available data from the industrial process at all times to be able to monitor and manage the process adequately and in a timely manner. This is important because of the nature of OT networks, where critical parts are controlled and where there is a risk of malfunction or danger to human health in the event of a process disturbance (nuclear power plants, thermal power plants, etc.). It is also necessary that data integrity is preserved, and only after these tears are preserved is the safety considered. IT and OT networks differ in the nature of the services they provide in terms of their importance. They differ in terms of priorities and especially in terms of the security of the data transmitted. They also differ in the subject/scope of the data transmitted. They also differ in the individual elements of the network. Another difference is the upgrades performed, where OT is significantly more complex than IT, as well as the replacement/upgrade of equipment (OT requires a higher lifetime).

2.1. Information Technology and Operational Technology Convergence

IT and OT convergence represent the current trend of interconnection of individual components, especially their availability via the Internet. This convergence involves the integration of existing OT networks and structures within the IT network. This convergence facilitates the use of the current trend of software as a service, especially for the processing and evaluation of available data, where this was often not possible before, and data could not leave the closed and isolated network. It is equally possible to remotely access and manage these data. While this brings a number of benefits, it also involves challenges that need to be addressed, particularly from the security perspective. The problem is the long-term enclosure of OT infrastructures, which has ensured security in terms of physical security. In order to access the assets, it was necessary to overcome physical security, and only then could the assets be accessed. It is convergence, however, that significantly alters this approach. There is no need to overcome physical security, and it is possible to access assets from a SW perspective without breaching the security perimeter (from a physical perspective).

Convergence increases the risk of a security incident compared to a closed approach [2]. Due to the long-term closed nature and reliance on physical security alone, security mechanisms and protocols are not at the same level as in IT networks. OT networks use industrial protocols for the transmission of individual data, which are specific protocols tailored for the transmission of sensor data and individual commands. However, these protocols often do not support confidentiality and integrity, and thus, various extensions and additional mechanisms have to be used. Thus, from a software perspective, OT networks represented insecurity by design. The challenges involved are to ensure the security of the unsecured protocol in such a way that the priorities of the requirements (availability first) are not affected. Thus, it is not possible to use current mechanisms from IT networks and apply them directly to the OT network environment without modification. Similarly, a secure separation of the IT and OT network must be implemented in such a way that the OT network is maximally separated from the rest of the network. This requires the use of firewalls, DMZ, IDS, and IPS mechanisms in conjunction with AI-enabled applications.

The impacts of the convergence of IT and OT networks include a significant proliferation of attack vectors. Convergence has made these networks "accessible" to the attacker, and physical security is no longer the main security measure. Thus, it is now (from a cyber-security perspective) a basic block that is as necessary as it used to be but no longer represents the main attack vector. Attackers can exploit the very interface that makes the connection between IT and OT networks. In particular, this may include internal services for managing and monitoring industrial processes [5]. In conjunction with these systems and devices, in general, within OT networks there are passphrases and inbuilt security measures. Insufficient quality/complexity of passphrases and excessive system measures also degrade cyber-security. The human factor is also a risk, especially in terms of social engineering or phishing attacks. According to [5], the first place in the attack vector is the compromise of IT systems, followed by the use of engineering workstations, and the third place is external remote services.

Protocol classification will help, especially with protocol security checks in the form of internal audits, etc. Knowledge of the protocols will also help with diagnostic data and obtaining an overview of the traffic occurring within the monitored OT networks. Finally, the development of a good industrial protocol classification method will help with the development of new devices. It is the automatic protocol recognition that will enable the creation of devices that automatically recognize the protocol in the network and can use this knowledge to, for example, automatically inspect and set firewall rules. In order to best secure the OT network, these approaches need to be combined. It is necessary to use tools for detecting security incidents, classifying the protocols used, as well as educating the human factor. The emergence of automated tools would enable effective control (auditing) and also the supervision of critical network elements. Industrial protocol classification can be used at individual industrial facilities (factories, plants, etc.), but also within various SaaS service providers, which can monitor and classify traffic within the network. Last but not least, this method can be used to perform non-invasive security checks of industrial protocols without the need to access the data themselves directly. It is thus possible to use the encrypted form of the messages and to perform protocol classification on this basis, including its cipher suite.

The early detection of security incidents helps to activate adequate countermeasures. Using the knowledge of the type of anomaly, it is possible to activate appropriate countermeasures so that the impact on the industrial process itself is minimized. This is related to the critical nature of the industrial processes themselves, where system shutdown can mean potential damage. It is thus advisable to perform a timely, safe system shutdown. However, the aim is to prevent such safety incidents. To do just that, it is advisable to use industrial protocol classification in the form of a security audit and implement appropriate countermeasures to minimize the likelihood of a security threat.

2.2. Operational Technology Hierarchy Model

The individual physical operations and related control and monitoring components are sorted according to IEC 62443 [6] (also known as the Purdue model) into individual layers (six in total). This division is made according to the purpose of each layer so that individual operations can be scaled and safety levels defined within the manufacturing process. Communication within the model is vertical between the layers to achieve effective control and monitoring of the process. The layers closer to the product itself (processed through the L0 layer) form the core and basic building blocks of OT networks. As the layers grow, they gain abstraction and gradually move into the IT network. The individual layers contain differently sensitive information, and therefore, it is necessary to maintain an adequate trust level (preferably zero-trust) [7]. A graphical visualization of such a model is shown in Figure 1, which shows the Purdue model as well as the basic blocks from the RAMI 4.0 model (right side). Level 0 (Field level) contains components directly dedicated to control, the actual execution of an activity using sensors (getting values) and actuators (executing activities).

Data sent to/from L0 is conducted from the L1 layer (Control level). This layer contains the individual Programmable Logic Controller (PLC), Distributed Control System (DCS), and PID devices. These are the components that acquire data from sensors and actuators (simplified as the first logic unit that evaluates the acquired data and can convert them into digital form). These units directly control the process through the connected actuators. The decision to intervene in the process can be initiated directly from L1 or by devices from L2 (Supervisory level) [4].

Within L2 there are parent PLCs that collect data from the slave PLCs and make process modifications based on the defined operations/schemes and settings. This layer (L2) also houses workstations (operator/attendant workstations) and the local Human Machine Interface (HMI), which is used to display the current status to the operator. The process can thus be controlled via the HMI, workstations, or status evaluation by the supervisor PLC from L2, then the data are passed to the PLCs on the L1 level, and they trigger the required actions on L0.

The fourth layer (L3—Planning level) serves mainly as a support layer for the whole system. Global HMI and other server services can be located within this layer. This may include Dynamic Host Configuration Protocol (DHCP), Domain Name System (DNS), Lightweight Directory Access Protocol (LDAP), and Network Time Protocol (NTP) servers. In addition, historian servers are often located at this level to provide specific services such as storing historical data (describing the behavior and state of the process over time), analyzing stored values, and archiving events/process states over time. This layer also contains Supervisory Control and Data Acquisition (SCADA) or DSC.

Both systems are used for data acquisition from the OT network and process control. The main objective of SCADA is data acquisition; networks consist of multiple Remote Terminal Units (RTUs) that are used to collect data back to the central control system where they can be used to make higher-level decisions (based on a global view of the data). DCS is mainly used for on-site process control, connecting PLCs, sensors/actuators state, and workstations. The main objective is to collect data and control the process from devices located closer to L0. The main difference between DCS and SCADA is, therefore, in their focus and application. DCS is more focused on automating and controlling manufacturing processes within a single facility or complex, while SCADA focuses on monitoring and controlling equipment spread over large areas with an emphasis on data collection and surveillance.

Layer L4, as well as L5 can be referred to as the management level. L4 is used to provide scheduling and provisioning of other local services (e.g., printing, web server, or domain controller), so it is the Plant operational level. This layer can also contain a historian mirror and a remote access server. In general, Manufacturing Execution Systems (MES) are software solutions that actively improve the quality and efficiency of manufacturing processes.

The L5 layer focuses on enterprise applications and Enterprise Resource Planning (ERP). However, the L4 and L5 layers are very intertwined.

This model can also be supplemented with a layer that vertically connects all the layers. This concept is referred to as NAMUR Open Architecture (NOA) [8]. The aim is to enable secure, flexible, and efficient interconnection of OT with IT without compromising the functioning of critical process control systems. This may involve the collection of data from additional sensors located on the equipment. Where these devices cannot directly compromise the process itself (there is no direct connection between the sensors and the OT infrastructure), there is a one-way data flow from OT to IT.

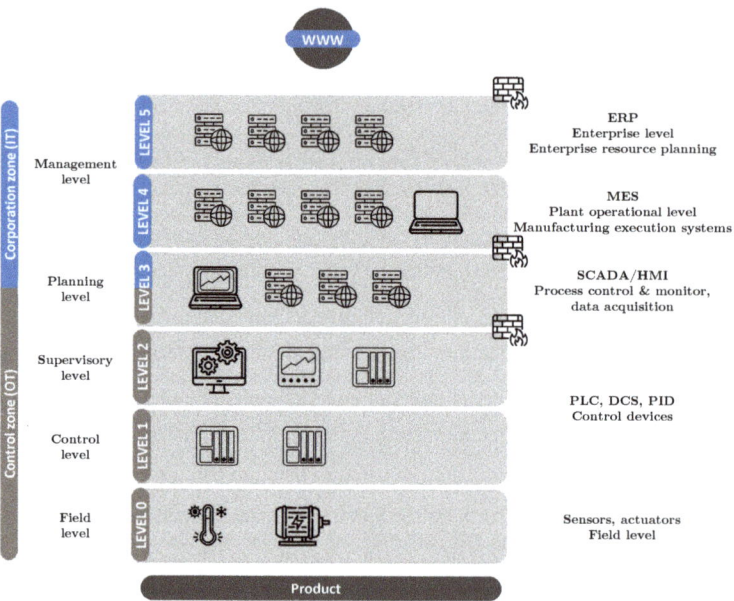

Figure 1. Hierarchical structure within OT networks expressed through the Purdue model.

For completeness, it should be noted that the term OT refers to hardware and software that directly monitors and controls physical equipment, processes and events in an industrial environment. OT includes Industrial Control Systems (ICS), which are specifically designed to control and automate industrial processes. ICS includes a variety of systems, including SCADA or DCS. OT networks have different requirements compared to IT networks. This is due to the nature of these networks and, in particular, their purpose. In the development of these networks, it is necessary to use up-to-date approaches such as ML and NN techniques, both for the detection of security incidents (traffic classification) and for the recognition and identification of the industrial protocols used. The convergence of IT and OT networks is putting pressure on the security of these networks, but it is always necessary to consider the appropriateness of individual measures in such a way that the functionality of the OT networks themselves is not compromised. The use of ML and NN techniques has the potential to enhance the security of OT networks and, in particular, can be used in such a way that they do not cause additional load to these networks. If used appropriately, a non-invasive way of using the available data can be achieved.

3. State of the Art

Protocol classification provides benefits, especially for automatic processing and automatic monitoring of data on the network. The use of classification in OT brings the benefits of enabling the development of protocol-independent approaches, especially in the area of cybersecurity. Therefore, it enables the automated management of data flows, the creation and modification of detection and mitigation rules, etc. Table 1 shows an overview of the current approaches to protocol recognition and traffic classification in both IT and OT industries. In general, supervised approaches, e.g., machine learning and neural networks, are required in classification. A common approach is the use of convolutional neural networks, where data streams, frames, or other data structures are visualized into image data and these are then identified through convolutional neural networks.

In general, traffic classification is also more common than protocol recognition. Protocol classification can be more challenging than traffic classification (this is evident from the success rates achieved by the models). Performing protocol classification in the OT sector is particularly important in the case of encrypted traffic. In the case of encryption, it is not possible to use common (generic) protocol identification methods, such as known port recognition at the transport layer level, or to use multiple parsers to find a match. Due to IT and OT convergence, it is also necessary to assume different masking techniques performed by the attacker, also for this reason, these classification methods are very important. Similarly, in the case of protocol recognition in OT, it is possible to recognize not only the industrial protocol itself but also other parameters, such as the type of cipher suite chosen.

In total, a comparison of 20 different approaches is made, where protocol recognition in OT networks is only addressed in a minimum of current literature, and most of them target IT networks. In the case of traffic classification, the ratio is more balanced. In the case of protocol recognition, OT networks are particular and present a significant challenge due to their distinct differences. Similarly, a small number of publicly available datasets focus on this issue. Finally, it often relies only on selected ports at the transport layer level. AI methods are not used in the case of protocol recognition in OT networks, even though these methods can represent a great cyber benefit (especially in connection with Industry 4.0+). A large number of works have focused on traffic classification in IT and OT networks. Most of the works focus on cyber-security with the aim of network anomaly detection/classification. This approach (traffic classification) thus represents the implementation of a classification of the data transmitted inside a chosen traffic protocol.

For classification reasons, a supervised approach is generally used, often in combination with convolutional neural networks (CNNs). This approach represents a method in which data blocks are expressed using visual representation, i.e., the conversion of information into image data. This may be processing at the level of data streams, packets, or other data units. Some papers also focus on the encrypted data stream (encoding column). This area presents great potential from the cybersecurity perspective, where it is possible to perform traffic recognition without having to decrypt the traffic. This can be particularly beneficial when processing large amounts of data, for example, at the network administrator level or for the purpose of monitoring whether industrial data are leaving specified sections. Also, most approaches do not focus on real-time classification, but delay-independent classification is performed. It is the low delay in the classification performed that allows the use of these methods (protocol recognition, traffic classification) in the control mechanisms performing the classification of the actual network traffic. Often, authors do not provide datasets, so the classification of the protocol or network traffic is performed on a dataset that is not publicly available. Thus, it is not possible to re-evaluate the results, directly relate the results to the obtained results, or compare different approaches for classification purposes. Custom (own) datasets that are no longer available bring significant limitations in the development and comparison of available tools and approaches.

Based on the analysis of the current state of the art, the main challenges can be identified as (i) the creation of suitable and publicly available datasets that are oriented towards industrial protocols. These datasets must also contain multiple industry protocols in order to validate the discriminative capabilities of each approach. Furthermore, (ii) focusing on the potential in the area of encrypted traffic (protocols) in OT networks. (iii) Comparing the different processing approaches of the developed dataset and identifying the main research direction.

Table 1. Comparison of relevant literature in protocol recognition and traffic classification from the perspective of IT and OT infrastructures.

Methods	Type	Year	Technique	Model	ML Type	Protocols	Encoding	Real-Time	Epochs	Layers	Accuracy [%]	Datasets	Ref.
Protocol recognition	OT	2021	CNN	AM-ADCNN + LSTM	Supervised	4	No	No	20	-	93.0	Own	[9]
		2023	DNN	PREIUD	Unsupervised	1	No	No	-	-	-	Own	[10]
		2011	Network Packet Inspection	Deterministic Finite-state Automaton	-	9	No	No	-	-	-	Own	[11]
		2012	Fingerprinting	-	-	4	No	Yes	-	-	95.0	Own	[12]
		2017	CNN + RNN	CNN + RNN-2a	Supervised	15	No	No	60–90	9	99.6	RedIRIS [13]	[14]
	IT	2020	CNN	PtrCNN	Supervised	4	No	Yes	20	8	96–100	DARPA [15]	[16]
		2020	CNN	-	Both	3	No	No	-	-	75.8–89.8	Own	[17]
		2021	Pattern matching algorithm	-	Supervised	4	No	No	-	-	93.8–100	DARPA [15]	[18]
		2021	CNN	ICLSTM	Supervised	12	Yes	No	-	-	97.5	ISCX 2016 [19]	[20]
		2023	CNN	-	Supervised	8	Yes	No	-	-	98.2	ISCX VPN-nonVPN [19]	[21]
		2019	ML	DT, KNN, SVM, NB	Supervised	1	Yes	No	-	-	95.0	Own	[22]
		2019	Traffic Fingerprinting	CART	-	-	No	No	-	-	94.8	SWaT [23], SCADA Network Data Sets for Intrusion Detection Research [24]	[25]
Traffic classification	OT	2020	ML	KNN, SVM, DT, NBG, BKNN, BT, RF, AdaBoost, GB	Both	1	No	No	-	-	99.7	Own	[26]
		2022	DNN	-	Supervised	1	Yes	No	100	10	94.5	Own	[27]
		2022	ML	DT	Supervised	2	No	No	-	-	99.9	Own	[28]
		2022	RNN	-	Supervised	1	No	No	-	-	97.5	Own	[29]
		2009	ML	C4.5, AdaBoost, NB, SVM, RIPPER	Supervised	8	Yes	No	-	-	98.4	DARPA [15], AMP [30], MAWI [31]	[32]
	IT	2017	CNN	1D-CNN	Supervised	12	Yes	No	40	7	99.5	ISCX VPN-nonVPN [19]	[33]
		2018	CNN	CNN-LSTM	Supervised	9	Yes	No	30	8	91.0	ISCX VPN-nonVPN [19]	[34]
		2021	Fuzzy Inference System	Fuzzy Inference System	-	6	Yes	Yes	-	-	90.9	ISCXVPN2016 [33]	[35]

A "-" indicates points that were not included in the publication.

4. Traffic Analysis Methods

Protocol Classification is a term typically used to describe the process by which network traffic is classified into different categories or classes based on the characteristics of the communication. Classification can be made based on factors such as ports, addresses, packet headers, or traffic patterns. Classification aims to understand network traffic better and allow different levels of network management policy to manage this traffic as needed.

Protocol Recognition is a term usually used to describe the process by which the characteristics of network communications are analyzed to identify the protocols in use. This process can be automated using a variety of techniques, including in-depth examination of network traffic and pattern matching against a database of known protocols. The goal is to identify what protocols are used within a given communication.

Protocol Identification is a term often used as a synonym for protocol recognition, but it can also be used in a more specific sense when referring to the process of determining specific attributes or properties of a protocol that are observed in a given network traffic. Protocol identification can be important for a number of purposes, including security analysis, network optimization, and performance tuning.

4.1. Traffic Classification Technique

Several methods for traffic classification exist, each handling traffic information differently. These techniques are port-based classification, payload-based classification, statistical-based classification, behavioral-based classification, and correlation-based classification [36,37].

The port-based classification method is widely used for classifying traffic using the ports of the corresponding applications. The method is based on examining packet headers and comparing port numbers of registered applications. Examining only the packet headers presents a fast and simple classification [36]. This type of classification is especially important for identifying network applications in large network traffic [36]. The false negative rate increases because of dynamic port numbers and the use of non-standard applications. Similarly, if applications are hidden behind a commonly known port, the false positive rate increases. In general, this classification method is fast and simple, provided the applications are used with their usual ports [37].

The payload-based classification method mainly uses the packet's data content for protocol recognition. The payload information contains characteristic patterns, messages, or protocol-specific data structures [36]. Payload-based classification can be divided into Deep Packet Inspection (DPI) and Stochastic Packet Inspection (SPI) [37]. DPI works with network traffic and packet content and achieves high accuracies in traffic classification, making it a well-known technique for traffic management, attack prevention, and overall network security analysis [37,38]. SPI is a technique complementary to DPI for classifying encrypted traffic. This method works with statistical payload information to create a pattern of protocol behavior and then automatically distinguish it from other protocols. This method achieves high accuracy in classifying encrypted data. However, it is complex and computationally intensive [38]. The method represents a slight improvement over the port-based classification method but does not achieve higher accuracy in high-speed networks. The significant disadvantage of this method is network privacy. Since the method uses data inside the packet, the confidentiality of the transmitted data and network security policies are violated.

The statistical-based classification method, unlike the packet-based method and the payload-based method, does not work with information inside the packet but measures statistical traffic parameters. Based on these statistical traffic parameters, it is possible to distinguish between different types of applications [36]. These parameters include the minimum packet size, the maximum packet size, the mean packet size, and the number of packets, etc. [37]. This method is also known as the rational-based classification method [36]. The advantage of this method is that it can efficiently recognize encrypted traffic without violating privacy. The disadvantage is a large number of parameters, which may be redundant for classification and introduce errors in training and testing machine learning models used for pattern search in large datasets [9].

The behavioral-based classification method is based on generating and analyzing host-side communication and traffic patterns. It performs classification by observing the host behavior in the network [36]. Assuming a large amount of data, this method achieves high classification accuracy [37].

The correlation-based classification method is based on creating correlations between individual data streams. Data flows are created by aggregating packets with the same attributes, such as source and destination IP address, source and destination port, and protocol used. This method is used in training and testing machine learning models to find relationships and data features. This method avoids the problem of the large number of features. However, it still poses a large computational cost [37].

4.2. Network Protocol Recognition and Identification Techniques

The basic principle in protocol recognition and identification is to extract important traffic information from the traffic, based on which the protocol can be identified. There are several methods that can be combined in protocol recognition and identification.

One division is into manual and automatic analysis. Manual analysis depends on the knowledge and experience of the person who performs the analysis [9]. Automatic analysis is based on the automatic extraction of protocol information from network traffic. Based on the extracted information, patterns of protocol behavior are created, and the techniques that enable automatic analysis create and operate on these patterns. Recognition by automatic analysis can be performed using several techniques, namely preset rules recognition, payload feature recognition, host behavior, and machine learning [9].

The preset rules recognition technique works with set rules such as port number. This method is not very reliable in terms of user customization of network settings. The payload features technique takes advantage of the deep packet inspection method, which means that it recognizes protocols using the data inside the packets. This method is very simple and easy to implement, but it cannot identify encrypted traffic and is computationally intensive. The host behavior technique works based on statistical parameters of network traffic. The method effectively avoids the process of extracting information from packets. However, the results are often inaccurate due to non-standard traffic parameters [37].

Machine learning is an important artificial intelligence technique that is used to analyze large-volume datasets based on features and associations between parameters [9]. Machine learning can be divided into shallow learning and deep learning. Shallow learning is used for modeling and analyzing. These are algorithms that cannot fully express complex nonlinear problems. At the same time, the quality of data preparation is crucial and affects the training and results of the model. Deep learning algorithms are able to solve more complex nonlinear problems. The disadvantage of classification based on shallow learning is that the feature extraction and learning process must be repeated after the dataset is changed. In deep learning-based classification, the model does not always need to be re-learned and takes advantage of the original parameters. Shallow learning algorithms include Support Vector Machine (SVM), Naive Bayes (NB), etc. Deep learning algorithms include deep neural networks, Long Short Term Memory algorithms [39], and Generative Adversarial Networks algorithms [16].

The use of deep learning methods has its application in IoT applications [40]. These methods can be used not only for anomaly detection within industrial networks but also for various operations requiring a high level of abstraction and the ability to understand complex structures.

4.3. Machine Learning Techniques for Traffic Classification

There are several types of learning: supervised learning, unsupervised learning, and reinforcement learning. In supervised learning, the processed data are labeled in advance to improve the learning process and improve the final model. In teacher-less learning, data are unlabeled and patterns are sought during the learning process by clustering the data. Feedback learning works with an agent that replaces human operators and helps determine the outcome (build a model) based on feedback [9,41].

Machine learning algorithms work with three types of data training, validation, and testing. Training and validation data form the dataset that is used to learn the model. With the help of training data, the model is created, and with the help of validation data, the model is tested during the learning process to improve the model. After the model is created/learned, the model is tested on the test dataset. Partitioning into these groups can be conducted, for example, by cross-validation. The dataset must be balanced to avoid incorrect model learning or lack of model validation [16].

Each algorithm analyzes the dataset in a different way using regression, classification, clustering, time series, association, or anomaly detection. Examples of such algorithms are linear or logistic regression, Naive Bayes algorithm, SVM, Random Forest algorithm (RF), Gradient Boosting (GB), K-Means, K-Nearest Neighbors (KNN) or Decision Tree (DT) [16].

K-means clustering is one of the popular machine-learning techniques. It belongs to the category of unsupervised learning and aims to identify unlabeled data in different clusters. The dataset and the number of clusters by which the data will be identified are essential for the proper functioning of this algorithm. Clustering consists of three parts, namely K-cluster, distance function, and new centroid. The advantage of this method is its simple implementation. The disadvantage is the sensitivity of the method to outliers [36].

K-Nearest Neighbors is a method used to determine the distance between features for classification and regression. This technique belongs to the category of supervised learning. The advantage of this method is that it is simple and suitable for problems with multiple classifications. The disadvantages of this technique are poor performance for unbalanced datasets and high computational cost.

Naive Bayes is a robust machine learning classifier for classification and belongs to the supervised category. The method is based on the Bayes Network Theorem and is used to solve complex classification and traffic identification problems. The method has many variations that use attributes for more accurate classification. The advantage of this method is high accuracy even with inaccurate data. The disadvantage is that the required attributes are independent of each other [36,37].

Support Vector Machine is another robust machine learning method. This technique is used to classify the traffic of large amounts of data. The technique is based on hyperplane separation to achieve binary classification and is classified as supervised learning. The advantage of this method is that it can solve nonlinear and high-dimensional problems. The disadvantage of this method is the high memory cost [37].

Decision Tree is a technique belonging to the supervised learning group. Decision Tree consists of a root node, several branches, and many leaves. C4.5 and ID3 machine learning classifiers are used to construct the Decision Tree. This technique is used to classify the target variable by determining the relationship and matching between attributes and creating new variables. The advantage of this method is fast classification with little computation. The disadvantage is the ease of overfitting the model when using high dimensional data because it does not correlate with these data [36].

Random Forest is a technique composed of many decision trees that fall into the same category as supervised learning. This method's advantages include a fast training phase and the fact that it is not easy to overfit due to the already mentioned large number of Decision Trees. The disadvantage is that it is unsuitable for low-dimensional and small datasets [36].

Logistic regression (LR) is a supervised learning technique. It is used for binary classification and uses general linear regression. The advantage of this method is the fast training phase and the possibility of dynamic adjustment of the classification threshold. The disadvantage of this method is easy overfitting [37].

AdaBoost is used to create a multi-classifier by integrating several weaker classifiers. By combining several classifiers and using their advantages together, the technique is able to achieve high classification accuracy. Additionally, there is no overfitting. However, the technique is sensitive to outliers [37].

Neural networks are based on the structure of the human nervous system. The basis of a neural network is a neuron or perceptron. These basic elements are interconnected and transmit signals to each other. Neurons form networks composed of layers. Networks are made up of an input layer, inner hidden layers, and an output layer. How inputs are converted to outputs depends on the value of weights, thresholds, transformation function, and network structure. The process in question is neural network learning. Neural network learning, as with machine learning, can be conducted with a teacher (supervised) or without a teacher (unsupervised). If a neural network has multiple layers, it is referred to as a Deep Neural Network (DNN). These algorithms include Convolutional Neural Networks (CNN) [41], Recurrent Neural Networks (RNN) [29], and Artificial Neural Networks (ANN) [16].

Table 2 makes a comparison of the most well-known and some of the most used ML approaches. These are mainly supervised approaches (this is due to the nature of having to perform partitioning into known, predefined classes). Each method has defined advantages and disadvantages. ML approaches represent an effective solution when classification needs to be performed, usually with sufficient recognition capabilities (metrics). The advantage over other approaches is the relative ease of use and the equally short time required to train the model. However, the individual results are strongly influenced by the chosen task/problem and equally strongly dependent on the chosen dataset (size, purity of records, etc.). The AdaBoost approach is deliberately not shown in the table, due to the fact that it is a combination of these approaches in order to achieve the highest quality results (metrics). Neural networks represent a more sophisticated approach that can achieve more quality metrics depending on the chosen task and, in particular, the quality of the dataset, thus creating a more robust model capable of representing more challenging structures. These approaches are well suited for large data volumes and more complex problems. However, this approach requires appropriate structure and individual parameter design (especially DNN approaches) and is also a more time and computationally intensive operation. Another advantage is that NN approaches are suitable for so-called transfer learning, where model "learning" and specific data (in this case industrial protocols) are performed. This results in a more robust model.

Table 2. Comparison of ML methods for protocol recognition.

Methods	Type	Description	Advantages	Disadvantages
K-mean	Unsupervised	Identify unlabeled data in different clusters	Simple implementation	Sensitivity to outliers
K-NN	Supervised	Determine the distance between features	Simple and suitable for classification	High computational cost
NB	Supervised	Bays Network Theorem; Complex classification	High accuracy	Required attributes are independent of each other
SVM	Supervised	Hyperplane separation for binary classification	Can solve nonlinear and high-dimensional problems	High memory cost
DT	Supervised	Classify the target variable	Fast classification	Ease of overfit
RF	Supervised	Algorithm composed of many decision trees	Fast training phase; Not easy to overfit	Unsuitable for low-dimensional and small datasets
LR	Supervised	General linear regression	Fast training phase; Not easy to overfit	Easy to overfit

4.4. Metrics for Machine Learning Model Evaluation

In order to evaluate machine learning models, it is necessary to use evaluation metrics [37,42]. These metrics numerically express the model's ability to perform defined activities, such as classification. The most basic case is binary classification, where a mapping of an input to just two outputs (0 or 1) is performed. If 1 is marked as a positive outcome (for example, a classified attack), four situations can occur:

- True Positive (TP)—(1 = 1)—the input is an attack, and the output of the model is classified as an attack,
- True Negative (TN)—(0 = 0)—the input is regular traffic, and the model output is classified as regular traffic,
- False Positive (FP)—(0 ≠ 1)—the input is regular traffic, and the output of the model is classified as an attack,
- False Negative (FN)—(1 ≠ 0)—the input is an attack, and the output of the model is classified as regular traffic.

These metrics are further used to calculate other auxiliary evaluation metrics [42]. Visualizations of the underlying metrics can be made in the form of a Confusion Matrix, which is used to provide a basic representation of the ratio of each group. Additional metrics are then typically calculated based on this matrix. Accuracy is a metric that defines the comprehensive success rate of the model and is defined as the ratio of TP and TN to the total number of classified entries; see Equation (1). This metric can be described as a definition of how good a model is and its recognition capabilities. Precision is a metric that is defined as the ratio of TP to the sum of TP and FP; see Equation (2). This metric is described as the accuracy of the model, i.e., whether the recognition capabilities are correct and whether it produces coherent results. Recall is a metric also referred to as True Positive Rate or Sensitivity and is the ratio of TP to the sum of TP and FN; see Equation (3). It is an indicator of the completeness of the model's detection of positive cases. Precision focuses on the accuracy of positive predictions, while Recall evaluates the ability of the model to detect as many true positive cases (TP) as possible. The F1 score metric provides a composite view of how accurate the model is, not only in its accuracy but also in its ability to identify TPs using the Precision and Recall metrics, see Equation (4). This metric aids model assessment, especially in cases where the dataset is unbalanced and where separate Precision and Recall values could be misleading.

$$Accuracy = \frac{TP + TN}{TP + FP + TN + FN} \; [-], \qquad (1)$$

$$Precision = \frac{TP}{TP + FP} \; [-], \qquad (2)$$

$$TPR; Sensitivity; Recall = \frac{TP}{TP + FN} \; [-], \qquad (3)$$

$$F1\ score = 2 \cdot \frac{Precision \cdot Recall}{Precision + Recall} \; [-]. \qquad (4)$$

Another metric used is the False Positive Rate (FPR) $\frac{FP}{FP+TN}$. This metric defines the false positive rate (FP) to all actually negative cases, how the model misinterprets negative cases as positives. False Negative Rate (FNR) $\frac{FN}{FN+TP}$. Metric defines the rate of false negative cases to all actually positive cases, how the model misinterprets positive cases as negatives. The True Negative Rate or also Specificity (TNR) metric $\frac{TN}{TN+FP}$ gives the ratio of actual negative cases to all true negative cases, and how well the model can detect negative situations or events.

The TPR and FPR indicators are further used to represent graphically in the form of a Receiver Operating Characteristic (ROC) curve of the model capabilities. FPR is plotted on the X-axis, and TPR is plotted on the Y-axis. The objective is to plot the threshold values to find a compromise between the high Sensitivity (TPR) and low FPR. The resulting Area Under the Curve (AUC) allows for the assessment of the model performance (a larger AUC implies a better AI model).

As the number of recognized classes increases (input data are classified into more groups, for example, identifying a specific type of attack), it is possible to approach accuracy from different perspectives [37]. Thus, it is possible to obtain an overall accuracy, which indicates the general ability of the classification model regardless of the specific class (number/measure of appropriately labeled samples regardless of the class). Class accuracy indicates the accuracy achieved relative to a specific class (some classes may achieve higher accuracy than others—this can identify strong/weak points of the model, hence the dataset). It is also possible to relate accuracy to the data flow itself (correlation-based classification methods) or byte accuracy. Byte accuracy focuses on individual bytes (even within a flow) [37].

5. Industrial Datasets Analysis

Datasets can be used for research in machine learning and neural networks. These datasets are used to train artificial intelligence tools and allow for the evaluation of different processing approaches [41].

This is possible just with a public dataset because it allows us to compare different approaches on an identical dataset. Thus, it is possible to identify suitable approaches such as the algorithm itself, its settings (hyperparameters), the preprocessing, or the representation of the dataset within AI processing.

AI development can also be performed on a custom dataset, but there is a risk of dataset deficiencies such as inconsistency (data may be recorded in an inappropriate way), incompleteness/diversity (not all possible states are included), duplication (dataset contains duplicate records), imbalance (representation of individual classes is not even), size (dataset is too small). Due to these problems/deficiencies, the developed AI algorithm can paradoxically achieve high portability, but in the case of practical use, such a tool is very limited (or overtraining may occur).

For this reason, datasets are published providing identical data on which the different approaches can be evaluated. However, published datasets often run into privacy issues. Thus, it is necessary to check the individual data within the dataset and ensure consent, anonymize the data, or generate the dataset in a closed/protected environment where sensitive information cannot be leaked.

Datasets can be stored in various data formats, the most common of which is the Comma-Separated Values (CSV) format or the network traffic record—PCAP format. Where the CSV format is more strict in terms of available information (features), the PCAP format allows parsing a wide range of information. Another important aspect of datasets is the documentation available. The documentation should include a complete description of the dataset, including a description of the main components (IP addresses, transport ports, etc.), in particular, the number of classes and the way the dataset is labeled, especially in the case of the CSV format. In the case of the PCAP format, it is important to uniquely identify the individual states that occurred in the record (especially in cyber-security)—e.g., identify the attacker, their IP address, ports, time horizon, type of attack, etc. Other useful data are the wiring/schema used to generate the dataset, tools used, etc.

Table 3 performs a comparison of publicly available datasets and makes comparisons from several perspectives. A comparison of the IT/OT focus of the dataset is made; the number of classes into which classification is made, the number of features (for CSV format only), and the format of the dataset is given. It also found whether the dataset is time-series data, whether the dataset is labeled, and the type of classification (anomalies—cyber-security attacks, protocol classification, OT anomalies). In addition, whether the dataset is cyber-security focused, the source is indicated, whether it is a real record or a simulation, and the protocol (IT represents common IT protocols). Last but not least, the number of records (CSV only) and whether documentation is available.

A total of 28 datasets were compared, where 17 datasets fall into the IT sector and 11 into the OT sector. Sixteen datasets are recorded as PCAP and 17 as CSV. Similarly, 17 datasets focus on time-series. The analysis also shows that a large part of the datasets focuses on the problem and anomalies as well as binary classification. The datasets directly targeting the problem of protocol analysis and classification form a very small part, with three datasets out of 17 in IT and only one dataset out of 11 in OT. The bulk is also not recorded directly in the real environment, which is due to the general focus on anomaly identification (or classification), but the recording is as close as possible to the real environment using simulated parts. All datasets contain documentation but often do not contain all the necessary information.

The analysis shows that the majority of available public datasets are focused on cybersecurity issues, while the classification of protocols is minimal. This may also be due to the distinct individuality of individual plants and industries. To this end, it is thus nontrivial to use the available datasets and to use only normal/regular data flow, thus reducing the dataset size considerably. Another aspect is the availability of public datasets, where some datasets are difficult to access, and it is necessary to be a subscriber.

In addition, datasets are available from the OT environment that contain only sensory data. Thus, these datasets cannot be directly used for the detection of industrial hazards but only for the detection or classification of security incidents within a given workplace. These datasets may include, among others, those mentioned in [43]. However, signal data cannot be used for protocol classification purposes, and anomaly detection may be strongly associated with a given workplace. It is necessary to train the AI model on just the specific states that can be "accepted"/assumed in a given environment.

Thus, based on the analysis performed, individual challenges were identified in order to classify the industrial protocols:

(i) create a representative and comprehensive dataset using an industrial protocol,
(ii) to use real industrial networks and devices to get closer to real applications,
(iii) to allow modification or change of the industrial protocol (within the dataset)—protocol diversity.

Fulfilling these challenges will thus enable research into methods to classify industrial protocols, the protocol versions used, and the cipher suites of encrypted protocol versions used. In the case of using the same workstation with only a change of industrial protocol, it is possible to focus only on the protocol itself, without the influence of the transmitted data on the industrial protocol classification performed (the protocol classification will not be directly influenced by the transmitted data).

A total of 28 datasets were compared in the analysis, with most of them focusing only on a specific part and, in particular, on areas of cyber security anomalies. The classification of the protocols themselves is very limited, especially in the OT area. In the case of the use of IT protocols, typical IT protocols such as HTTP, HTTPS, DNS, FTP, ICMP, IMAP, POP3, etc., are often used. In the case of OT protocols, these are typically Modbus, IEC 60870-5-104, and DNP3. There is also a range of sensor data (data obtained from the L0 Purdue model—data obtained from sensors and actuators). However, these data are intended for anomaly detection in terms of the behavior of individual states and do not contain the protocol itself (they are only application data or values of individual variables). In terms of size (records, volume parameter in Table 3), the individual datasets vary considerably, and in the case of the PCAP source, this value is variable depending on what data are parsed. Dataset balance has not been considered in the table because many datasets do not provide predefined training and test sets (separate datasets). It is the train/test split parameter that may be crucial and, as such, it may be a target of research.

Table 3. Overview of the most relevant datasets for machine learning and neural network research.

Link	Name of Dataset	Year	IT/OT	Classes	Feature Count	Format	Time-Series	Labeled	Classification of	Cyber-sec.	Source	Protocol	Volume	Docu.
[15]	DARPA	1998	IT	2	NR	PCAP	Yes	No	Anomaly	Yes	Real *	IT	-	Yes
[44]	KDD Cup 1999	1999	IT	5	41	CSV	No	Yes	Anomaly	Yes	Simulated	-	4,000,000	Yes *
[31]	MAWI/Wide/Keio	2000	IT	?	NR	PCAP	Yes	Yes *	Protocol	No	Real *	IT	-	Yes *
[45]	CAIDA	2008	IT	?	NR	PCAP	Yes	No	Protocol	No	Real	IT	-	Yes *
[46]	NSL-KDD	2009	IT	2	41	CSV	No	Yes	Anomaly	Yes	Simulated	-	148,000	Yes
[47]	MAWILab	2010	IT	4	NR	PCAP	Yes	Yes	Anomaly	Yes	Real *	IT	-	Yes
[48]	ISCX-IDS-2012	2012	IT	2	NR	PCAP	Yes	Yes	Anomaly	Yes	Real *	IT	-	Yes
[49]	CTU-13	2014	IT	3	NR	PCAP; BIGARUS	Yes	Yes	Anomaly	Yes	Real *	IT	-	Yes
[50]	ISCX-Bot-2014	2014	IT	2	NR	PCAP	Yes	Yes	Anomaly	Yes	Real *	IT	-	Yes
[51]	UNSW-NB15	2015	IT	10	49	CSV	No	Yes	Anomaly	Yes	Real *	IT	2,500,000	Yes
[52]	CTU-Mixed (capture 1–8)	2015	IT	2	NR	PCAP; BIGARUS	Yes	No	Anomaly	Yes	Real	IT	-	Yes
[53]	USTC-TFC2016	2016	IT	20	NR	PCAP	Yes	Yes	Protocol; Anomaly	Yes	Real *	IT	-	Yes
[54]	CIC-IDS-2017	2017	IT	2	78	CSV	No	Yes	Anomaly	Yes	Real *	IT	692,703	Yes
[55]	CAN 2017	2017	IT	4	11	TXT	No	Yes *	OT anomaly	Yes	Real *	CAN	4,613,909	Yes
[54]	CSE-CIC-IDS2018	2018	IT	7	80	CSV	No	Yes	Anomaly	Yes	Real *	IT	16,233,002	Yes
[56]	CIRA-CIC-DoHBrw-2020	2020	IT	2	34	CSV	No	Yes	Anomaly	Yes	Real *	IT	371,836	Yes
[57]	NSS Mirai	2021	IT	11	12	CSV	No	Yes	Anomaly	Yes	Real *	IT	64,025	Yes *
[58]	Electra dataset	2010	OT	4	10	CSV	No	Yes	OT anomaly	Yes	Simulated	Modbus; S7comm	1,048,575	Yes *
[23]	SWAT	2015	OT	2	NR	PCAP; CSV	Yes	Yes	OT anomaly	Yes	Real	Senzoric data	-	Yes *
[19]	ISCX VPN-nonVPN	2016	IT/OT	14	NR	PCAP; CSV	Yes	Yes	Protocol	No	Real *	IT	-	Yes
[59]	Batadal	2016	OT	2	45	CSV	Yes	Yes *	OT anomaly	Yes	Real *	Senzoric data	23,788	Yes *
[24]	Providing SCADA Network Data Sets for Intrusion Detection Research	2016	OT	2	NR	PCAP; CSV	Yes	Yes *	OT anomaly	Yes	Real	Modbus; Senzoric data	-	Yes *
[60]	WADI	2017	OT	2	NR	PCAP; CSV	Yes	Yes	OT anomaly	Yes	Real	Senzoric data	1,221,372	Yes *
[61]	BoT-IoT	2019	OT	5	46	CSV	No	Yes	Anomaly	Yes	Real *	IT	72,000,000	Yes
[62]	DNP3 Intrusion Detection Dataset	2022	OT	?	NR	PCAP; CSV	Yes	Yes	OT anomaly	Yes	?	DNP3	-	Yes *
[63]	CIC Modbus dataset 2023	2023	OT	?	NR	PCAP	Yes	No	Anomaly	Yes	Simulated	Modbus	-	Yes
[64]	IEC 60870-5-104 Intrusion Detection Dataset	2023	OT	?	NR	PCAP; CSV	Yes	Yes	OT anomaly	Yes	?	IEC 60870-5-104	-	Yes *
[65]	HIL-based augmented ICS security	2023	OT	53	225 (HAIEnd)	CSV	No	Yes	OT anomaly	Yes	Real	Senzoric data	?	Yes *

* indicates incomplete fulfilment of the criterion; NR = Not Relevant; ? = unable to find.

6. Discussion

The purpose of this paper was to answer the two main scientific questions presented in the introduction. How can industrial protocol classification be achieved? What publicly available datasets can currently be used specifically to classify these protocols? Classification, recognition, and identification of protocols are closely related techniques that use the same methods. The most commonly used methods for traffic classification and protocol recognition have been presented and compared. Each method has its specific use and depends on the purpose for which it is to be used. Among the state-of-the-art methods are machine learning algorithms and especially neural networks. These algorithms allow for fast traffic classification and protocol recognition and provide high-quality metrics. However, these algorithms are limited in terms of input data. An analysis of the state of the art revealed that the majority of research is in the IT domain. Similarly, research is not targeted at encrypted versions of protocols.

The available datasets often do not achieve the qualities needed for good and accurate classification, such as the number of records, the diversity of records, or the number of logs in the dataset. Currently, the number of datasets from IT environments exceeds the number of datasets. Although it is possible to use some IT protocols in OT systems from the point of view of the convergence of IT and OT networks, it is not advisable to rely on this fact alone. OT networks require specific protocols and requirements that are not as strict in IT networks. Based on the analysis of publicly available datasets, key requirements for future research were identified. Namely, the creation of a representative dataset containing industrial protocols using real industrial devices. Currently, no suitable dataset has been found for protocol recognition research in OT. It is the creation of such a dataset that would enable follow-up research and the comparison of different methods from the ML and NN domains.

7. Conclusions

The issue of protocol recognition and traffic classification is a broad area with overlap from IT to OT networks. In conjunction with the convergence of IT and OT networks, it is necessary to focus on cyber-security within OT networks and to use current techniques from IT and implement them in the OT domain in order to increase the current level of security. Similarly, with the trend of Industry 4.0+, data (not only IT but also OT) are leaving isolated networks for processing on remote servers or for using software as a service. For this reason, this paper has focused on the analysis of different methods and processing of data flow (or other units) for the purpose of protocol recognition and traffic classification in connection with OT specifics. Furthermore, publicly available datasets have been compared in terms of their contribution, usability, etc. The output of this work is thus a comparative analysis of approaches specifically to protocol recognition and traffic classification. The analysis shows that there is currently only a very limited number of publicly available datasets that would allow development in the area of protocol recognition and traffic classification in OT networks. Thus, it is necessary to build on the IT networks and the knowledge gained in the area of protocol recognition and traffic classification in IT networks and, on the basis of a good and robust dataset, to compare these approaches, to make modifications and, in particular, to evaluate them in OT networks.

Author Contributions: Conceptualization, E.H., R.F. and J.M.; methodology, E.H. and R.F.; validation, E.H., R.F. and J.M.; formal analysis, E.H. and R.F.; investigation, E.H.; resources, E.H.; data curation, E.H. and R.F.; writing—original draft preparation, E.H.; writing—review and editing, E.H., R.F. and J.M.; visualization, E.H. and R.F.; supervision, R.F. and J.M.; project administration, R.F. and J.M.; funding acquisition, R.F. All authors have read and agreed to the published version of the manuscript.

Funding: This article is a result of the project FW07010004, which was supported by the Technology Agency of the Czech Republic in the Program TREND.

Data Availability Statement: Data are contained within the article.

Conflicts of Interest: The authors declare no conflicts of interest.

References

1. Santos, M.F.O.; Melo, W.S.; Machado, R. Cyber-Physical Risks identification on Industry 4.0. In Proceedings of the 2022 IEEE International Workshop on Metrology for Industry 4.0 & IoT (MetroInd4.0&IoT), Trento, Italy, 7–9 June 2022; pp. 300–305. [CrossRef]
2. Santos, S.; Costa, P.; Rocha, A. IT/OT Convergence in Industry 4.0. In Proceedings of the 2023 18th Iberian Conference on Information Systems and Technologies (CISTI), Aveiro, Portugal, 20–23 June 2023; pp. 1–6. [CrossRef]
3. Duan, L.; Da Xu, L. Data Analytics in Industry 4.0: A Survey. *Inf. Syst. Front.* 2021, ahead of print. [CrossRef]
4. Knapp, E.D.; Langill, J.T. Chapter 8—Risk and Vulnerability Assessments. In *Industrial Network Security*, 2nd ed.; Knapp, E.D., Langill, J.T., Eds.; Syngress: Boston, MA, USA, 2015; pp. 1–439.
5. Parsons, D. *SANS ICS/OT Cybersecurity Survey: 2023's Challenges and Tomorrow's Defenses, Sans.org*; SANS Institute: Rockville Pike, MD, USA, 2023; pp. 1–19.
6. *ISA-99—Industrial Automation and Control Systems Security*; International Society of Automation (ISA): Pittsburgh, PA, USA, 2007.
7. Perducat, C.; Mazur, D.C.; Mukai, P.; Sandler, S.N.; Anthony, M.J.; Mills, J.A. Evolution and Trends of Cloud on Industrial OT Networks. *IEEE Open J. Ind. Appl.* 2023, 4, 291–303. [CrossRef]
8. Grüner, S.; Trosten, A. A Cloud-Native Software Architecture of NAMUR Open Architecture Verification of Request using OPC UA PubSub Actions over MQTT. In Proceedings of the 2023 IEEE 28th International Conference on Emerging Technologies and Factory Automation (ETFA), Sinaia, Romania, 12–15 September 2023; pp. 1–8. [CrossRef]
9. Zhai, L.; Zheng, Q.; Zhang, X.; Hu, H.; Yin, W.; Zeng, Y.; Wu, T. Identification of Private ICS Protocols Based on Raw Traffic. *Symmetry* 2021, 13, 1743. [CrossRef]
10. Ning, B.; Zong, X.; He, K.; Lian, L. PREIUD: An Industrial Control Protocols Reverse Engineering Tool Based on Unsupervised Learning and Deep Neural Network Methods. *Symmetry* 2023, 15, 706. [CrossRef]
11. Chen, C.; Wang, F.; Lin, F.; Guo, S.; Gong, B. Fast Protocol Recognition by Network Packet Inspection. *Neural Inf. Process.* 2011, 7063, 37–44. [CrossRef]
12. Liu, Q.; Zhang, J.; Zhao, B. Traffic Classification Using Compact Protocol Fingerprint. In Proceedings of the 2012 International Conference on Industrial Control and Electronics Engineering, Xi'an, China, 23–25 August 2012; pp. 147–151. [CrossRef]
13. Vulnerability Databases. *Rediris.es* 2001. Available online: https://www.rediris.es/cert/links/vuldb.html.en (accessed on 21 March 2024).
14. Lopez-Martin, M.; Carro, B.; Sanchez-Esguevillas, A.; Lloret, J. Network Traffic Classifier With Convolutional and Recurrent Neural Networks for Internet of Things. *IEEE Access* 2017, 5, 18042–18050. [CrossRef]
15. Lippmann, R.; Haines, J.W.; Fried, D.J.; Korba, J.; Das, K. Analysis and Results of the 1999 DARPA Off-Line Intrusion Detection Evaluation. *Recent Adv. Intrusion Detect.* 2000, 1907, 162–182. [CrossRef]
16. Feng, W.; Hong, Z.; Wu, L.; Fu, M.; Li, Y.; Lin, P. Network protocol recognition based on convolutional neural network. *China Commun.* 2020, 17, 125–139. [CrossRef]
17. Xue, J.; Chen, Y.; Li, O.; Li, F. Classification and identification of unknown network protocols based on CNN and T-SNE. *J. Phys. Conf. Ser.* 2020, 1617, 012071. [CrossRef]
18. Shi, J.; Yu, X.; Liu, Z.; Niu, B. Nowhere to Hide. *Secur. Commun. Netw.* 2021, 2021, 6672911. [CrossRef]
19. Draper-Gil, G.; Lashkari, A.H.; Mamun, M.S.I.; Ghorbani, A.A. Characterization of Encrypted and VPN Traffic using Time-related Features. In Proceedings of the 2nd International Conference on Information Systems Security and Privacy, Rome, Italy, 19–21 February 2016; pp. 407–414. [CrossRef]
20. Lu, B.; Luktarhan, N.; Ding, C.; Zhang, W. ICLSTM. *Symmetry* 2021, 13, 1080. [CrossRef]
21. Zhu, P.; Wang, G.; He, J.; Chang, Y.; Kong, L.; Liu, J. Encrypted Traffic Protocol Identification Based on Temporal and Spatial Features. In Proceedings of the 2023 4th International Seminar on Artificial Intelligence, Networking and Information Technology (AINIT), Nanjing, China, 16–18 June 2023; pp. 255–262. [CrossRef]
22. de Toledo, T.; Torrisi, N. Encrypted DNP3 Traffic Classification Using Supervised Machine Learning Algorithms. *Mach. Learn. Knowl. Extr.* 2019, 1, 384–399. [CrossRef]
23. Mathur, A.P.; Tippenhauer, N.O. SWaT. In Proceedings of the 2016 International Workshop on Cyber-Physical Systems for Smart Water Networks (CySWater), Vienna, Austria, 11 April 2016; pp. 31–36. [CrossRef]
24. Lemay, A.; Fernandez, J.M. Providing SCADA Network Data Sets for Intrusion Detection Research. In Proceedings of the 9th Workshop on Cyber Security Experimentation and Test (CSET 16), Austin, TX, USA, 8 August 2016.
25. Sheng, C.; Yao, Y.; Yang, W.; Liu, Y.; Fu, Q. How to Fingerprint Attack Traffic against Industrial Control System Network. In Proceedings of the 2019 1st International Conference on Industrial Artificial Intelligence (IAI), Shenyang, China, 23–27 July 2019; pp. 1–6. [CrossRef]
26. Lan, H.; Zhu, X.; Sun, J.; Li, S. Traffic Data Classification to Detect Man-in-the-Middle Attacks in Industrial Control System. In Proceedings of the 2019 6th International Conference on Dependable Systems and Their Applications (DSA), Harbin, China, 23–27 July 2020; pp. 430–434. [CrossRef]

27. Holasova, E.; Fujdiak, R. Deep Neural Networks for Industrial Protocol Recognition and Cipher Suite Used. In Proceedings of the 2022 IEEE International Carnahan Conference on Security Technology (ICCST), Valec, Czech Republic, 7–9 September 2022; pp. 1–7. [CrossRef]
28. Yu, C.; Zhang, Z.; Gao, M. An ICS Traffic Classification Based on Industrial Control Protocol Keyword Feature Extraction Algorithm. *Appl. Sci.* **2022**, *12*, 11193. [CrossRef]
29. Wang, W.; Zhang, B.; Yu, Z.; Gao, X. Anomaly Detection Method of Unknown Protocol in Power Industrial Control System Based on RNN. In Proceedings of the 2022 5th International Conference on Renewable Energy and Power Engineering (REPE), Beijing, China, 28–30 September 2022; pp. 68–72. [CrossRef]
30. Zhang, F.; Wei, K.; Slowikowski, K.; Fonseka, C.Y.; Rao, D.A.; Kelly, S.; Goodman, S.M.; Tabechian, D.; Hughes, L.B.; Salomon-Escoto, K.; et al. Defining inflammatory cell states in rheumatoid arthritis joint synovial tissues by integrating single-cell transcriptomics and mass cytometry. *Nat. Immunol.* **2019**, *20*, 928–942. [CrossRef] [PubMed]
31. Cho, K. MAWI Working Group Traffic Archive. Available online: http://mawi.wide.ad.jp/mawi/ (accessed on 20 March 2024).
32. Alshammari, R.; Zincir-Heywood, A.N. Machine learning based encrypted traffic classification. In Proceedings of the 2009 IEEE Symposium on Computational Intelligence for Security and Defense Applications, Ottawa, ON, Canada, 8–10 July 2009; pp. 1–8. [CrossRef]
33. Wang, W.; Zhu, M.; Wang, J.; Zeng, X.; Yang, Z. End-to-end encrypted traffic classification with one-dimensional convolution neural networks. In Proceedings of the 2017 IEEE International Conference on Intelligence and Security Informatics (ISI), Beijing, China, 22–24 July 2017; pp. 43–48. [CrossRef]
34. Zou, Z.; Ge, J.; Zheng, H.; Wu, Y.; Han, C.; Yao, Z. Encrypted Traffic Classification with a Convolutional Long Short-Term Memory Neural Network. In Proceedings of the 2018 IEEE 20th International Conference on High Performance Computing and Communications; IEEE 16th International Conference on Smart City; IEEE 4th International Conference on Data Science and Systems (HPCC/SmartCity/DSS), Exeter, UK, 28–30 June 2018; pp. 329–334. [CrossRef]
35. Kim, S.W.; Kim, K.C. Traffic Type Recognition Method for Unknown Protocol—Applying Fuzzy Inference. *Electronics* **2021**, *10*, 36. [CrossRef]
36. Sheikh, M.S.; Peng, Y. Procedures, Criteria, and Machine Learning Techniques for Network Traffic Classification: A Survey. *IEEE Access* **2022**, *10*, 61135–61158. [CrossRef]
37. Zhao, J.; Jing, X.; Yan, Z.; Pedrycz, W. Network traffic classification for data fusion. *Inf. Fusion* **2021**, *72*, 22–47. [CrossRef]
38. Xu, C.; Chen, S.; Su, J.; Yiu, S.M.; Hui, L.C.K. A Survey on Regular Expression Matching for Deep Packet Inspection: Applications, Algorithms, and Hardware Platforms. *IEEE Commun. Surv. Tutor.* **2016**, *18*, 2991–3029. [CrossRef]
39. Zhao, H.; Li, Z.; Wei, H.; Shi, J.; Huang, Y. SeqFuzzer: An Industrial Protocol Fuzzing Framework from a Deep Learning Perspective. In Proceedings of the 2019 12th IEEE Conference on Software Testing, Validation and Verification (ICST), Xi'an, China, 22–27 April 2019; pp. 59–67. [CrossRef]
40. Elhanashi, A.; Dini, P.; Saponara, S.; Zheng, Q. Integration of Deep Learning into the IoT. *Electronics* **2023**, *12*, 4952. [CrossRef]
41. Krupski, J.; Graniszewski, W.; Iwanowski, M. Data Transformation Schemes for CNN-Based Network Traffic Analysis: A Survey. *Electronics* **2021**, *10*, 2042. [CrossRef]
42. Yan, J. A Survey of Traffic Classification Validation and Ground Truth Collection. In Proceedings of the 2018 8th International Conference on Electronics Information and Emergency Communication (ICEIEC), Beijing, China, 15–17 June 2018; pp. 255–259. [CrossRef]
43. Jourdan, N.; Longard, L.; Biegel, T.; Metternich, J. Machine Learning for Intelligent Maintenance and Quality Control: A Review of Existing Datasets and Corresponding Use Cases. In Proceedings of the Conference on Production Systems and Logistics: CPSL 2021, Hannover, Germany, 25–28 May 2021; Volume 2. [CrossRef]
44. Salvatore, S.; Wei, F.; Wenke, L.; Andreas, P.; Philip, C. *KDD Cup 1999 Data*; UCI Machine Learning Repository: Irvine, CA, USA 1999. [CrossRef]
45. UCSD C. *The CAIDA Anonymized Internet Traces Dataset (April 2008–January 2019)*; CAIDA: La Jolla, CA, USA, 2018.
46. Tavallaee, M.; Bagheri, E.; Lu, W.; Ghorbani, A.A. A detailed analysis of the KDD CUP 99 data set. In Proceedings of the 2009 IEEE Symposium on Computational Intelligence for Security and Defense Applications, Ottawa, ON, Canada, 8–10 July 2009; pp. 1–6. [CrossRef]
47. Fontugne, R.; Borgnat, P.; Abry, P.; Fukuda, K. MAWILab. In Proceedings of the 6th International COnference, New York, NY, USA, 26–28 August 2010; pp. 1–12. [CrossRef]
48. Shiravi, A.; Shiravi, H.; Tavallaee, M.; Ghorbani, A.A. Toward developing a systematic approach to generate benchmark datasets for intrusion detection. *Comput. Secur.* **2012**, *31*, 357–374. [CrossRef]
49. García, S.; Grill, M.; Stiborek, J.; Zunino, A. An empirical comparison of botnet detection methods. *Comput. Secur. J.* **2014**, *45*, 100–123. [CrossRef]
50. Beigi, E.B.; Jazi, H.H.; Stakhanova, N.; Ghorbani, A.A. Towards effective feature selection in machine learning-based botnet detection approaches. In Proceedings of the 2014 IEEE Conference on Communications and Network Security, San Francisco, CA, USA, 29–31 October 2014; pp. 247–255. [CrossRef]
51. Moustafa, N.; Slay, J. UNSW-NB15. In Proceedings of the 2015 Military Communications and Information Systems Conference (MilCIS), Canberra, ACT, Australia, 10–12 November 2015; pp. 1–6. [CrossRef]
52. Garcia, S. Malware Capture Facility Project, 2018. Available online: https://stratosphereips.org (accessed on 20 March 2024).

53. Wang, W.; Zhu, M.; Zeng, X.; Ye, X.; Sheng, Y. Malware traffic classification using convolutional neural network for representation learning. In Proceedings of the 2017 International Conference on Information Networking (ICOIN), Da Nang, Vietnam, 11–13 January 2017; pp. 712–717. [CrossRef]
54. Sharafaldin, I.; Lashkari, A.H.; Ghorbani, A.A. Toward Generating a New Intrusion Detection Dataset and Intrusion Traffic Characterization. In Proceedings of the 4th International Conference on Information Systems Security and Privacy, Funchal, Portugal, 22–24 January 2018; pp. 108–116. [CrossRef]
55. Lee, H.; Jeong, S.H.; Kim, H.K. OTIDS. In Proceedings of the 2017 15th Annual Conference on Privacy, Security and Trust (PST), Calgary, AB, Canada, 28–30 August 2017; pp. 57–5709. [CrossRef]
56. MontazeriShatoori, M.; Davidson, L.; Kaur, G.; Lashkari, A.H. Detection of DoH Tunnels using Time-series Classification of Encrypted Traffic. In Proceedings of the 2020 IEEE International Conference on Dependable, Autonomic and Secure Computing, International Conference on Pervasive Intelligence and Computing, International Conference on Cloud and Big Data Computing, International Conference on Cyber Science and Technology Congress (DASC/PiCom/CBDCom/CyberSciTech), Calgary, AB, Canada, 17–22 August 2020; pp. 63–70. [CrossRef]
57. Kalupahana Liyanage, K.S.; Divakaran, D.M.; Singh, R.P.; Gurusamy, M. NSS Mirai Dataset. Available online: https://ieee-dataport.org/documents/nss-mirai-dataset (accessed on 20 March 2024).
58. Electra Dataset: Anomaly Detection ICS Dataset. Available online: http://perception.inf.um.es/ICS-datasets/ (accessed on 20 March 2024).
59. Taormina, R.; Galelli, S.; Tippenhauer, N.O.; Salomons, E.; Ostfeld, A.; Eliades, D.G.; Aghashahi, M.; Sundararajan, R.; Pourahmadi, M.; Banks, M.K.; et al. Battle of the Attack Detection Algorithms. *J. Water Resour. Plan. Manag.* **2018**, *144*, 1–11. [CrossRef]
60. Ahmed, C.M.; Palleti, V.R.; Mathur, A.P. WADI. In Proceedings of the 3rd International Workshop on Cyber-Physical Systems for Smart Water Networks, Pittsburgh, PA, USA, 21 April 2017; pp. 25–28. [CrossRef]
61. Koroniotis, N.; Moustafa, N.; Sitnikova, E.; Turnbull, B.P. Towards the Development of Realistic Botnet Dataset in the Internet of Things for Network Forensic Analytics: Bot-IoT Dataset. *arXiv* **2018**, arXiv:1811.00701.
62. Radoglou-Grammatikis, P.; Kelli, V.; Lagkas, T.; Argyriou, V.; Sarigiannidis, P. DNP3 Intrusion Detection Dataset. 2022. Available online: https://ieee-dataport.org/documents/dnp3-intrusion-detection-dataset (accessed on 20 March 2024).
63. Boakye-Boateng, K.; Ghorbani, A.A.; Lashkari, A.H. Securing Substations with Trust, Risk Posture, and Multi-Agent Systems. In Proceedings of the 2023 20th Annual International Conference on Privacy, Security and Trust (PST), Copenhagen, Denmark, 21–23 August 2023; pp. 1–12. [CrossRef]
64. Radoglou-Grammatikis, P.; Rompolos, K.; Lagkas, T.; Argyriou, V.; Sarigiannidis, P. IEC 60870-5-104 Intrusion Detection Dataset. 2022. Available online: https://ieee-dataport.org/documents/iec-60870-5-104-intrusion-detection-dataset (accessed on 20 March 2024).
65. Shin, H.K.; Lee, W.; Yun, J.H.; Kim, H. HAI 1.0: HIL-based Augmented ICS Security Dataset. In Proceedings of the 13th USENIX Workshop on Cyber Security Experimentation and Test (CSET 20), Online, 10 August 2020; USENIX Association: Berkeley, CA, USA, 2020.

Disclaimer/Publisher's Note: The statements, opinions and data contained in all publications are solely those of the individual author(s) and contributor(s) and not of MDPI and/or the editor(s). MDPI and/or the editor(s) disclaim responsibility for any injury to people or property resulting from any ideas, methods, instructions or products referred to in the content.

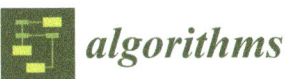

Article

A Biased-Randomized Discrete Event Algorithm to Improve the Productivity of Automated Storage and Retrieval Systems in the Steel Industry

Mattia Neroni [1], Massimo Bertolini [1] and Angel A. Juan [2,*]

[1] "Enzo Ferrari" Engineering Department, University of Modena and Reggio Emilia, 41125 Modena, Italy; massimo.bertolini@unimore.it (M.B.)

[2] Research Center on Production Management and Engineering, Universitat Politècnica de València, 03801 Alcoy, Spain

* Correspondence: ajuanp@upv.es

Abstract: In automated storage and retrieval systems (AS/RSs), the utilization of intelligent algorithms can reduce the makespan required to complete a series of input/output operations. This paper introduces a simulation optimization algorithm designed to minimize the makespan in a realistic AS/RS commonly found in the steel sector. This system includes weight and quality constraints for the selected items. Our hybrid approach combines discrete event simulation with biased-randomized heuristics. This combination enables us to efficiently address the complex time dependencies inherent in such dynamic scenarios. Simultaneously, it allows for intelligent decision making, resulting in feasible and high-quality solutions within seconds. A series of computational experiments illustrates the potential of our approach, which surpasses an alternative method based on traditional simulated annealing.

Keywords: automated storage and retrieval system; makespan minimization; simulation optimization; discrete event simulation; biased-randomized algorithms

Citation: Neroni, M.; Bertolini, M.; Juan, A.A. A Biased-Randomized Discrete Event Algorithm to Improve the Productivity of Automated Storage and Retrieval Systems in the Steel Industry. *Algorithms* **2024**, *17*, 46. https://doi.org/10.3390/a17010046

Academic Editors: Nuno Fachada and Nuno David

Received: 1 January 2024
Revised: 16 January 2024
Accepted: 18 January 2024
Published: 19 January 2024

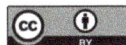

Copyright: © 2024 by the authors. Licensee MDPI, Basel, Switzerland. This article is an open access article distributed under the terms and conditions of the Creative Commons Attribution (CC BY) license (https://creativecommons.org/licenses/by/4.0/).

1. Introduction

Warehousing involves the storage of raw materials, components, work in progress (WIP), and finished goods. It has consistently been recognized as a crucial element within the supply chain and within logistics. A well-designed and effectively managed warehousing system can yield significant benefits, such as reducing the risk of running out of stock, mitigating the bullwhip effect, and decreasing the lead time of the final products [1]. Over recent decades, advancements in automation have led to the proliferation of fully automated solutions like automated storage and retrieval systems (AS/RSs) and automated vehicle storage and retrieval systems (AVS/RSs) across various industrial environments [2]. An AS/RS comprises two essential components: (i) a storage area that can be subdivided and (ii) multiple automated machines responsible for material movement within and outside the storage area. Compared to traditional manual warehouses, AS/RSs offer undeniable advantages, including labor savings, an increased storage capacity, a reduced throughput time, and a decreased occurrence of errors, damage, and risks for operators. However, the success of AS/RS implementation relies on the efficiency and alignment of the control policies with the needs of the industrial system. A well-designed AS/RS must autonomously address various challenges, such as scheduling retrieval and storage operations, assigning stock items to customer orders, allocating delivery trucks to output points, and determining routing for operations involving storage and retrieval machines, among others [3].

Despite their complexity, and owing to their numerous benefits, AS/RSs have rapidly gained traction across diverse sectors in recent decades. One industry where AS/RSs are becoming increasingly prevalent is the steel industry. According to an analysis by the World Steel Association (https://www.worldsteel.org/, accessed on 15 January 2024), this industry is at the heart of global development. In 2017, the steel industry achieved sales of USD 2.5 trillion and generated USD 500 billion in value. For every USD 1 added within the steel industry, an additional USD 2.50 of value-added activity is supported across other sectors of the global economy due to purchases of raw materials, goods, energy, and services. This generates over USD 1.2 trillion in value. In terms of employment, this analysis study confirmed that the steel industry employs more than 6 million people, and for every 2 jobs in the steel sector, 13 more jobs are supported throughout its supply chain, resulting in a total of around 40 million jobs. AS/RSs used in the steel sector significantly differ from those implemented in other environments, such as AS/RSs for pallets [2], miniloads [4], shuttle-based AS/RSs [5], etc. These differences predominantly stem from the fact that, in the steel sector, the systems are designed to handle unconventional stock-keeping units and typically heavier and bulkier items (e.g., slabs, blooms, billets, tubes and bundles, metal sheet bundles, etc.). Consequently, solutions proposed for other AS/RSs are often impractical for systems intended for the steel sector. One of the most prevalent AS/RSs in the steel sector is the shuttle–lift–crane (SLC)-based AS/RS (SLC-AS/RS) (Figure 1): a fully automated system specifically designed for storing bundles of long metal bars or tubes, wherein the stored items themselves act as the unit loads (i.e., the bundles themselves).

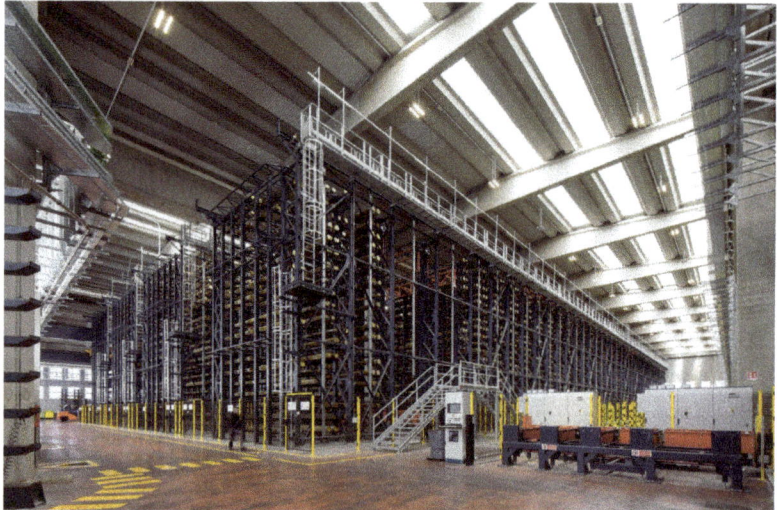

Figure 1. A picture of a shuttle–lift–crane AS/RS.

To the best of the authors' knowledge, the SLC-AS/RS has received limited attention in the scientific literature despite its significance in this industry. Thus, this paper contributes to partially filling this gap. Managing the handling of metal bar bundles involves several constraints related to the weight and quality of goods, complicating operational decisions. Previous work by Bertolini et al. [6] addressed the allocation problem using simulated annealing (SA), albeit limited to improving the retrieval phase. In this paper, the authors expand on the aforementioned work by enhancing both the retrieval and storage operations. Here, the problem is approached using a simulation optimization methodology that combines discrete event simulation (DES) principles with a biased-randomized (BR) algorithm [7]. While the DES component handles intricate time dependencies among different events, the BR component facilitates intelligent decision making. The resulting BR-DES is then integrated into a multi-start framework, enabling the generation of multiple high-quality solutions within short computing times.

The remainder of this paper is organized as follows: Section 2 provides an overview of related work. Section 3 offers a detailed description of the AS/RS under analysis. Section 4 introduces the optimization problem to be solved. Section 5 details the deterministic heuristic used by the authors to evaluate solutions. The proposed biased-randomized algorithm, along with its integration into a multi-start framework, is described in Section 6. The obtained solutions for different instances are compared with those generated by previous approaches in Section 7. Finally, conclusions and future research directions are presented in Section 8.

2. Related Work

Automated storage and retrieval systems have long been a focal point in the scientific community. A comprehensive overview of AS/RS literature was first presented by Roodbergen and Vis [2] after over 30 years of research in the field. These authors were the first to spotlight design and control issues addressed in AS/RSs, encompassing design decisions, storage assignment, batching, dwell location, sequencing of storage and retrieval requests, and performance measurement. Recently, Bertolini et al. [8] extended the review, focusing on papers published between 2009 and 2019. Over the years, numerous aspects related to AS/RSs have been meticulously studied, while new areas of interest, such as environmental aspects and energy consumption, have emerged [9,10]. Moreover, as AS/RSs have become more widespread across different sectors, many challenges initially addressed in classical AS/RSs for pallets have now been extended to modern systems. These new systems introduce new issues due to varying physical designs, collaborative machine operations, and limitations associated with handled unit loads. Among the most researched AS/RS typologies are shuttle-based AS/RSs [5], mini-loads [11], autonomous vehicle AS/RSs [12], split platform AS/RSs [13], and tier-to-tier AS/RSs [14]. Thus, Ekren and Heragu [15] discusses the significance of material handling, specifically focusing on unit load storage and retrieval systems. The paper highlights the evolution of crane-based automation technologies since the 1970s, leading to the widespread use of AS/RSs in distribution and production environments. Roy et al. [16] analyze the adoption of autonomousvehicle-based AS/RSs as an alternative to traditional automated systems for unit-load operations. These authors model the system as a multi-class semi-open queuing network with class switching and propose a decomposition-based approach to evaluate system performance. Ekren et al. [12] employ a matrix-geometric method to model and analyze an autonomous vehicle AS/RS as a semi-open queuing network. Their model accounts for waiting times, and it can solve the network and derive key performance measures. Liu et al. [17] focus on the travel time analysis of a split-platform AS/RS with a dual command cycle operating mode and an input/output dwell point policy. The study introduces a continuous travel time model and validates its accuracy through computer simulations. Liu et al. [13] investigate travel time models for split-platform AS/RSs, where machines employ independent horizontal shuttles and vertical lifts. The paper presents two dual command travel time models, which are validated through computer simulations. Hu et al. [18] analyze the travel time of a novel AS/RS designed for extra heavy loads like sea container cargo, where conventional stacker cranes may be insufficient. A travel time model is presented under the stay dwell point policy and validated through computer simulations. In addition, the authors provide guidelines for optimizing the design of a rectangular-in-time AS/RS rack. Cai et al. [19] model and evaluate an autonomous vehicle AS/RS with tier-to-tier vehicles utilizing a semi-open queuing network. Various storage/retrieval requests are represented as different customer classes in the model. Due to the time-consuming nature of analyzing multiple configurations through computer simulations, this paper employed analytical methods. This research also compared two synchronization policies. Finally, Zou et al. [14] also model and analyze tier-captive autonomous vehicle storage and retrieval systems, introducing a parallel processing policy where arrival transactions can simultaneously request both the lift and the vehicle. An approximation method, based on decomposing the fork-join network, is developed to estimate system performance. Simulation models validated the effectiveness of analytical models, showing that the fork-join network accurately estimates system performance under the parallel processing policy. Although other typologies, like the adoption of two storage and retrieval machines sharing the same path, have been highlighted [20], the steel sector has been notably neglected throughout this technical and scientific evolution. Noteworthy contributions specifically aimed at improving AS/RS performance in the steel sector include works by Bertolini et al. [6] and Zammori et al. [21].

This work introduces novelty in two key areas: (i) the system considered and (ii) the proposed algorithm. The system under consideration is known as the shuttle–lift–crane automated storage and retrieval system (SLC-AS/RS), widely deployed in the steel industry and occasionally used in the wood industry to preserve tree trunks. A detailed system description is provided in Section 3. Apart from the aforementioned works by Bertolini et al. [6] and Zammori et al. [21], we are pioneers in offering an optimization technique for such systems. The proposed solution, described in Section 6, is based on a discrete-event heuristic (DEH). The DEH combines a swift heuristic algorithm for decision making with discrete event simulation to evaluate the impact of decisions within a complex system characterized by high levels of parallelism and resource interaction. While similar approaches have proven efficient in various contexts, such as those seen in Arnau et al. [22], the application of a DEH to automated storage and retrieval systems is novel.

3. Modeling an Automated Warehouse in the Steel Sector

The shuttle–lift–crane automated storage and retrieval system is a prevalent storage solution in the steel industry, specifically designed to store bundles of long metal bars or tubes ranging from ten to twelve meters in length and weighing between 1000 and 5000 kg. Notably, this system does not involve picking individual bundles. Rather, each bundle enters and exits the warehouse without any alterations. As a result, the SLC-AS/RS does not employ loading units or boxes to store items since the bundles themselves serve as the unit loads. Typically, the overall storage area of an SLC-AS/RS is divided into several bearing metal structures known as racks. Each rack can reach heights of up to 20 to 25 m, widths of 12 m (depending on the stored tubes or bars' length), and lengths exceeding 100 m. To facilitate understanding this complex system, a schematic representation is provided in Figure 2, displaying a system comprising three racks and two input and two output locations.

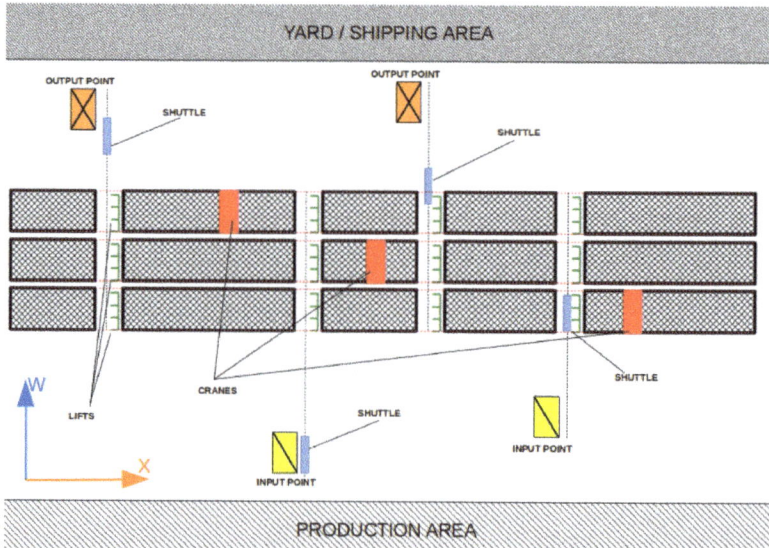

Figure 2. Schematic representation of ann SLC-AS/RS.

Unlike standard AS/RSs for pallets, each rack in the SLC-AS/RS is divided into perpendicular aisles, crossing the rack lengthwise (x-axis) and splitting it into multiple sections. Storage locations, composed of metal shelves, line both sides of these aisles, accommodating multiple bundles of varying types and lengths, as depicted in Figure 3. Consequently, these storage locations are not standardized, and previous allocations can affect the possibility of utilizing specific storage spaces. This unique aspect of the SLC-AS/RS could be formulated as a one-dimensional cutting stock problem to minimize the number of storage locations used.

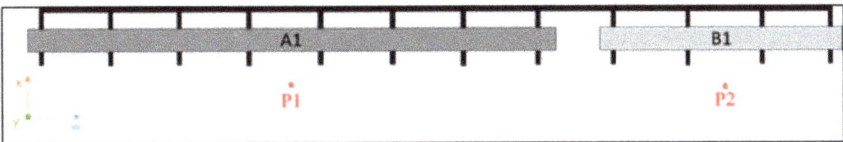

Figure 3. Example of bundle allocation in a single storage location.

Resource-wise, an SLC-AS/RS encompasses four categories: (i) input/output (I/O) points; (ii) shuttles; (iii) lifts; and (iv) cranes. Each shuttle serves all racks but only one I/O point, while each lift serves a single crane and shuttle. Conversely, each crane serves every lift within its rack. A detailed breakdown of these machines is provided below:

- I/O points: Chain conveyors serve as buffers between the system and external processes, such as truck loading or production lines. Input points, equipped with sensors for bundle alignment and weight control, are also depicted in Figure 4A.
- Shuttles: Vehicles handle horizontal movements, transporting bundles between I/O points and racks. They can transport one or two bundles, depending on single-depth or double-deep storage, as illustrated in Figure 4B.
- Lifts: Responsible for vertical movements and transporting bundles between shuttles and the top of racks or cranes. Figure 4C showcases an example of these lifts.
- Cranes: Essential for storage and retrieval operations, moving bundles between lifts and shelves or vice versa. Each rack houses one crane capable of three-axis movements, as detailed in Figure 4D.

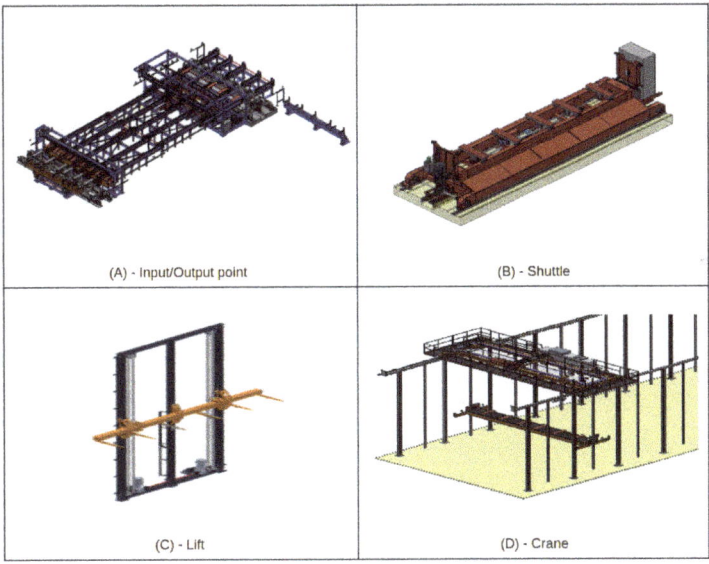

Figure 4. Main elements of a shuttle–lift–crane AS/RS.

For a comprehensive understanding of the SLC-AS/RS operations and cycle time computation, refer to Zammori et al. [21]. In this work, we focus on the behavior and interactions of machines during input and output operations. The operation begins when the entering bundle reaches an input point. If the shuttle is not near the input point, it is recalled, the bundle is loaded upon arrival, and then proceeds to the assigned rack. Once the bundle is loaded onto the lift, it is transported to the top of the rack and requested by the crane for storage. The crane then moves the bundle to the designated storage location. Similarly, we will consider the process for retrieval or output operations. The operation is sent to the crane, which retrieves the required bundle from the storage location and transports it to the corresponding lift for output.

4. Detailed Problem Description

This section provides an accurate description of the problem being studied in this paper, which includes the main assumptions and description of the stock-keeping units, a description of the customers' orders and storage facilities, and a formal model.

4.1. Main Assumptions and Stock-Keeping Units Description

We consider an SLC-AS/RS with single, deep storage locations, featuring one single crane on each rack and only one shuttle for each I/O point. Due to the latter two aspects, there is no need to consider anti-collision policies. Additionally, since each shuttle is associated with exactly one I/O point, shuttles linked to an input point solely perform input operations, while those connecting racks to an output point exclusively execute output operations. As previously mentioned, the stock-keeping units (SKUs) comprise bundles of metal bars, hereafter denoted as $i \in B$. Each SKU i is defined by the following attributes: (i) a unique code, c_i; (ii) a specific quality level, q_i, influenced by factors like the geometric dimensional tolerances of the bar, chemical purity of the material, and the presence of surface damages; (iii) a weight w_i and length L_i; and (iv) the rack r_i where the bundle is located, along with its position inside the rack, denoted as p_i.

4.2. Customers' Orders and Storage Requests

All customer orders, denoted as output requests, $k \in R^{\text{out}}$, possess the following attributes: (i) an arrival time, ρ_k; (ii) a required product identified by a unique code, c_k; (iii) a specified required quantity, w_k; (iv) a minimum quality level of the material, q_k; and (v) an indicator specifying the I/O point used, s_k. Distinguishing customer orders $k \in R^{\text{out}}$ from storage orders (input requests $k \in R^{\text{in}}$) involves an additional attribute, t_k. In the former case, t_k holds a value of zero, whereas in the latter case, it holds a value of one. The interpretation of the remaining attributes varies based on t_k. For instance, in a customer order, c_k, w_k, and q_k signify the product, quantity, and required quality level, respectively. Conversely, in a storage request, they represent the product, weight, and quality of the incoming bundle, respectively.

In an SLC-AS/RS, processing customers' orders differs slightly from traditional AS/RS setups for pallets. Typically, customers specify a particular product type, along with a quantity in kilograms and a desired quality level. The fulfillment of this request necessitates one or more bundles, ensuring that the overall quantity and quality of retrieved bundles closely match the required specifications. This resembles a knapsack problem embedded within the larger issue at hand.

4.3. Mathematical Formalization and Scope of the Algorithm

The primary objective of the proposed approach is to minimize the makespan, denoted as the time required to complete a given set of operations. Here, $j \in J = \{1, 2, \ldots, N\}$ represents the operations to fulfil requests, $m \in M$ denotes the set of machines (such as shuttles, lifts, and cranes), and $END_m(j)$ signifies the time at which machine $m \in M$ finishes operation j. The objective function can be formally defined as:

$$\min\ A \qquad (1)$$

where A is a newly introduced variable subject to the following constraints:

$$A \geq END_m(j), \quad \forall j \in J, \forall m \in M \qquad (2)$$

For each storage request, represented by $k \in R^{in}$, we define an input operation. Similarly, for each customer order $k \in R^{out}$, one or more retrieval operations are defined based on the required quantity and stock availability. The algorithm does not handle the assignment of input/output points to requests, as this decision relies on external factors. Specifically, the input point depends on the production line from which the entering bundle originates, while the output point is chosen by the truck driver, typically opting for the first available one. The sequence in which requests are processed is highly constrained. For input requests, rearranging the order of entry bundles once they have reached the input point and placed on the conveyor is time-consuming due to their substantial weight (over five tons) and length (up to twelve meters). Altering the sequencing of input requests involves significant expenses, typically requiring at least two operators and a forklift or a bridge crane. Hence, changing the sequence of input requests should be minimized. Regarding output requests, due to the bulkiness of the bundles, they cannot be temporarily stored in a loading area or yard (as with classic pallets). Therefore, output requests should generally adhere to first-in-first-out (FIFO) logic. Postponing an output request is rare and only considered when the required product (in the required quantity) is not in stock.

The constraints for assigning bundles to output operations and empty spaces to input operations can be formalized as follows. For a storage operation $j \in R^{in}$, the only requirement is that the space accommodating the entering bundle b_j must be of sufficient length. Thus, if L_j represents the length of b_j, L_σ denotes the length of a generic space, and $z_{\sigma,j} \in 0,1$ is a decision variable equal to one only if space σ is assigned to operation j, the following constraint must be satisfied:

$$L_j * z_{\sigma,j} \leq L_\sigma, \quad \forall j \in J, \forall \sigma \in S \qquad (3)$$

Conversely, for a customer order, quantity and quality constraints are essential. For each customer order $k \in R^{out}$, the difference between the required and retrieved quantities must fall within certain limits:

$$w_k - \triangle \leq \sum_{i \in B_k} w_i \leq w_k + \triangle, \quad \forall k \in R^{out} \qquad (4)$$

where B_k represents the set of in-stock bundles selected to fulfil customer order k, and $\triangle$ denotes an acceptable deviation from the required quantity. Regarding the quality constraint, B_k must have an average quality level equal to or higher than the required quality q_k:

$$q_k \leq \frac{\sum_{i \in B_k} q_i}{|B_k|}, \quad \forall k \in R^{out} \qquad (5)$$

where $|B_k|$ refers to the cardinality of set B_k.

5. Evaluation of the Solutions

The solution generated by the proposed algorithm includes a set of operations $j \in J$, encompassing both input and output operations aimed at fulfilling the requests. Each input operation corresponds to an empty storage location where the entry bundle will be stored. Similarly, every output operation is linked to a bundle in stock for retrieval. Sorting the operations by their scheduled execution time enables the computation of the makespan through a discrete event simulation. This simulation can accommodate stochastic processing times and is applicable irrespective of the system's complexity. Notably, the deterministic simulation considered here naturally extends to a stochastic one. During each simulation run, deterministic processing times can be substituted with randomly generated times using corresponding probability distributions. The specific probability distributions employed to model these random processing times are derived from fitted historical data. To elucidate the computation of the makespan analytically, a simple example is provided below, showcasing machines and operations:

- r_j, s_j, and l_j represent the crane, shuttle, and lift necessary for operation j, dependent on its associated operation and the bundle it involves.
- $j^*_{r,s,l}$ denotes the most recent operation involving machines r, s, and l. Similarly, j^*_r signifies the most recent operation involving only r, while $j^*_{r,s}$ indicates the most recent operation involving crane r and shuttle s.

Key events occurring during the simulation of each operation are defined as follows:

- $AVAIL_m(j)$ represents the moment when operation j becomes available for machine m.
- $START_m(j)$ signifies the start time when machine m initiates work on operation j.
- $END_m(j)$ indicates the completion time when machine m finishes work on operation j.
- $P1_j$ and $P2_j$ denote the first and second positions that crane r_j must visit to execute operation j. If j is an input operation, $P1_j$ represents the interchange point between lift l_j and crane r_j, while $P2_j$ denotes the storage location. Conversely, for an output operation, $P1_j$ corresponds to the storage location, while $P2_j$ indicates the interchange point between lift l_j and crane r_j.

An illustration of the SLC-AS/RS under consideration is depicted in Figure 5. The layout assumes a configuration with one crane and two lifts within the rack (with one lift designated for each I/O point). The warehouse comprises ten aisles, each spanning a length of one meter. For the input shuttle, traversal of the rack occurs through the fourth aisle, while the output shuttle navigates along the eighth aisle. Within each aisle, storage consists of three levels, each standing at a height of one meter. The crane's movement follows a uniform, linear trajectory, covering one meter per second in both length and height. The unidirectional travel time for the lifts is presumed to be 3 s, while the upload and download times are estimated at 5 s. Additionally, the one-way travel time for shuttles to reach the rack is set at 6 s. The operations to be executed include:

- $t_1 = OUTPUT$; $\rho_1 = 3$; $P1_1 = (5,1)$; $P2_1 = (8,0)$.
- $t_2 = INPUT$; $\rho_2 = 4$; $P1_2 = (4,0)$; $P2_2 = (7,2)$.
- $t_3 = INPUT$; $\rho_3 = 10$; $P1_3 = (4,0)$; $P2_3 = (1,3)$.
- $t_4 = OUTPUT$; $\rho_4 = 11$; $P1_4 = (7,2)$; $P2_4 = (8,0)$.
- $t_5 = OUTPUT$; $\rho_5 = 20$; $P1_5 = (7,1)$; $P2_5 = (8,0)$.

In a properly executed simulation, the timing for each event (in seconds) is detailed in Table 1. Additionally, a Gantt chart depicting the sequence of operations is presented in Figure 6.

Table 1. Timing of the events (in seconds) associated with each of the operations in the showcased simulation.

		Operations		
Operation 1	Operation 2	Operation 3	Operation 4	Operation 5
$AVAIL_{r_1}(1) = \rho_1 = 3$	$START_{s_2}(2) = 4$	$START_{s_3}(3) = 26$	$AVAIL_{r_4}(4) = 11$	$AVAIL_{r_5}(5) = 20$
$START_{r_r}(1) = 3$	$AVAIL_{r_2}(2) = 23$	$AVAIL_{r_3}(3) = 45$	$START_{r_4}(4) = 77$	$START_{r_5}(5) = 92$
$END_{r_1}(1) = 17$	$END_{s_2}(2) = 26$	$END_{s_3}(3) = 48$	$END_{r_4}(4) = 90$	$END_{r_5}(5) = 109$
$START_{s_1}(1) = 17$	$START_{r_2}(2) = 27$	$START_{r_3}(3) = 50$	$START_{s_4}(4) = 90$	$START_s(5) = 112$
$END_{l_1}(1) = 28$	$END_{r_2}(2) = 42$	$END_{r_3}(3) = 66$	$END_{l_4}(4) = 101$	$END_l(5) = 123$
$END_{s_1}(1) = 39$			$END_{s_4}(4) = 112$	$END_s(5) = 134$

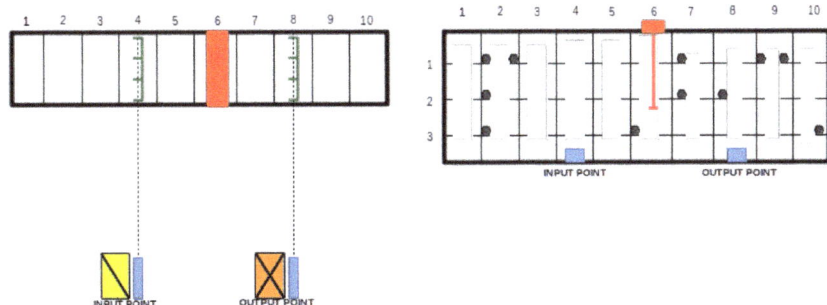

Figure 5. Planar (**left**) and frontal (**right**) view of the SLC-AS/RS considered.

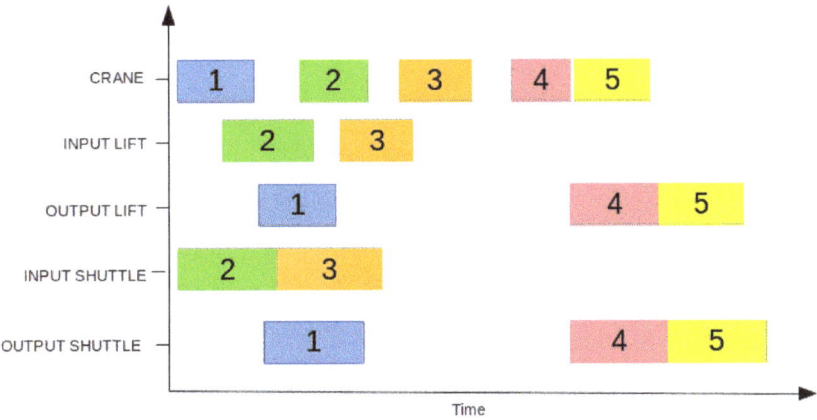

Figure 6. Schematic representation of operations in the presented example.

6. The Proposed Simulation Optimization Algorithm

This section delineates the hybrid algorithmic approach utilized to address the aforementioned problem. This approach combines biased randomization with discrete-event heuristics; consequently, both concepts are described in the following subsections.

6.1. Biased-Randomized Heuristics

The algorithm proposed can be classified as a biased-randomized heuristic. BR algorithms are part of the family of random search methods extensively employed for addressing large-scale NP-hard optimization problems. As described by Dominguez et al. [7], in a BR algorithm, solution-building elements are arranged in a list based on logical criteria specific to the optimization problem at hand. Subsequently, during each iteration of the solution-construction process, a new element is selected from this list according to a probability distribution. The probability of selection increases with a higher position of the element in the sorted list. This approach aims to introduce slight modifications to the greedy constructive path, facilitating exploration beyond local optima by traversing 'similar' paths (retaining most of the heuristic logic) within shorter computing times.

Two of the earliest biased-randomized procedures were proposed by Arcus [23] and Tonge [24], known as biased random sampling (BRS), and used to bias the selection of randomly generated solutions. Subsequently, numerous priority-rule-based heuristics have been developed. Before the advent of BR techniques utilizing skewed probability distributions like the geometric one, probabilistic tabu search (PTS) was introduced by Glover [25] and expanded upon again by Glover [26]. Another metaheuristic framework implementing similar concepts is ant colony optimization (ACO), pioneered by Dorigo and Gambardella [27]. However, many of these approaches define probabilities using empirical distributions. An alternative approach advocates employing theoretical probability distributions. Consequently, some authors have advocated for the implementation of skewed theoretical probability distributions to devise BR algorithms. Overall, the primary advantages of utilizing a theoretical probability distribution over empirical ones include: (i) the reduced computing times required for generating random numbers (employing analytical expressions instead of loops); and (ii) simplification of the fine-tuning process (which might become intricate when using empirical probability distributions due to the numerous parameters and their ranges). Among the most commonly used theoretical probability distributions in BR algorithms is the geometric distribution, chosen likely due to its flexibility, simplicity, and dependence on a single parameter. The algorithm's dependence on a single parameter streamlines the fine-tuning process, avoiding time-consuming complexities.

6.2. Adding Discrete Event Simulation Principles to BR

To synchronize the various events within the warehouse, the BR heuristic is enhanced with a discrete event simulation. Employing DES allows for a consistent and reliable evaluation of the impacts of BR decisions. Given the system's high parallelism and synchronization complexities, measuring the makespan of a set of operations would be infeasible without DES. Consequently, during the deterministic discrete event simulation of the system, a BR process is employed at each decision stage to select the next building element from a list of candidates. This hybrid BR-DES approach facilitates the rapid generation of a range of feasible solutions (in terms of event synchronization) guided by the logic of the constructive heuristic, ensuring potentially favorable solutions in terms of quality. The integration of BR with DES is depicted in Figure 7. The entire algorithm can be visualized as a multi-start framework, where, until the computational time does not surpass a predefined threshold, new, random but oriented solutions are continually generated from scratch. This architecture comprises two distinct components: the BR heuristic, which includes a Monte Carlo simulation that makes random but oriented decisions, and the discrete event simulation. Each new solution is created by running the simulation, delegating decisions to BR within what we term the algorithm simulation loop. Subsequently, the new solution is compared with the best solution obtained so far and this is replaced if superior.

Within the simulation loop, key decisions made by BR include the sequencing of input and output operations, the selection of retrieved bundles to fulfil customer orders, and the allocation of storage locations for entering bundles. Specifically, input and output requests are jointly processed using an FIFO criterion. For each request, the algorithm strives to deliver a satisfactory and feasible solution—such as assigning a storage location for input operations or a set of bundles for output operations. If the solution found is deemed infeasible, the request is postponed, and the subsequent input request is processed. For instance, when $k \in R^{in}$ represents an input request and the solution is infeasible, all subsequent input requests originating from the same input point s_k are deferred. This strategy minimizes changes to the input request queue, crucial due to the complexities of handling large metal bar bundles, as detailed in Section 4. Specifically, if the non-feasible input request involves storing a bundle of type c_k, all subsequent inputs are postponed until after the next output request requiring retrieval of the same bundle type. This action, as exemplified in Table 2, ensures sufficient space is created by the output request, guaranteeing fulfillment of the previously postponed non-feasible request k.

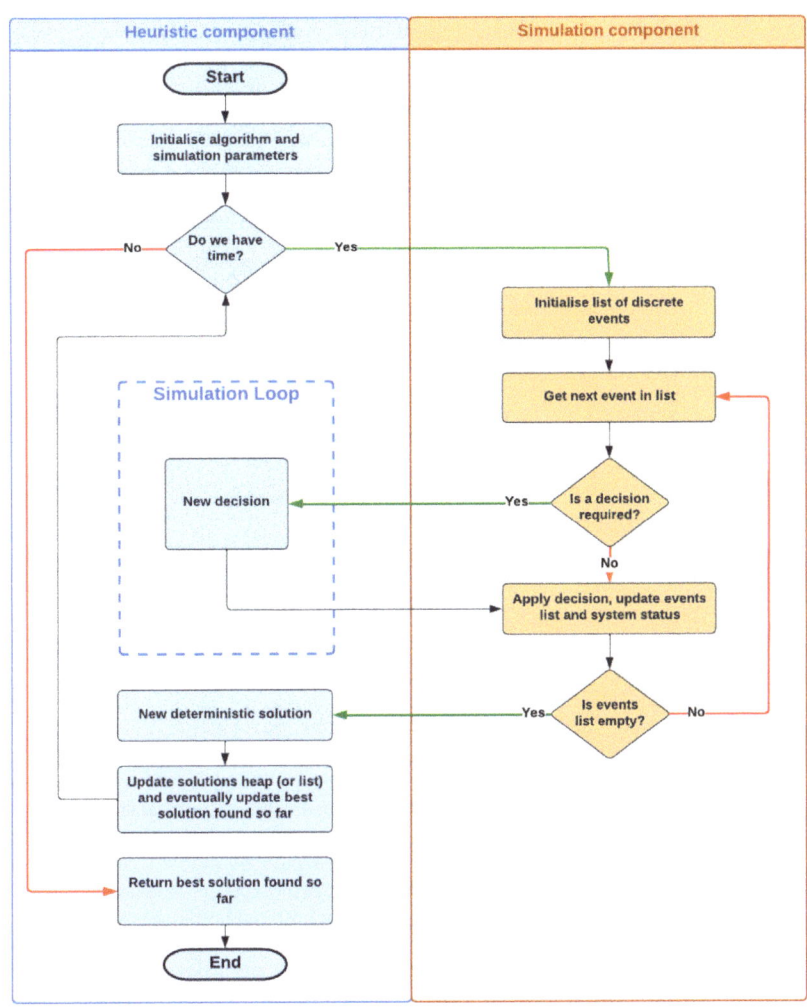

Figure 7. Flowchart of a generic discrete-event heuristic.

Table 2. List of requests before (left) and after (right) the postponement process.

Request k	Type t_k	I/O Point s_k	Bundle Type c_k	Request k	Type t_k	I/O Point s_k	Bundle Type c_k
1	IN	1	A	2	IN	2	B
2	IN	2	B	4	OUT	3	B
3	IN	1	C	5	OUT	3	A
4	OUT	3	B	1	IN	1	A
5	OUT	3	A	3	IN	1	C
6	IN	2	C	6	IN	2	C

If the non-feasible request pertains to an output, it is deferred until after the subsequent input that introduces the required product type into the system. The pseudo-code outlining the overall BR-DES algorithm is presented in Algorithm 1. The parameters within the algorithm should be interpreted as follows: *requests* denotes the list containing both input and output orders to be processed; *racks* signifies the list of warehouse racks; and *beta* represents the vector of parameters utilized for the geometric distributions employed in the various BR processes.

Algorithm 1 Pseudo-code of the proposed BR-DES algorithm.

```
input: requests, racks, beta
solution ← NULL                                              ▷ init final solution
while length(requests) > 0 do
    nextr ← getNextRequest(requests)
    reqSol ← NULL                                  ▷ init solution to current request
    if type(nextr) == Input then
        sol ← processInput(nextr, solution, racks, beta)
    else if type(nextr) == Output then
        sol ← processOutput(nextr, solution, racks, beta)
    end if
    if isFeasible(sol) then
        postponementProc(nextr, requests)                    ▷ request postponed
    else
        solution ← add(solution, sol)
    end if
end while
return solution
```

For an input operation, the objective is to identify an available space within the warehouse to accommodate the incoming bundle. The space must be sufficiently long, aligning with the bundle's type (code). To determine a viable solution, all racks are taken into consideration. During each iteration, racks are prioritized based on the availability of their respective cranes, with one of these racks chosen through a BR procedure. This phase is crucial for ensuring an equitable distribution of workload among all cranes. Specifically, the BR procedure incorporates a geometric probability distribution, as proposed in Hatami et al. [28]. If x denotes the position occupied by a candidate in the previously sorted list and β represents the parameter of the geometric probability distribution, then the probability $f(x)$ of selecting candidate x is calculated as follows:

$$f(x) = (1 - \beta)^x \qquad (6)$$

When the chosen rack contains feasible storage locations, one of them is randomly selected using a uniform distribution. The decision is recorded in the emerging solution, and a new operation is scheduled to update the system's state. However, if the selected rack lacks feasible space, it is eliminated from the list of potential racks, and the BR rack-selection process is reiterated. If the list of potential racks becomes empty without finding a solution, a non-feasible solution is returned. In such cases, the BR-DES procedure postpones the input request. The pseudo-code for processing input operations is presented in Algorithm 2.

Algorithm 2 Pseudo-code for input processing

input: *nextr, solution, racks, beta*
$pRacks \leftarrow \textbf{copy}(racks)$ ▷ list of racks to consider
$sol \leftarrow NULL$ ▷ solution to the current request
while $sol == NULL$ **and** $length(pRacks) > 0$ **do**
  $pRacks \leftarrow \textbf{sort}(pRacks, key : craneAvailability)$ ▷ sort racks prioritizing the busiest ones
  $rack \leftarrow \textbf{findBR}(pRacks, beta)$ ▷ select a rack by using BR
  $pPlaces \leftarrow \textbf{feasiblePlaces}(rack)$ ▷ feasible storage locations
  if $length(pPlaces) > 0$ **then**
    $place \leftarrow \textbf{randomUniformChoice}(pPlaces)$ ▷ pick a random storage location
    $sol \leftarrow \textbf{new}InputOperation(nextr, rack, place)$
    $\textbf{scheduleOperation}(solution, sol)$ ▷ schedule the new operation to carry out
  else ▷ if rack has no feasible solution, remove it
    $pRacks \leftarrow \textbf{remove}(pRacks, rack)$
  end if
end while
return *sol*

For output operations, constructing a solution involves selecting multiple bundles. Upon choosing a bundle, the system's state must be updated to accurately select the subsequent bundle. However, the solution cannot be deemed feasible until all required bundles have been retrieved. Therefore, before initiating solution construction, the system's state is saved to enable restoration to a previous state if the solution is found to be non-feasible. The construction process operates iteratively. If, at any stage, quantity constraints are violated and no feasible bundles remain, the process is halted, the system state is restored, and a non-feasible warning is issued. Similarly, if the construction process adheres to quantity constraints but violates quality constraints, the system state is restored and a non-feasible warning is issued. For a bundle to be considered feasible, its weight, in addition to the weight of the current solution, must not surpass a predefined threshold. Bundles from prior input operations are only considered if the respective input operation has concluded. If no feasible bundles exist in the selected rack, the rack is eliminated from the list of potential racks, and the process begins anew with another rack. Conversely, if feasible bundles are available, they are arranged by decreasing the weight and then by the difference between their quality and the required quality level. Bundles with quality levels closer to the required level are given priority. Once the bundles are sorted, one of them is selected using a new geometric distribution (note that the β parameter value used here may differ from the one used for rack selection). Subsequently, the solution's weight, total quality, and the count of retrieved items are updated. The system state is also updated, and the list of possible racks is reset. This process continues iteratively until a feasible solution is achieved. The pseudo-code for processing output operations is detailed in Algorithm 3.

Algorithm 3 Pseudo-code for output processing.

input: $nextr, solution, racks, beta$
$sSolution \leftarrow \mathbf{copy}(solution)$ ▷ save the state of the solution
$sol \leftarrow NULL$ ▷ solution to the current request
$pRacks \leftarrow \mathbf{copy}(racks)$ ▷ list of racks to consider
$w \leftarrow 0$ ▷ total weight of retrieved bundles
$q \leftarrow 0$ ▷ total quality of retrieved bundles
$n \leftarrow 0$ ▷ number of retrieved bundles
while $w < weightRequired(nextr) - acceptedError(nextr)$ **and** $length(pRacks) > 0$ **do**
　　$pRacks \leftarrow \mathbf{sort}(pRacks, key : craneAvailability)$ ▷ sort racks prioritizing the busiest ones
　　$rack \leftarrow \mathbf{findBR}(pRacks, beta)$ ▷ select a rack by using BR
　　$pBundles \leftarrow \mathbf{feasibleBundles}(rack, w, nextr)$ ▷ feasible bundles in rack
　　if $length(pBundles) > 0$ **then**
　　　　$pBundles \leftarrow \mathbf{sort}(pBundles, key : increasingWeight)$ ▷ sort bundles by weight
　　　　$pBundles \leftarrow \mathbf{sort}(pBundles, key : deltaQuality)$ ▷ sort bundles by quality
　　　　$bundle \leftarrow \mathbf{findBR}(pBundles, beta)$ ▷ select a bundle by using BR
　　　　$w \leftarrow w + weight(bundle)$ ▷ update weight
　　　　$q \leftarrow q + quality(bundle)$ ▷ update quality
　　　　$n \leftarrow n + 1$ ▷ update number of retrieved bundles
　　　　$op \leftarrow \mathbf{new}\ OutputOperation(nextr, rack, bundle)$ ▷ instantiate a retrieve
　　　　$\mathbf{scheduleOperation}(solution, op)$ ▷ schedule a retrieval operation
　　　　$sol \leftarrow \mathbf{add}(sol, op)$
　　　　$pRacks \leftarrow \mathbf{copy}(racks)$ ▷ restore the set of possible racks
　　else
　　　　$pRacks \leftarrow \mathbf{remove}(pRacks, rack)$
　　end if
end while

7. Computational Experiments

The BR-DES algorithm was implemented in Python 3.7 and executed using the CPython interpreter. The testing was conducted on a standard personal computer equipped with an Intel QuadCore *i7* CPU running at 2.4 GHz and 8 GB RAM with the Ubuntu 18.04 operating system. When constructing the experimental data sets, the quality level of each bundle was randomly generated using a uniform probability distribution between 1 (minimum level) and 10 (maximum level). Then, the quality of a solution was computed as the average of the quality of the retrieved bundles. The input quantity was randomly generated using a uniform probability distribution between 700 and 1300, expressed in kilograms. We assume that two bundles enter together as input, each with an average weight of 500 kg. Finally, since a customer might require many bundles, the output quantity was randomly generated using a uniform probability distribution between 700 and 10,000, expressed in kilograms. Table 3 displays the data corresponding to Instance 1, where type 0 represents an input point and type 1 refers to an output point. Both the desired quality and quantity are provided as reference values. These reference values will be compared with those associated with the solution provided by each algorithm to calculate the mismatch. Similar data for the remaining instances, as well as the algorithm code, are available at https://github.com/mattianeroni/Shuttle-Lift-Crane-AS-RS (accessed on 15 January 2024).

Table 3. Example of an instance data set—Instance 1.

Type	Bay	Desired Quality	Desired Quantity	Length (in Shelves)
0	1	9	900	5
0	0	4	1200	4
0	1	8	800	5
0	0	1	800	6
0	1	7	900	6
0	1	5	1200	5
0	0	2	1000	5
0	1	9	1000	4
0	0	7	1100	6
1	2	9	3056	4
1	2	10	766	3
1	3	4	3719	3
1	3	10	6682	4
1	2	6	6788	6
1	3	2	8165	6
1	2	10	4257	6
1	2	4	9901	5
1	2	10	1449	3
1	2	7	6592	4
1	2	10	7505	4
1	3	5	6394	3
1	3	5	1922	6
1	3	9	6943	5
1	3	6	1615	3
1	2	3	2567	4
1	3	5	1268	4
1	2	6	6621	5
1	3	2	8400	5
1	2	7	9665	6
1	3	4	8262	3

As can be seen in Tables 4 and 5, our algorithm demonstrates an efficient performance, since it is capable of providing competitive solutions in just a few seconds, while other approaches require noticeably longer times without reaching the same solution quality. To validate the proposed methodology, a comparison with three distinct approaches is presented. The selected benchmark approaches are as follows: (i) a random algorithm utilizing a uniform probability distribution to select from different possibilities at each step of the solution-construction process; (ii) a greedy heuristic that consistently chooses the top-listed element in the candidates' list, sorted based on a minimum time criterion; and (iii) the simulated annealing method proposed by Bertolini et al. [6] for a similar problem, adapted for the specific problem considered in this study by incorporating new constraints. The random approach serves as a lower-bound benchmark and was obtained by implementing the proposed BR-DES while substituting the geometric distribution with a uniform distribution. This adjustment was achieved by setting the beta value to 0 in the BR-DES algorithm. However, when employing such low beta values, the algorithm often failed to find a feasible solution. To address this limitation, we utilized a geometric probability distribution with a slightly higher beta value of 0.3, allowing the algorithm to discover feasible solutions in most test scenarios, although not all. On the other hand, the greedy algorithm presents a practical solution for warehouse system managers and was acquired by implementing the proposed BR-DES with a beta value of 1. The SA algorithm by Bertolini et al. [6] is currently the only algorithm explicitly tailored for this type of automated warehouse system (i.e., an SLC-AS/RS). While theoretically serving as a solid benchmark, the original SA algorithm did not consider any constraints regarding the sequence of request processing. To ensure a fair comparison, we integrated these constraints into the SA algorithm.

For the comparison, we employed the actual layout of an SLC-AS/RS consisting of three racks, each containing 500 storage locations, with two input and two output points. In the computational experiments, 12 different request lists were used, each varying in size (30, 60, 90, and 150 requests). Every algorithm was executed three times on each request list to monitor both its average performance and its variability. The comparison primarily focuses on the total makespan, expressed in minutes (Table 4), and computational time (Table 5). Additionally, we monitored the overall mismatch between the quantities and quality levels required by customers (Table 6). The parameters of the proposed algorithm, namely the betas of the geometric distribution used in the selection of racks (β_r) and bundles (β_b), were adjusted in each iteration according to trimmed Gaussian distributions. The means of these Gaussian distributions ($\mu_r = 0.7$ and $\mu_b = 0.9$) were determined through a series of empirical experiments, exploring combinations of $\mu_r \in (0,1)$ and $\mu_b \in (0,1)$ with a step of 0.1. Both were set with a standard deviation of 0.025. Regarding SA, the same parameter values as proposed in Bertolini et al. [6] were employed. All BR-DES and SA results were acquired after exploring 1000 solutions. The makespan results are presented in Table 4. As anticipated, our proposed algorithm consistently outperforms the greedy and random approaches, as well as the SA algorithm, in all instances. Notably, the random and greedy approaches often fail to find feasible solutions, whereas our algorithm consistently obtains feasible solutions in all scenarios.

Table 4. Comparison of makespans (in minutes) achieved by the greedy, random, BR-DES, and SA approaches for each instance (row).

Instance	Number of Requests	Greedy	Random (Beta = 0.3)		BR-DES		SA	
			Avg.	St.Dev.	Avg.	St.Dev.	Avg.	St.Dev.
1	30 (9 in/21 out)	37.24	48.36	2.29	32.04	0.15	43.22	4.52
2	30 (12 in/18 out)	35.34	39.41	0.48	31.03	0.32	37.12	3.28
3	30 (12 in/18 out)	40.53	49.47	4.87	38.02	0.18	44.97	0.01
4	60 (9 in/51 out)	55.46	71.95	3.76	51.19	0.89	59.03	0.74
5	60 (12 in/48 out)	52.20	69.00	5.82	44.63	2.08	54.25	2.17
6	60 (26 in/34 out)	52.24	72.04	0.93	48.93	0.55	52.10	1.75
7	90 (42 in/48 out)	112	132.43	-	105.02	3.9	110.84	10.23
8	90 (28 in/62 out)	89.29	115.24	4.18	88.32	1.52	89.20	3.33
9	90 (35 in/55 out)	108.36	132.14	4.70	107.50	1.84	110.34	2.21
10	150 (38 in/112 out)	-	-	-	230.96	100.23	257.12	23.04
11	150 (73 in/77 out)	-	255.67	-	227.94	7.90	241.23	0.34
12	150 (59 in/91 out)	-	-	-	195.89	6.64	201.32	6.43

Table 5. Computational times (in seconds) associated with each of the approaches (greedy, random, BR-DES, and SA) for each instance (row).

Instance	Number of Requests	Greedy	Random (Beta = 0.3)		BR-DES		SA	
			Avg.	St.Dev.	Avg.	St.Dev.	Avg.	St.Dev.
1	30 (9 in/21 out)	0.001	0.001	0	1.002	0.002	5.234	0.122
2	30 (12 in/18 out)	0.001	0.001	0	1.034	0.004	8.032	0.392
3	30 (12 in/18 out)	0.001	0.002	0	1.009	0	6.003	3.211
4	60 (9 in/51 out)	0.001	0.001	0	1.023	0.002	6.023	0.045
5	60 (12 in/48 out)	0.001	0.003	0	1.206	0.034	5.998	1.520
6	60 (26 in/34 out)	0.001	0.003	0	1.115	0.078	5.104	2.174
7	90 (42 in/48 out)	0.002	0.005	0	1.904	0.022	19.047	2.348
8	90 (28 in/62 out)	0.001	0.019	0	1.821	0.103	18.222	2.011
9	90 (35 in/55 out)	0.003	0.004	0	2.338	0.088	22.304	8.327
10	150 (38 in/112 out)	-	-	-	2.904	0.155	35.120	2.664
11	150 (73 in/77 out)	-	0.027	-	3.011	0.095	33.979	2.884
12	150 (59 in/91 out)	-	-	-	2.992	0.121	34.014	6.092

An additional noteworthy aspect is the greater variability exhibited by the SA algorithm when compared to the BR-DES algorithm. This variability is due to the SA algorithm's exploration of infeasible solutions across numerous iterations, as it is not guided by a discrete event list. In contrast, BR-DES operates based on a discrete event list, allowing for feasibility and making informed decisions at each stage. Consequently, it requires considerably less computational time to achieve comparable or superior solutions compared to those generated by the SA algorithm. Computational times are displayed in Table 5. Notably, our BR-DES consistently outperforms the SA algorithm in terms of solution quality as well as computational efficiency. Throughout the tests, we closely monitored the deviation, encompassing both quantity and quality indicators, between the optimal solution derived by the algorithms and the customer-requested specifications. Table 5 presents the aggregate discrepancy observed after fulfilling all the requests. Each algorithm underwent three executions for each instance. In these terms, BR-DES emerges as the superior approach. The top solutions obtained by BR-DES for each instance are significantly approximate to the customers' specified requirements, both in terms of quality and quantity. Following closely, the SA algorithm constitutes the second-best alternative. At times, the greedy algorithm produces commendable solutions. However, this achievement often prolongs the makespan. Minimizing the divergence between the proposed solution and the customers' stipulations holds immense significance. Even as the primary objective revolves around reducing the makespan, meticulous adherence to the aforementioned quality and quantity requisites significantly augments customer satisfaction.

Table 6. Mismatches in quantity (kilograms) and quality levels between the required and retrieved items for each approach (greedy, random, BR-DES, and SA) and instance (row).

Instance	Greedy		Random (Beta = 0.3)		BR-DES		SA	
	Quantity Mismatch	Quality Mismatch	Quantity Mismatch	Quality Mismatch	Quantity Mismatch	Quality Mismatch	Quantity Mismatch	Quality Mismatch
1	2373	3.70	9219	16.40	1326	9.59	2881	40.21
2	1890	8.42	6084	36.89	860	14.91	1421	28.91
3	1134	14.19	7470	16.72	931	21.95	1721	22.21
4	3468	16.94	23,205	112.86	3809	67.58	5580	93.21
5	8880	15.78	12,432	56.66	3143	12.28	5772	88.28
6	2418	29.62	7832	84.69	2539	50.36	4103	18.22
7	4896	38.63	19,296	13.96	4752	20.17	5193	33.22
8	9610	15.42	21,204	55.61	3640	41.71	3698	17.03
9	8525	13.27	4850	146.91	5225	42.46	4433	31.99
10	-	-	-	-	6272	19.15	9003	198.02
11	-	-	12,936	15.44	6006	14.14	8633	92.26
12	-	-	-	-	7189	120.45	8874	6.31

Figures 8 and 9 visually juxtapose the considered approaches with regards to makespan and quantity mismatch. Since the greedy and random approaches fail to produce feasible solutions for Instances 10 to 12, only Instances 1 to 9 are considered in these figures. Notice that the BR-DES algorithm outperforms all other approaches both in terms of the makespan and the quantity mismatch.

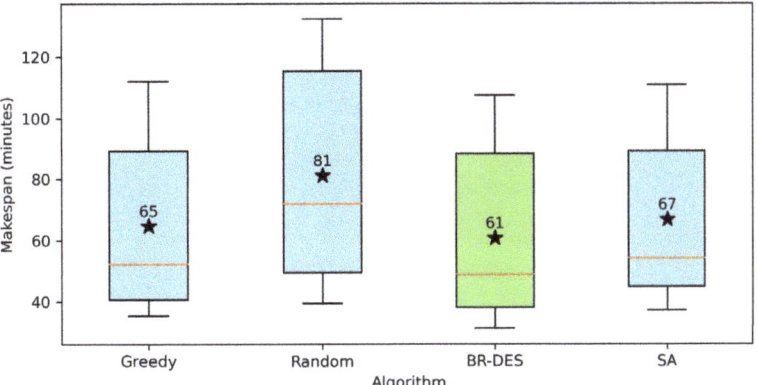

Figure 8. Makespan comparison of different approaches.

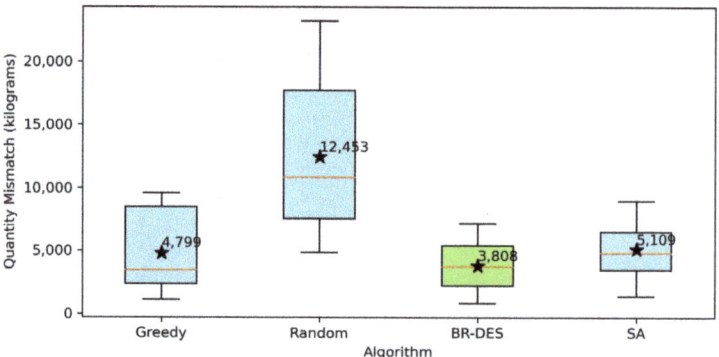

Figure 9. Quantity mismatch comparison of different approaches.

8. Conclusions and Future Perspectives

This paper has discussed a complex and realistic warehouse automated storage and retrieval system (AS/RS) in the steel industry sector. The peculiar characteristics of this sector, notably the considerable size and weight of items and bundles stored and retrieved, alongside stringent quality constraints, constitute a challenge when enhancing the system performance. Traditional approaches such as developing a simulation model or employing classical optimization methods, albeit viable, present limitations to providing optimal solutions within reasonable computational time frames. Hence, this paper advocates a novel hybrid simulation optimization algorithm. It combines the precision of discrete event simulations, crucial in managing time dependencies within the system's sequential operations, with a biased-randomized heuristic. This combination, encapsulated within a multi-start framework, swiftly generates a multitude of promising, high-quality solutions in seconds, outperforming the more traditional simulated annealing (SA) metaheuristic. Although the SA algorithm is a robust approach, it struggles to adequately address the intricate time dependencies among events in the warehouse system.

Our approach boasts adaptability, a key advantage for accommodating novel scenarios. Based on simulation principles, it holds the potential to evolve into a simheuristic [28], adept at tackling stochastic versions of the problem. This adaptability extends to various AS/RS configurations, thus illustrating its versatility. Furthermore, the computational experiments conducted confirm the capacity of our approach in providing feasible and high-quality solutions for optimization problems characterized by complex constraints, especially those entailing intricate time dependencies among decisions.

From a managerial perspective, the proposed approach can enhance decision-making processes, particularly in managing the complexities of AS/RS operations characterized by time-dependent sequences and stringent constraints. The BR-DES algorithm is specifically tailored to the challenges of steel storage systems, including large item sizes, substantial weights, and strict quality constraints. From a business impact perspective, the algorithm contributes to improving the operational efficiency by rapidly generating high-quality solutions, resulting in a reduced makespan and optimized resource utilization. This, in turn, can lead to savings in labor, energy, and equipment usage. The algorithm's focus on reducing the discrepancy between the proposed solutions and customer specifications ensures an enhanced customer satisfaction, thereby positively impacting customer relations.

The following points outline the potential directions for future research: (i) extending our approach to achieve full automation, enabling the algorithm to make decisions autonomously without human intervention; (ii) improving the algorithm's handling of weight and quality constraints, particularly in more constrained scenarios, to enhance its effectiveness even further; and (iii) expanding the approach to encompass scenarios involving random times and stochastic availability of items, broadening its applicability to diverse, less deterministic environments.

Author Contributions: Conceptualization, M.B. and M.N.; methodology, A.A.J. and M.N.; software, M.N.; writing—original draft preparation, M.N., A.A.J. and M.B.; writing—review and editing, A.A.J. and M.B. All authors have read and agreed to the published version of the manuscript.

Funding: This work was partially funded by the Horizon Europe program (HORIZON-CL4-2022-HUMAN-01-14-101092612 SUN and HORIZON-CL4-2021-TWIN-TRANSITION-01-07-101057294 AIDEAS), as well as by the Generalitat Valenciana (PROMETEO/2021/065).

Institutional Review Board Statement: Not applicable.

Informed Consent Statement: Not applicable.

Data Availability Statement: All data and code is available at https://github.com/mattianeroni/Shuttle-Lift-Crane-AS-RS (last accessed on 15 January 2024).

Conflicts of Interest: The authors declare no conflicts of interest.

References

1. Zhang, G.; Lai, K. Combining path relinking and genetic algorithms for the multiple-level warehouse layout problem. *Eur. J. Oper. Res.* **2006**, *169*, 413–425. [CrossRef]
2. Roodbergen, K.J.; Vis, I.F. A survey of literature on automated storage and retrieval systems. *Eur. J. Oper. Res.* **2009**, *194*, 343–362. [CrossRef]
3. Chen, L.; Langevin, A.; Riopel, D. The storage location assignment and interleaving problem in an automated storage/retrieval system with shared storage. *Int. J. Prod. Res.* **2010**, *48*, 991–1011. [CrossRef]
4. Foley, R.D.; Hackman, S.T.; Park, B.C. Back-of-the-envelope miniload throughput bounds and approximations. *IIE Trans.* **2004**, *36*, 279–285. [CrossRef]
5. Kosanić, N.Ž.; Milojević, G.Z.; Zrnić, N. A survey of literature on shuttle based storage and retrieval systems. *FME Trans.* **2018**, *46*, 400–409. [CrossRef]
6. Bertolini, M.; Esposito, G.; Mezzogori, D.; Neroni, M. Optimizing retrieving performance of an automated warehouse for unconventional stock keeping units. *Procedia Manuf.* **2019**, *39*, 1681–1690. [CrossRef]
7. Dominguez, O.; Juan, A.A.; Faulin, J. A biased-randomized algorithm for the two-dimensional vehicle routing problem with and without item rotations. *Int. Trans. Oper. Res.* **2014**, *21*, 375–398. [CrossRef]
8. Bertolini, M.; Neroni, M.; Uckelmann, D. A survey of literature on automated storage and retrieval systems from 2009 to 2019. *Int. J. Logist. Syst. Manag.* **2023**, *44*, 514–552. [CrossRef]
9. Liu, S.; Wang, Q.; Sun, J. Integrated optimization of storage allocations in automated storage and retrieval system of bearings. In Proceedings of the 25th Chinese Control and Decision Conference, Guiyang, China, 25–27 May 2013; pp. 4267–4271.
10. Wang, W.; Tang, X.; Shao, Z. Study on energy consumption and cable force optimization of cable-driven parallel mechanism in automated storage/retrieval system. In Proceedings of the Second International Conference on Soft Computing and Machine Intelligence, Dubai, United Arab Emirates, 23–25 November 2016; pp. 144–150.
11. Lerher, T.; Sraml, M.; Potr, I. Simulation analysis of mini-load multi-shuttle automated storage and retrieval systems. *Int. J. Simul. Model.* **2015**, *14*, 48–59. [CrossRef]
12. Ekren, B.Y.; Heragu, S.S.; Krishnamurthy, A.; Malmborg, C.J. Matrix-geometric solution for semi-open queuing network model of autonomous vehicle storage and retrieval system. *Comput. Ind. Eng.* **2014**, *68*, 78–86. [CrossRef]
13. Liu, T.; Gong, Y.; De Koster, R.B. Travel time models for split-platform automated storage and retrieval systems. *Int. J. Prod. Econ.* **2018**, *197*, 197–214. [CrossRef]
14. Zou, B.; Xu, X.; Gong, Y.; De Koster, R. Modeling parallel movement of lifts and vehicles in tier-captive vehicle-based warehousing systems. *Eur. J. Oper. Res.* **2016**, *254*, 51–67. [CrossRef]
15. Ekren, B.; Heragu, S. *A New Technology for Unit-Load Automated Storage System: Autonomous Vehicle Storage and Retrieval System*; Springer: London, UK, 2012; pp. 285–339.
16. Roy, D.; Krishnamurthy, A.; Heragu, S.S.; Malmborg, C.J. Performance analysis and design trade-offs in warehouses with autonomous vehicle technology. *IIE Trans.* **2012**, *44*, 1045–1060. [CrossRef]
17. Liu, T.; Xu, X.; Qin, H.; Lim, A. Travel time analysis of the dual command cycle in the split-platform AS/RS with I/O dwell point policy. *Flex. Serv. Manuf. J.* **2016**, *28*, 442–460. [CrossRef]
18. Hu, Y.H.; Huang, S.Y.; Chen, C.; Hsu, W.J.; Toh, A.C.; Loh, C.K.; Song, T. Travel time analysis of a new automated storage and retrieval system. *Comput. Oper. Res.* **2005**, *32*, 1515–1544. [CrossRef]
19. Cai, X.; Heragu, S.S.; Liu, Y. Modeling and evaluating the AVS/RS with tier-to-tier vehicles using a semi-open queueing network. *IIE Trans.* **2014**, *46*, 905–927. [CrossRef]

20. Carlo, H.J.; Vis, I.F.A. Sequencing dynamic storage systems with multiple lifts and shuttles. *Int. J. Prod. Econ.* **2012**, *140*, 844–853. [CrossRef]
21. Zammori, F.; Neroni, M.; Mezzogori, D. Cycle time calculation of shuttle-lift-crane automated storage and retrieval system. *IISE Trans.* **2021**, *54*, 40–59. [CrossRef]
22. Arnau, Q.; Barrena, E.; Panadero, J.; de la Torre, R.; Juan, A.A. A biased-randomized discrete-event heuristic for coordinated multi-vehicle container transport across interconnected networks. *Eur. J. Oper. Res.* **2022**, *302*, 348–362. [CrossRef]
23. Arcus, A.L. A computer method of sequencing operations for assembly lines. *Int. J. Prod. Res.* **1965**, *4*, 259–277. [CrossRef]
24. Tonge, F.M. Assembly line balancing using probabilistic combinations of heuristics. *Manag. Sci.* **1965**, *11*, 727–735. [CrossRef]
25. Glover, F. Tabu search—Part I. *ORSA J. Comput.* **1989**, *1*, 190–206. [CrossRef]
26. Glover, F. Tabu search—Part II. *ORSA J. Comput.* **1990**, *2*, 4–32. [CrossRef]
27. Dorigo, M.; Gambardella, L.M. Ant colony system: A cooperative learning approach to the traveling salesman problem. *IEEE Trans. Evol. Comput.* **1997**, *1*, 53–66. [CrossRef]
28. Hatami, S.; Calvet, L.; Fernandez-Viagas, V.; Framinan, J.M.; Juan, A.A. A simheuristic algorithm to set up starting times in the stochastic parallel flowshop problem. *Simul. Model. Pract. Theory* **2018**, *86*, 55–71. [CrossRef]

Disclaimer/Publisher's Note: The statements, opinions and data contained in all publications are solely those of the individual author(s) and contributor(s) and not of MDPI and/or the editor(s). MDPI and/or the editor(s) disclaim responsibility for any injury to people or property resulting from any ideas, methods, instructions or products referred to in the content.

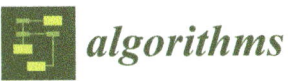 algorithms

Article

Efficient Multi-Objective Simulation Metamodeling for Researchers

Ken Jom Ho *, Ender Özcan and Peer-Olaf Siebers *

School of Computer Science, University of Nottingham, Jubilee Campus, Nottingham NG8 1BB, UK; ender.ozcan@nottingham.ac.uk
* Correspondence: psxkh1@nottingham.ac.uk (K.J.H.); peer-olaf.siebers@nottingham.ac.uk (P.-O.S.)

Abstract: Solving multiple objective optimization problems can be computationally intensive even when experiments can be performed with the help of a simulation model. There are many methodologies that can achieve good tradeoffs between solution quality and resource use. One possibility is using an intermediate "model of a model" (metamodel) built on experimental responses from the underlying simulation model and an optimization heuristic that leverages the metamodel to explore the input space more efficiently. However, determining the best metamodel and optimizer pairing for a specific problem is not directly obvious from the problem itself, and not all domains have experimental answers to this conundrum. This paper introduces a discrete multiple objective simulation metamodeling and optimization methodology that allows algorithmic testing and evaluation of four Metamodel-Optimizer (MO) pairs for different problems. For running our experiments, we have implemented a test environment in R and tested four different MO pairs on four different problem scenarios in the Operations Research domain. The results of our experiments suggest that patterns of relative performance between the four MO pairs tested differ in terms of computational time costs for the four problems studied. With additional integration of problems, metamodels and optimizers, the opportunity to identify ex ante the best MO pair to employ for a general problem can lead to a more profitable use of metamodel optimization.

Keywords: discrete multiple objective; simulation; metamodel; optimization; test environment

Citation: Ho, K.J.; Özcan, E.; Siebers, P.-O. Efficient Multi-Objective Simulation Metamodeling for Researchers. *Algorithms* **2024**, *17*, 41. https://doi.org/10.3390/a17010041

Academic Editors: Nuno Fachada and Nuno David

Received: 31 December 2023
Revised: 14 January 2024
Accepted: 15 January 2024
Published: 18 January 2024

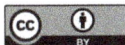

Copyright: © 2024 by the authors. Licensee MDPI, Basel, Switzerland. This article is an open access article distributed under the terms and conditions of the Creative Commons Attribution (CC BY) license (https://creativecommons.org/licenses/by/4.0/).

1. Introduction

A simulation model of a physical and/or social system of interest can unlock useful experimental capabilities [1]. Not only are the costs of simulation experimentation in general much lower than an equivalent series of real-world experiments, but there are also scenarios where the latter are simply unfeasible—for example, if the system does not yet exist. However, there always exists a frontier where computational costs limit viable use cases [2].

An Agent-Based Simulation (ABS) usually features decision-making entities who interact with their environment and, directly or indirectly, with one another. When the decisions of many so-called "agents" are critical to system dynamics, utilizing an ABS approach for extending standard models would be a good option, but also a computationally expensive one.

Complicating problem-solving further, many real-world problems, from designing ships to chemical engineering or saving energy, cannot be neatly simplified into a single objective to be maximized or minimized [3]. If one option performs worse in all objectives compared to another option, the first one is "dominated" and would never be worth picking even when both are feasible. At the same time, it is possible to have two options such that neither dominates the other; in this scenario, the decision between them is external to the optimization that produced the options. A collection of all the non-dominated options is most commonly known as a Pareto front but also as Pareto frontier, and Pareto set [4], and as in the two-option case above, does not allow improvements in any objective(s) without having to suffer a worsening of other objective(s). This presents distinctive challenges [5], in particular, the need to thoroughly explore a greater proportion of the input space to generate a Pareto front [6] compared to the single objective problem.

Fortunately, for many optimization problems, a "model of a model", commonly referred to as a metamodel, can enable experimentation and thus optimization that is less costly than directly using a simulation model. Metamodels are "a mathematical approximation to the implicit input-output function of a simulation model" [7]. They have been adopted in various domains, and depending on the context are referred to as surrogate models, response surface models, or proxy models. Some domains have a rich literature on the use of metamodels within their context [8], but such findings do not necessarily apply to other domains in terms of the most effective use of a metamodel and optimizer. A more general way to make comparisons is by using benchmark problems [9] which may involve a mathematical function [10], domain-specific models [11] or data sets [12]. However, the issue still remains when moving outside domains or problems that are "similar" to these, which led to some siloing and duplication of effort in terms of optimization research in general [13], although there have been efforts to compile this work in a more practitioner-salient form [14].

1.1. Simulation Optimization

The use of simulation in optimization has a long history of development and deployment, and there are a variety of simulation-capable or focused platforms. AnyLogic [15,16] is a popular choice in Operations Research (OR), and options are available for ABS-focused applications [17]. Platforms with more general capabilities like R [18] can also be employed in this role.

Simulation-optimizer methodologies (also known as simheuristics or metaheuristics [19]) are the most direct way to employ a simulation model and optimizer to solve problems, with packages integrating these components like OptQuest and Witness Optimizer being commercially available [20] and open-source options such as SimOpt [21] enabling more user-driven development.

1.2. Metamodeling

When a good balance is struck between efficient exploration of the input space ("learning" the behavior of the system) and focusing on potential areas of optimization interest, a metamodel allows to minimize the use of any costly simulation model evaluations, as described in the work of [22]. Additionally, techniques reviewed by [23] such as variable screening, dimensionality reduction, and use of multiple metamodels can further extend the legs of metamodels, increasing the number of scenarios where they can be profitably employed.

Similar to simulation optimization, methodologies employing metamodels and comparisons between them exist [24]. However, the points of comparison such as between setups, problem types and domains, or specifics of the simulation models used differ between the observed case studies, making it hard to draw fully generalizable conclusions regarding performance or cost characteristics.

Of course, some domains have long-established and well-explored metamodels. For example, the domain of energy prediction models [25] extends standard surrogate energy prediction models by incorporating household preferences into the underlying simulation model and using an artificial neural network metamodel. In engineering designs, kringing regression is popular, as demonstrated in applications such as vacuum/pressure swing adsorption systems [26]. Polynomial-based surrogates are also seeing advancements in engineering applications [27]. These are not the only options, as metamodeling does not have a "one size fits all" methodology. Technique selection comes with various trade-offs. Ref. [28] compares a number of these trade-offs for the scenario of building design optimization while [29,30] do the same for the water resources modeling case.

There is a growing number of studies on deep learning to fully exploit the power of neural networks. Deep learning has been applied to many real-world problems successfully, however, two main issues, among others, raised by [31] are relevant to consider. First of all, deep learning techniques require a large amount of data. As one of the goals of this work is a methodology that minimizes the use of expensive simulation model evaluation, gathering this data to train a deep learning system would not be ideal. Secondly, deep learning models can have high memory and computational requirements. As a result, while deep learning can provide a high level of flexibility, when simpler metamodels, where the best is selected from a variety of options, can achieve good final Pareto front performance, the approach that requires less data and incurs lower computational costs might be more appropriate.

1.3. Optimizers

Implicit in the above discussion is the need for an optimizer heuristic to decide which experiments to run and at which level of model; evolutionary methodologies [32] like genetic algorithms are a popular choice. The ability to algorithmically test and evaluate various Metamodel Optimizer (MO) pairs would also bring benefits for researchers and practitioners in terms of reproducibility and avoiding reliance on excessive problem- or domain-specific tuning; finely tailored heuristics can exhibit improved performance but with less visible costs of requiring specific knowledge or reducing the generalizability of the solution method, something pointed out by the review of [13].

1.4. Aim

The aim of this paper is to introduce a comprehensive methodology designed to facilitate the systematic application and evaluation of metamodeling and optimization heuristics. While platforms exist to handle setups utilizing metamodels, such as OPTI-MIZE [33], these focus more on enabling users without specialist optimization knowledge to employ metamodeling to solve optimization problems. In contrast, our methodology enables researchers to compare setups experimentally, determining which MO pair is the best performer at each tested time limit for a given problem, in a way that allows drawing specific and in some cases general conclusions about the optimal MO pairs.

2. Test Environment and Methods

The primary feature of the test environment is to enable researchers to run experiments on discrete multiple objective optimization problems using a simulation model and metamodel. These experiments evaluate the relative performance of MO pairs on a time and solution quality basis. As many such experiments may need to be conducted and the main goal of employing a metamodel is to economize on simulation model costs, the test environment utilizes a specific method for generating and storing simulation model Full Evaluations (FEs), or FE, for all future users. For each problem, corresponding to a simulation model, an exhaustive list of input–output data (including evaluation times) allows for faster-than-FE lookup, and reproducible FEs. In addition, this mechanism takes a stochastic simulation model and provides all future users with a deterministic response to any set of inputs, namely the mean of the simulation repetitions for that specific set of inputs.

The components of the test environment interact as illustrated in Figure 1. Notably, while the external simulation models are evaluated on another platform (AnyLogic or SimOpt), users will use the FE record, meaning that only R needs to be actively executed for experiments. This record is separate from what the optimizer has in "memory" for each experiment run, which only consists of FEs it has already requested and "paid for" in terms of time costs and any Quick Evaluations (QEs) it has made via the latest updated metamodel.

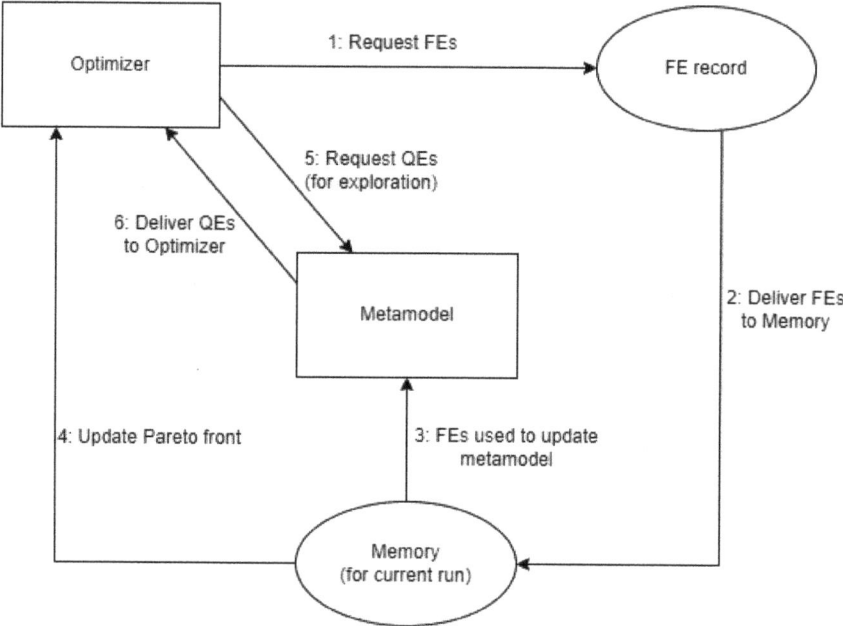

Figure 1. MO test environment components.

The overall sequence followed to complete an experiment run is as follows:
1. Optimizer requests FEs;
2. Requested FEs are delivered to memory;
3. All FEs in memory are used to update the metamodel;
4. Optimizer updates its current Pareto front, using all FEs in memory;
5. Optimizer requests QEs from metamodel (this is an exploration step);
6. Metamodel delivers QEs to the optimizer;
7. If any of the QEs would be part of the Pareto front, they will be listed and requested by returning to step 1.

For each experiment run, the first time step 1 occurs, the FEs requested correspond to the initial sample. Step 4 can be considered the exploitation step each time it occurs except the first time, as this is when the Pareto front actually improves. Although QEs are used to identify potential additions to the Pareto front, the objective values from a QE must be "confirmed" with FEs for those inputs.

If an experiment run reaches the time limit while going through a list of requested FEs, only the FEs that would have been done before the time limit can be part of the final Pareto front. Otherwise, reaching the time limit means that the most recent Pareto front is the one that is stored and evaluated.

For each problem investigated, a set of experiments is run on the simulation model, using different combinations of metamodel, optimizer and time limits. Each experiment run produces a Pareto front as output, which will be stored for later use. Once the experiment is completed, all Pareto fronts can be evaluated using the metrics detailed below. This allows the user to compare the evolution of solution quality against the time limit for each MO pair.

2.1. Metamodels

Two different popular metamodeling methodologies are integrated into the test environment. The first is based on Gaussian regressions, and the second is using a neural network approach. It should be noted that the solution Pareto fronts will only contain points that have been obtained through FE.

2.1.1. Gaussian Regression (GR) Metamodel

This metamodel employs the "GPFDA" package (https://github.com/gpfda/GPFDA-dev, accessed on 23 May 2023) for R [34] and treats outputs as independent, though this is not a restriction on all Gaussian regressions.

For an objective x, the FEs in memory relate values of the objective to values of the inputs, so if there are n FEs in memory, we can express $Memory = \{(x_1, t_1), (x_2, t_2), \ldots (x_n, t_n)\}$ where t_j is a vector of input values corresponding to x_j.

The Gaussian regression model for x is then:

$$x_i = f(t_i) + \epsilon_i, \; i = 1, \ldots, n$$
$$e_i \sim i.i.d.N(0, \sigma_\epsilon^2) \quad (1)$$
$$f(.) \sim GP(\mu(.), k(.,.)) \; where \; k(t_i, t_j) = COV(f(t_i), f(t_j))$$

The mean function used is $\mu(.) = 0$, which means the covariance function of a Gaussian process is the only item that has to be estimated in order to characterize that Gaussian process.

The Matern covariance function is used here, so:

$$k(t_i, t_j) = v_0 \frac{(d\sqrt{2v})^v}{\Gamma(v)2^{v-1}} K_v(d\sqrt{2v}) \quad (2)$$
$$d = |t_i - t_j|^2$$

where K_v is the modified Bessel function of order v, and $v = 1.5$ is used.

2.1.2. Neural Network (NN) Metamodel

This metamodel employs the "neuralnet" package (https://github.com/bips-hb/neuralnet, accessed on 23 May 2023) for R [35] and uses a back propagation algorithm. Specifically, the neural network used here consists of input neurons $x_{IN,1}, x_{IN,2}, \ldots, x_{IN,n_{IN}}$ corresponding to the inputs, output neurons $x_{OUT,1}, x_{OUT,2}, \ldots, x_{OUT,n_{OUT}}$ corresponding to the number of objectives, and n_H layers of hidden neurons, where $x_{i,j}$ correspond to the jth neuron on the ith hidden layer. Input neurons interact only with neurons on the first hidden layer, and neurons on each hidden layer interact only with neurons on the following hidden layer, with neurons on the final hidden layer interacting with the output neurons.

As a result, in a system with N_H hidden layers, where the ith hidden layer has n_i neurons, the value of the first output neuron (dropping the $OUT, 1$ notation for clarity) might be expressed as:

$$x = f(w_0 + \sum_{j=1}^{n_{N_H}} w_j * x_{N_H}). \quad (3)$$

Every neuron has a weight for each neuron on the previous layer, and a constant neuron. The weighted sum of neuron values on the previous layer (for output neurons, the previous layer is the N_Hth hidden layer) is the input to $f()$, the activation function. In this case, the activation function is the logistic function: $f(u) = \frac{1}{1+e^{-u}}$ as it gives final outputs in the interval $[0, 1]$ and the metamodel works on inputs and objectives scaled to this interval.

In keeping with the design intent to minimally adjust component settings, the main default options are used for training the model. In particular, the algorithm used is the resilient backpropagation with weight backtracking by [36] on two layers of hidden neurons (five in the first layer and three in the second).

2.2. Optimizers

The two implemented optimizers make use of a metamodel to explore potential solutions before deciding which ones to request FEs for. At the start of each run, the optimizer starts off with no FEs and thus cannot train a metamodel. This is why the first step for all optimizers is to draw an initial sample of FEs from the input space in proportion to its size. For our experiments, the initial sample size is always fixed at 5% of the input space. Other than this initial sample, optimizers only request FEs for solutions that are expected to improve their Pareto front. When the time limit is reached, optimizers will stop and record the Pareto front from all the obtained FEs.

2.2.1. Basic (B) Optimizer

The algorithm is as follows:

1. Perform initial sampling;
2. Using the list of all prior FEs, train metamodel;
3. Populate the full list of candidate solutions by requesting QEs;
4. Remove all Pareto-dominated solutions to generate a potential Pareto front;
5. If any solutions of the Pareto front are from a QE, request FEs, store the results and return to step 2, else;
6. If all solutions on the Pareto front are from FEs, the optimizer terminates successfully.

If step 6 is reached, the optimizer has no FEs to request. This means there is no new data to update the metamodel, and as it already in step 3 used the metamodel exhaustively for QEs, the input space is fully explored. As a result, it will terminate even if the time limit has not yet been reached.

2.2.2. Genetic Algorithm (GA) Optimizer

The algorithm is as follows:

1. Perform initial sampling;
2. Using the list of all prior FEs, train metamodel;
3. Remove all Pareto-dominated solutions to generate a Pareto front—this is the "parent population";
4. Generate new "children" solutions;
5. Request QEs for all children solutions;
6. Generate a new Pareto front from the combined parents and children population;
7. If any solutions of the Pareto front are from a QE, request FEs, store the results and return to step 2, else;
8. If all solutions on the Pareto front are from FEs, return to step 4.

The population for the genetic algorithm consists of all solutions on the Pareto front. These always consist of FEs. Children are generated by randomly selecting two parent individuals at random. Each time step 4 occurs, up to twice the number of the parent population or the number of the initial sample size (whichever is greater) of children will be generated.

There is a 10% chance for each input to undergo crossover, and a 10% chance for each input to mutate by 1, subject to input constraints. In step 8, all "children" from the previous step 4 become part of the next "parent" generation. This optimizer always utilizes the full allowed time limit, even if it constantly generates new "children" that do not meet expected improvements.

2.2.3. Normalized Hypervolume

The hypervolume measure is calculated by defining a section of the problem's output space bounded by each objective's minimum and maximum as observed from the optimal Pareto front, the set $A \subset \mathbb{R}^d$ (d is the number of objectives). Any Pareto front is a set of points, B, with each point $b \in B$ dominating a portion of A, the set $D(b, A) \subset A$. The hypervolume of the Pareto front B is thus:

$$HV_B = \Lambda(\cup_{b \in B} D(b, A)) \tag{4}$$

where Λ is the Lebesgue measure.

The hypervolume measure is normalized by dividing the hypervolume of a Pareto front by the hypervolume of the optimal Pareto front. The maximum is 1. Thus, a *higher* normalized hypervolume indicates a better-quality solution.

2.2.4. Normalized Hausdorff Distance

The Hausdorff distance [37] measures how close two sets are to each other. For finite sets (which the Pareto fronts here all are due to the discrete problem construction) the Hausdorff distance between sets X and Y can be expressed as:

$$dist_H = max[\max_{x \in X} d(x, Y), \max_{y \in Y} d(y, X)] \tag{5}$$

where $d(a, B)$ is the minimum Euclidean distance between a point a and any member of set B. The Hausdorff distance is normalized by dividing the Hausdorff distance between a Pareto front and the optimal Pareto front by the maximum Hausdorff distance between any Pareto front from the experiment set and the optimal Pareto front. The minimum (between a set and itself) is 0. Thus a *lower* normalized Hausdorff distance indicates a better-quality solution.

2.2.5. Normalized Crowding Distance

The crowding distance [38] measures how close points on a Pareto front are to each other. In the case where there are N_o objectives and N_p Points on the Pareto front, every point on the Pareto front will have a series of rankings $(x_1, x_2, \ldots x_j, \ldots x_{N_o})$ where each x_j is its ranking in objective j ($x_j \in [1, 2 \ldots N_p]$). Let $I[a].b$, $b \in [1, 2 \ldots N_o]$ denote the objective value of element a in the ranking corresponding to objective b.

For every non-boundary point (not at the maximum or minimum for any one objective as observed on the Pareto front) with the per-objective rankings as above, we can define its crowding distance as:

$$CD_{point} = \sum_{j=1}^{N_o} \frac{I[x_j + 1] \cdot j - I[x_j - 1] \cdot j}{max_j - min_j} \tag{6}$$

where max_j and min_j are the maximum and minimum values for objective j.

The crowding distance for the whole Pareto front is then calculated as the average of the crowding distances across all non-boundary points. The crowding distance is normalized by dividing the crowding distance of a Pareto front by the crowding distance of the optimal Pareto front. A *lower* normalized crowding distance implies points on the Pareto front are closer to one another, which indicates a better-quality solution.

3. Experimentation

3.1. Simulation Models

For our experimentation, we have chosen four OR simulation models as part of the test environment, which are deployed together with the FE records in the Supplementary Material: A student services model and a telecom model [39] models—which were run in AnyLogic as well as a Continuous News Vendor model and a dual sourcing model [21], which run in the Python-based SimOpt package (https://pypi.org/project/simoptlib/, accessed on 23 May 2023).

3.1.1. Student Services Simulation

This model represents a trio of student service centers that face a stochastic distribution of incoming students in each location. These students require different types of service: one general service and two specific services. The two objectives being examined are the total labor costs of hiring three different classes of employees corresponding to service types (specialists can handle their specific specialist enquiries as well as general enquiries, while non-specialists can only handle general enquiries) and the total time cost, faced by students on average.

The student traveling, queuing and service processes correspond to a classic discrete event simulation with stochastic elements, while the simulation model's main agent-based features are the students, using a "smart app" that gives students information about queue length and average waiting times, allowing them the decision to select between different centers. A student using the smart app will select the service center with the lowest expected time cost to them, considering not only the expected queuing times but also travel time, which depends on the distance of the student from a service center as well as the student's travel speed.

Students start in one of three locations, with each location being close to one service center (5 distance units away) and far from the other two service centers (15 distance units away). The distribution of student starting locations is not uniform each day, but instead one service center will see half of the students starting near it, and the other two service centers will see one quarter of the students starting near each of them. Students have stochastic travel speeds, with a mean of one distance unit per minute. Even with the smart app, students do not know the exact time they will be queuing at the time they start, but this is estimated by multiplying a moving average of waiting times for their enquiry type by the queue length for their enquiry type at the time they make their decision. The expected service time after traveling and queuing is the same across all centers for any given student enquiry type (which they are aware of).

3.1.2. Telecom Simulation

This model is a publicly available AnyLogic example model [39] of a telecom company operating in a market with competitors. The inputs of interest are call price per minute and aggressiveness (referring to marketing effectiveness). The objectives of interest are as follows: voice revenue (which is specific to people paying to make calls), "value added" service revenue (which covers other items besides calls), as well as aggressiveness itself, as the cost of the required marketing strategy to reach a certain level of effectiveness is not represented within the model. In this model, aggressiveness affects the addressable market share, but users decide which company to support based on the prices they observe. This behavior is implemented in the model by referencing tables that presumably represent statistical market research on the probabilities involved.

The Telecom simulation allows for dynamic adjustment of the inputs, which will result in a transition to a new market equilibrium. For the case study, selected inputs were applied at the start of the simulation. The experimental inputs do not correspond to the initial market state. This requires the simulation to be run until it reaches the new equilibrium, at which time the objectives can be measured.

3.1.3. Continuous News Vendor Simulation

This model is included in the SimOpt distribution and represents a newsvendor who orders a quantity of stock, and decides on a price to sell it to customers. However, the day's demand is randomly drawn from a Burr Type XII distribution, where the cumulative distribution is given by:

$$F(x) = 1 - (1 + x^\alpha)^{-\beta} \qquad (7)$$

with $\alpha = 2$ and $\beta = 20$.

The two inputs of interest relate to stock quantity and selling price decisions, while the two objectives of interest are the news vendor's profits and the quantity of stock actually sold.

3.1.4. Dual Sourcing Simulation

This model is included in the SimOpt distribution and represents a manufacturing location purchasing its input via regular or expedited suppliers with different ordering costs and delays while facing stochastic demand. Regular deliveries cost 100 per unit and take 2 days to arrive, while expedited deliveries cost 110 per unit but take 0 days to arrive. One simulation run will simulate 1000 days of operation.

There are storage costs when the location carries stock from one day to the next day, and a penalty "cost" per unit of shortage whenever there is a lack of stock to meet demand. Satisfied demand has no benefit other than zero penalty, which implies that location is a substitute for a cost center that aims to minimize costs and penalties.

The strategy followed by the location can be summarized as follows: It consists of having two inventory target levels, one for the regular supplier and one for the expedited supplier. The location will place an order with a specific supplier whenever the stock level falls below its associated threshold value. Although the goods being ordered are homogeneous when in stock, goods that are yet to arrive are not considered against the target level for the expedited supplier as they will only arrive after the expedited delivery.

The two inputs of interest are these two threshold levels. The three objectives of interest are the three main types of costs to be considered: ordering costs, holding costs and penalties for running out of stock.

3.2. Procedural Steps

We compare the performance of MO pairs on each simulation model separately, as each such case study corresponds to a different scenario. There are four scenarios in total. Each case study used four time limits, so from an optimization standpoint, there are four problem instances per case study, for sixteen total across all case studies. Each individual experiment specification is run fifty times with the same setup, as is required for stochastic experimentation.

More specifically, each case study covers all possible combinations of the following:

- Two metamodel options (Gaussian regression, Neural network);
- Two optimizer options (Basic, Genetic algorithm);
- Four time limits (as determined for each simulation problem).

The selection of time limits is different for each simulation model. The lowest time limit corresponds to the time required to carry out the FEs corresponding to the initial sample. For all experiments, initial sample sizes are 5% of the simulation model's input space, although this can be user-defined. The initial sample is uniformly and randomly distributed via Latin hypercube sampling.

The experiments are run sequentially, from the initial sampling until the time limit is reached or, for the Basic optimizer only, if the stopping condition is reached before the time limit. As the test environment uses FE records instead of obtaining objective values from running the simulation model directly for each required set of inputs, the real-world time taken for an experiment will be shorter than the time limit, as the time limit accounts for the full FE time costs. For each completed experiment, the final Pareto front is stored. All Pareto fronts for a given case study are evaluated as a set, as the metrics used to evaluate MO pair performance are all normalized.

Three metrics, normalized hypervolume, normalized Hausdorff distance and normalized crowding distance, are used to evaluate the obtained Pareto fronts, which, for consistency, use as a reference the Pareto front generated from the exhaustive FE record. This optimal Pareto front, corresponding to the specific simulation model problem, remains the same whenever the simulation model is referenced, ensuring that all metrics have a common benchmark across different sets of experiments.

3.3. System Configuration and General Experimental Setup

All experiments were run on a laptop with a dual-core 11th Gen Intel(R) Core(TM) i5-1135G7 (2.40 GHz, 2.42 GHz) CPU and 20 GB of RAM (Intel, Santa Clara, CA, USA). This same system was used to generate the FE records.

4. Results

When identifying specific MO pairs, the acronyms for metamodels (Gaussian Regression: GR, Neural Network: NN) and optimizers (Basic: B, Genetic Algorithm: GA) are used to identify MO pairs in that order (metamodel optimizer). For example, GR-B corresponds to experiments using the Gaussian regression metamodel and Basic optimizer.

For each of the four time limits, we identified the best-performing MO pair with respect to the mean normalized hypervolume, denoted as μ_{norm}, considering each case study. We applied a paired Wilcoxon signed-rank test to determine if the best-performing and each of the other MO pairs have a statistically significant performance difference within a confidence interval of 95%. Tables 1–4 summarize the results obtained by repeating each experiment for fifty trials, providing μ_{norm} associated with the standard deviation, indicated as σ- and p-values for each pair-wise statistical performance comparison of the best and associated MO pairs.

Before we come to presenting the individual results, there is one more point to clarify. While one would expect the mean quality of Pareto fronts for a given MO pair to always stagnate or increase with higher time limits, we found that the mean quality in this case sometimes decreases. The explanation for this behavior is that experiments with different specified time limits are not direct "progressions" from one another and there is variance of results, even when individual time limits are higher.

4.1. Student Services Simulation Case Study

As mentioned in Section 3.1.1, the goal of this case study is to optimize the operations of three student service centers that handle stochastic student arrivals and offer both general and specialized services. Figure 2 shows the relationship between normalized hypervolume and time limits for the Student Services problem. The symbols between the two lines of each MO pair represent the mean value, while the lines represent the limits of the associated confidence interval. The graph suggests that the Student Services problem is relatively easy to solve, as all MO pairs, even with low time limits, can achieve a high normalized hypervolume (above 0.98).

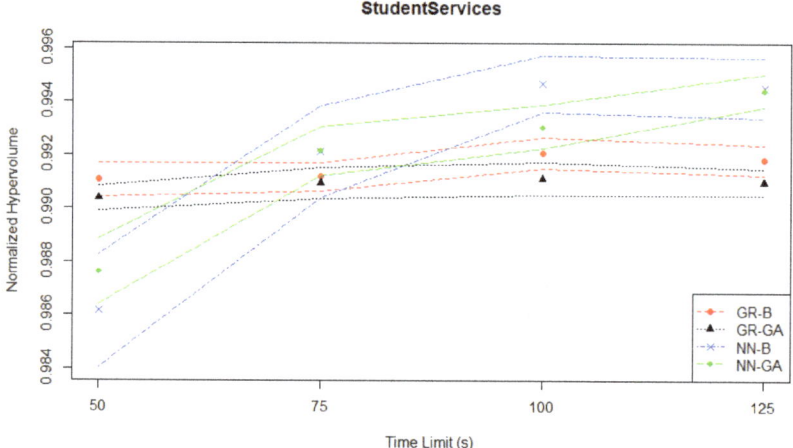

Figure 2. Student services experiments—hypervolume evaluation—time series.

Table 1 summarizes the results for the Student Services experiments based on the mean normalized hypervolume performance (μ_{norm}s) of each MO pair with the best-performing one at each time limit. The results show that at the lowest time limit of 50 s, GR-B turns out to be the best-performing approach while GR-GA delivers a similar performance based on the statistical test. As the time limit is increased to 75 s, NN-GA becomes the best approach, where the performance difference is statistically significant with p-values being less than 0.05 when compared to both GR-based methods. NN-B delivers a similar, but slightly worse performance than NN-GA. As the computational budget is increased further to 100 s and 125 s, NN-B outperforms the other MO pairs, while NN-GA ranks the second best method with a similar performance to NN-B, except for 100 s. The GR-B and GR-GA pairs once again turn out to be the worst methods of all. The performance difference between NN-B and GR-based methods is statistically significant at the 95% confidence level for the time limits greater than 50 s. Regardless of the given time limit, all methods produce a μ_{norm} about 0.99.

Table 1. Student services experiments—normalized hypervolume performance comparison of each MO pair with the best-performing one at each time limit.

Time Limit (s)	MO Pair	μ_{norm}	σ	p-Value
50	GR-B	0.991049	3.23×10^{-4}	Best
	GR-GA	0.990360	2.35×10^{-4}	8.61×10^{-2}
	NN-B	0.986146	1.08×10^{-3}	1.57×10^{-4}
	NN-GA	0.987603	6.28×10^{-4}	1.37×10^{-5}
75	GR-B	0.991151	2.71×10^{-4}	3.76×10^{-2}
	GR-GA	0.990927	2.88×10^{-4}	8.04×10^{-3}
	NN-B	0.992102	8.78×10^{-4}	3.97×10^{-1}
	NN-GA	0.992128	4.74×10^{-4}	Best
100	GR-B	0.992058	2.95×10^{-4}	1.93×10^{-5}
	GR-GA	0.991106	3.16×10^{-4}	1.94×10^{-6}
	NN-B	0.994665	5.34×10^{-4}	Best
	NN-GA	0.993041	4.19×10^{-4}	4.96×10^{-3}
125	GR-B	0.991801	2.92×10^{-4}	3.17×10^{-4}
	GR-GA	0.990969	2.52×10^{-4}	3.94×10^{-6}
	NN-B	0.994517	5.65×10^{-4}	Best
	NN-GA	0.994415	3.06×10^{-4}	1.29×10^{-1}

One interesting detail is that for the 75 s time limit case, the best Pareto front (Figure 3) and the worst Pareto front (Figure 4) are both from the NN-B pair, which has the largest standard deviation across all MO pairs and time limits. The reason for the difference between them is that the metamodel in the worst case has underestimated the performance of solutions that would have otherwise been located in the top left corner of the Pareto front, where wages are low and student inquiry time is high. In this case, that means it had an excessively high estimate for student time cost or employee wages. The explanation for this is that the Basic optimizer uses the metamodel evaluations to check every possible solution and does not identify them as possible candidates for inclusion.

The general pattern of slow improvements in the two Gaussian regression-based pairs, leading to them being out-performed by the neural network-based pairs is also reflected in the normalized Hausdorff distance plot in Figure 5.

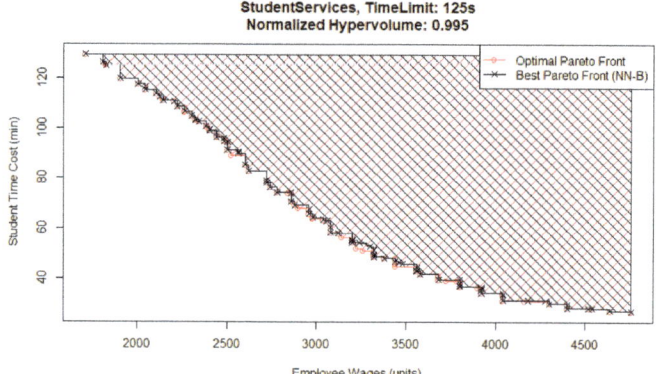

Figure 3. Student services experiment—optimal and best Pareto front.

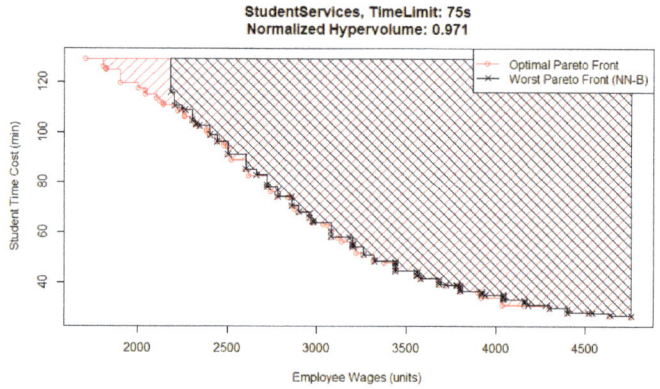

Figure 4. Student services experiment—optimal and worst Pareto front.

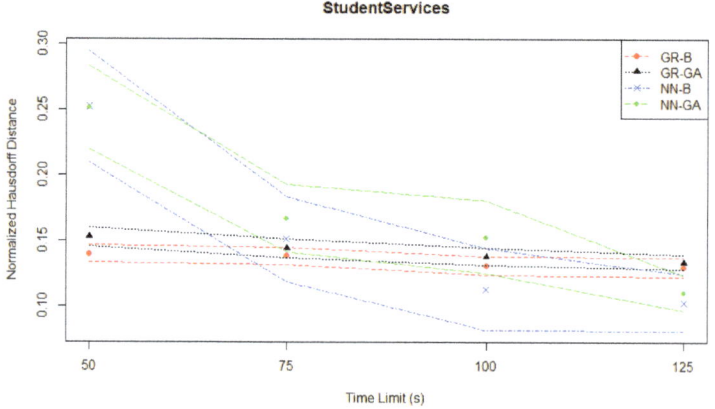

Figure 5. Student services experiments—Hausdorff distance evaluation—time series.

The crowding distances depicted in Figure 6 confirm the previously identified patterns of behavior.

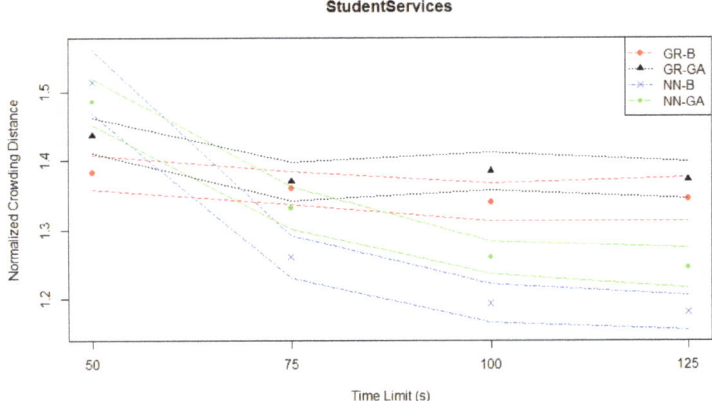

Figure 6. Student services experiments—crowding distance evaluation—time series.

4.2. Telecom Simulation Case Study

As mentioned in Section 3.1.2, the goal of this case study is to optimize the operations of a telecom company in a competitive market, considering call price, marketing aggressiveness, and revenue components. There is a dramatic improvement in normalized hypervolume initially, as well as a later clear separation of performance between the different MO pairs seen in Figure 7 which depicts the hypervolume evaluation. For example, between the two NN-based pairs (and overall between all four pairs) the NN-GA pair underperforms in terms of not improving from between the time limits of fifty to one hundred seconds, with the second-worst being the GR-GA pair.

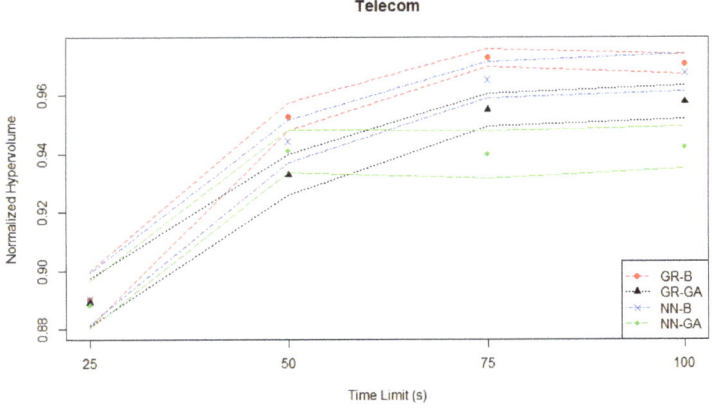

Figure 7. Telecom experiments—hypervolume evaluation—time series.

Table 2 summarizes the results for the Telecom experiments based on the mean normalized hypervolume performance (μ_{norm}s) of each MO pair with the best-performing one at each time limit. At a time limit of 25 s, the NN-B pair performs the best among all MO pairs without statistical significance. At the time limits of 50 s, 75 s and 100 s, the "top two MO pairs" in this Telecom case study are different from the Student Services case study, as the GR-B pair outperforms the others. For all these increasing time limits, the NN-B pair delivers a similar performance to GR-B, while the performance differences between GR-B and both GR-GA and NN-GA pairs are statistically significant having p-values less than 0.05. The μ_{norm} produced by GR-B increases from 0.953 to 0.971 as the time limit is doubled.

Table 2. Telecom experiments—normalized hypervolume performance comparison of each MO pair with the best-performing one at each time limit.

Time Limit (s)	MO Pair	μ_{norm}	σ	p-Value
25	GR-B	0.890518	4.84×10^{-3}	6.22×10^{-1}
	GR-GA	0.889344	4.16×10^{-3}	9.85×10^{-1}
	NN-B	0.890610	4.50×10^{-3}	Best
	NN-GA	0.888545	4.13×10^{-3}	9.15×10^{-1}
50	GR-B	0.952749	2.41×10^{-3}	Best
	GR-GA	0.932791	3.53×10^{-3}	5.26×10^{-5}
	NN-B	0.944377	3.67×10^{-3}	1.08×10^{-1}
	NN-GA	0.941043	3.70×10^{-3}	1.60×10^{-2}
75	GR-B	0.972904	1.56×10^{-3}	Best
	GR-GA	0.955054	2.82×10^{-3}	1.90×10^{-6}
	NN-B	0.965317	3.06×10^{-3}	6.88×10^{-2}
	NN-GA	0.939940	4.08×10^{-3}	1.10×10^{-7}
100	GR-B	0.970620	1.71×10^{-3}	Best
	GR-GA	0.957607	2.92×10^{-3}	6.67×10^{-4}
	NN-B	0.967764	3.26×10^{-3}	7.72×10^{-1}
	NN-GA	0.942319	3.62×10^{-3}	2.67×10^{-7}

There is a small decrease in mu_norm from a time limit of 75 s to 100 s for GR-B. When testing if this difference is statistically significant, the p-value is 0.447, so the decrease is not statistically significant at the 95% confidence level.

Plotting the best-performing Pareto front from the 100 s case in Figure 8 highlights where losses in quality occur relative to the optimal Pareto front. Where both Pareto fronts overlap, the color is black, corresponding to the best Pareto front. Thus, any red points plotted correspond to points only found on the optimal Pareto front. The right-side edge of the Pareto fronts is where the majority of these points are seen. However, as this best Pareto front has a high normalized hypervolume of 0.997, the quality losses from not including the red points are not major, which implies the Pareto front already captures most of the trade-off solutions by hypervolume.

We can compare the previous situation to the worst-performing 100 s Pareto front (normalized hypervolume of 0.880) plotted in Figure 9. There is a more visually obvious presence of red points on the left and right edges of the worst Pareto front.

In this case study, the two best-performing MO pairs are the GR-B and NN-B pairs. Thus the main decider of performance is the optimizer rather than the metamodel. This contrasts with the Student Services case where the two best-performing MO pairs are the NN-B and NN-GA pairs which would suggest the main decider of performance is the metamodel rather than the optimizer. If we consider the normalized Hausdorff distances plotted in Figure 10, the two best-performing MO pairs are still the GR-B and NN-B pairs, but the distinctive under-performance of the NN-GA pair relative to the other three MO pairs seen in the hypervolume evaluation at time limits of 75 s or 100 s is not observed in the Hausdorff distance evaluation.

By contrast, when considering the normalized crowding distances plotted in Figure 11, the GR-GA pair has a noticeably higher crowding distance from the other three MO pairs at 75 s and 100 s, although as previously noted it is not the worst-performing in the hypervolume evaluation.

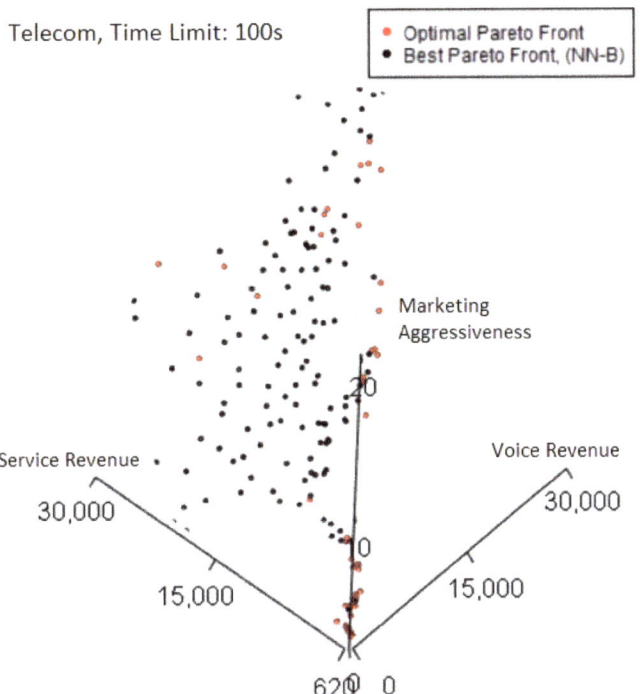

Figure 8. Telecom experiments—optimal and best Pareto front.

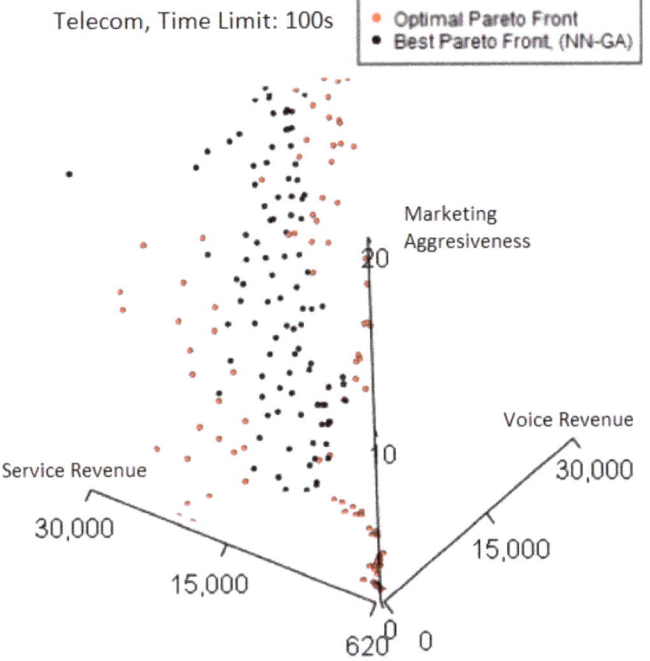

Figure 9. Telecom experiments—optimal and worst Pareto front.

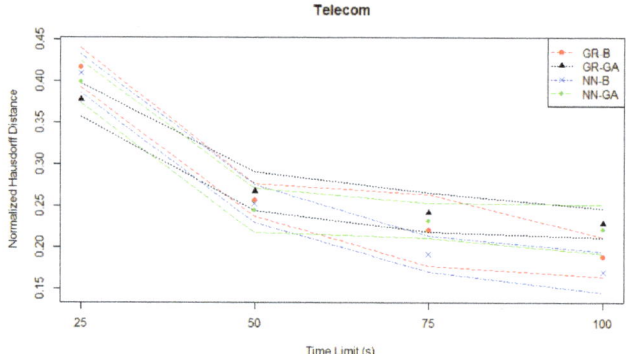

Figure 10. Telecom experiments—Hausdorff distance evaluation—time series.

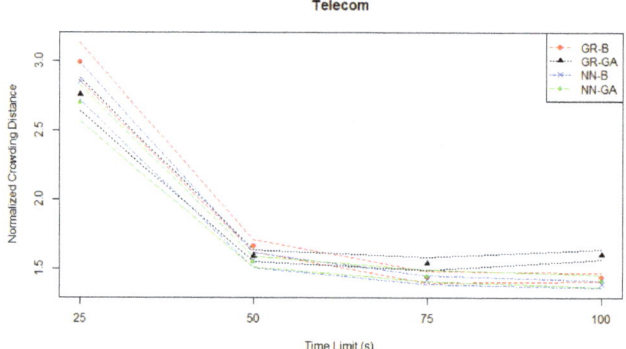

Figure 11. Telecom experiments—crowding distance evaluation—time series.

4.3. Continuous News Vendor Simulation Case Study

As mentioned in Section 3.1.3, the goal of this case study is to optimize a news vendor's stock quantity and selling price, considering random daily demand. In both the hypervolume evaluation plotted in Figure 12 and the Hausdorff distance evaluation plotted in Figure 13, the NN-GA pair is a consistent worst-performer when compared to the other three MO pairs.

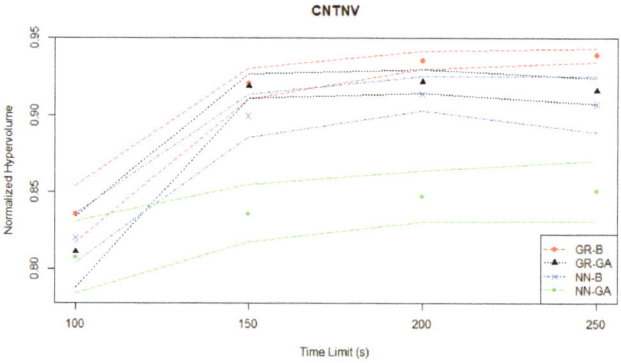

Figure 12. Continuous News Vendor experiments—hypervolume evaluation—time series.

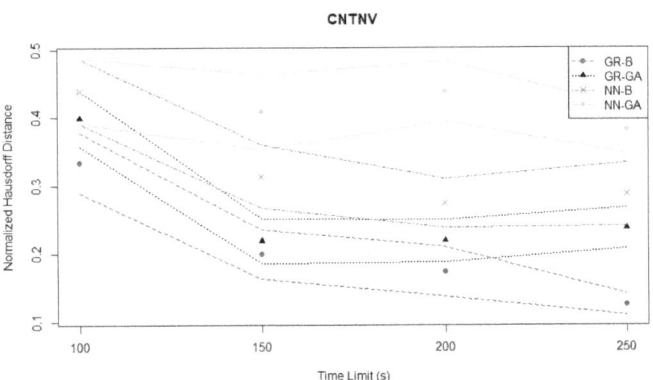

Figure 13. Continuous News Vendor experiments—Hausdorff distance evaluation—time series.

Table 3 summarises the results from the Continuous News Vendor experiments based on the mean normalized hypervolume performance (μ_{norm}s) of each MO pair with the best-performing one at each time limit. For any given time limit, the GR-B pair outperforms the rest of the methods. At the 100 s time limit, all methods deliver a similar performance to GR-B, although their μ_{norm}s are slightly worse. This observation persists for the time limit of 150 s, while NN-GA performs significantly worse than GR-B. As the time limit increases above 200 s, the performance differences between GR-B and each of the other MO pairs become statistically significant with p-values less than 0.05, and GR-GA ranks the second best-performing method among all. The μ_{norm}s of GR-B increases from 0.836 to 0.939 as the time limit increases by a factor of 2.5.

Table 3. Continuous News Vendor experiments—normalized hypervolume performance comparison of each MO pair with the best-performing one at each time limit.

Time Limit (s)	MO Pair	μ_{norm}	σ	p-Value
100	GR-B	0.835878	9.33×10^{-3}	Best
	GR-GA	0.811036	1.17×10^{-2}	1.45×10^{-1}
	NN-B	0.820163	8.09×10^{-3}	1.32×10^{-1}
	NN-GA	0.807869	1.20×10^{-2}	7.89×10^{-2}
150	GR-B	0.920727	5.03×10^{-3}	Best
	GR-GA	0.918869	4.00×10^{-3}	4.96×10^{-1}
	NN-B	0.899821	7.03×10^{-3}	1.18×10^{-2}
	NN-GA	0.836305	9.49×10^{-3}	7.18×10^{-8}
200	GR-B	0.935907	3.00×10^{-3}	Best
	GR-GA	0.921874	3.95×10^{-3}	9.02×10^{-3}
	NN-B	0.914207	5.74×10^{-3}	2.30×10^{-3}
	NN-GA	0.847465	8.43×10^{-3}	2.91×10^{-9}
250	GR-B	0.939361	2.22×10^{-3}	Best
	GR-GA	0.915885	4.24×10^{-3}	9.44×10^{-5}
	NN-B	0.907325	9.17×10^{-3}	1.21×10^{-3}
	NN-GA	0.850925	9.84×10^{-3}	8.26×10^{-9}

One feature of the Continuous News Vendor optimization problem is that relatively few sets of inputs will correspond to a point on the Pareto front: an exhaustive search encompasses 651 potential input combinations of which only eleven make up the optimal Pareto front. Solution Pareto fronts had between four to fifteen points across all the experiments.

To further analyze the potential effect this causes in solution quality, we consider the Pareto fronts from experiments with a time limit of 150 s. The best-performing Pareto front from a 150 s time limit experiment is plotted in Figure 14 (and is from a GR-GA pair) and can be compared with the best Pareto front from a 150 s time limit experiment specifically from a NN-GA pair, shown plotted in Figure 15. In these figures, the Pareto front of interest and the optimal Pareto front from the FE records are plotted, with the dominated area for each shaded in the appropriate color.

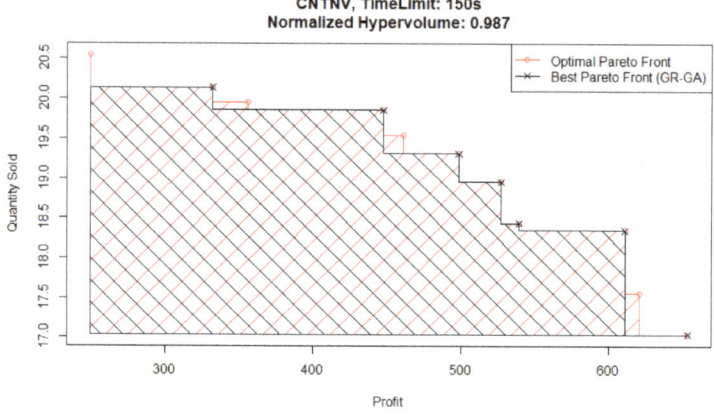

Figure 14. Continuous News Vendor experiments—optimal and best Pareto front.

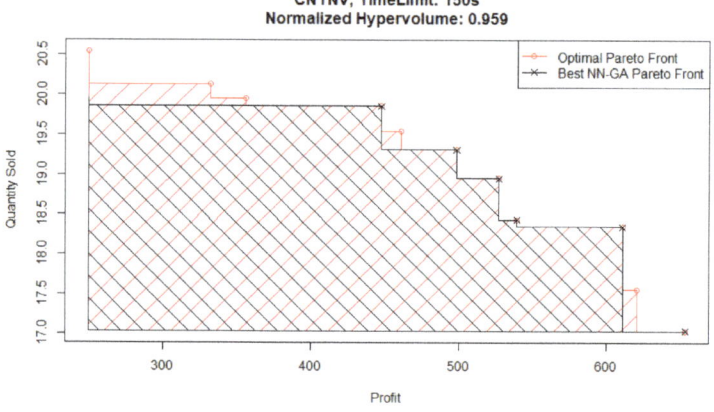

Figure 15. Continuous News Vendor experiments—optimal and best NN-GA Pareto front.

The main area of difference between the two Pareto front solutions is the area corresponding to high quantities sold and low profits. To follow up on this, consider the best NN-GA Pareto front from an experiment with a higher time limit of 250 s plotted in Figure 16. Although the Pareto front from this experiment captures the corner corresponding to high quantities sold and low profits, it does not capture part of the medium quantities sold and medium profits area.

These findings can indicate an issue faced by the genetic algorithm optimizer relative to the Basic optimizer when parent populations are relatively small due to Pareto fronts having only a few points in them. It is harder to identify ex ante which metamodel would under-perform in this situation. However, the hypervolume evaluation shows that the GR-B pair performs the best and the NN-GA pair performs the worst for this problem.

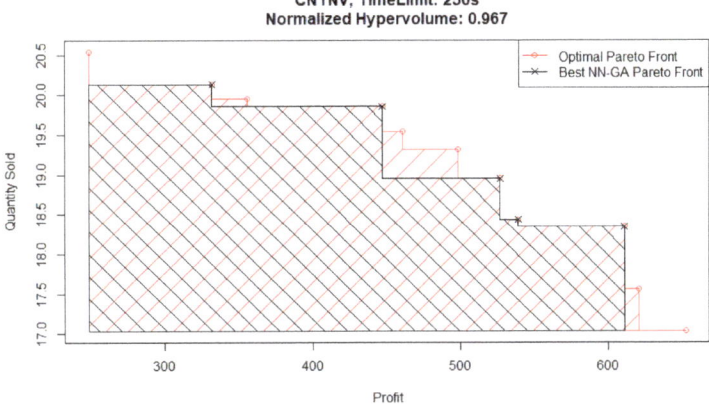

Figure 16. Continuous News Vendor experiments—optimal and best NN-GA Pareto front.

The crowding distance evaluation plotted in Figure 17 confirms that the NN-GA pair has the most widely spaced Pareto fronts of the four pairs, while the GR-B has the closest spacing. Additionally, at a time limit of 250 s, there are GR-B Pareto fronts with normalized crowding distances below 1.

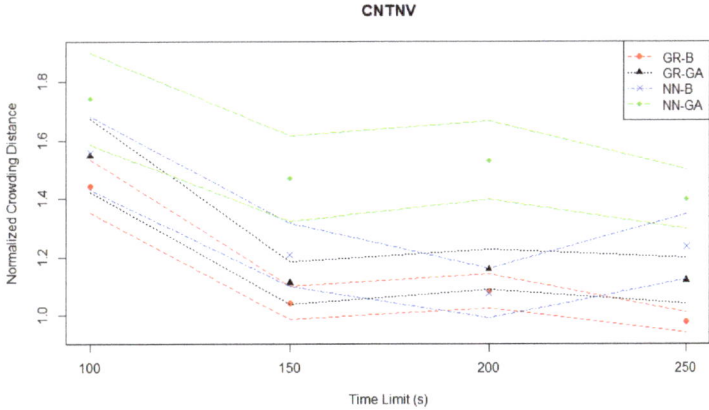

Figure 17. Continuous News Vendor experiments—crowding distance evaluation—time series.

4.4. Dual Sourcing Simulation Case Study

As mentioned in Section 3.1.4, the goal of this case study is to minimize costs and penalties for a manufacturer present in multiple locations, involving procurement from regular or expedited suppliers with varied costs and delays. The Dual Sourcing experiments provide an important contrast with those of the Continuous News Vendor, as the proportion of total input combinations that would be on the Pareto front is much higher (861 of 1681). While solution Pareto fronts have between 383 to 694 points across all experiments, the hypervolume evaluation plot in Figure 18 shows that all MO pairs perform very well, similar to what was observed in the Student Services experiments.

Table 4 summarizes the results from the Dual Sourcing experiments based on the mean normalized hypervolume performance (μ_{norm}s) of each MO pair with the best-performing one at each time limit. In all time limits (240 s, 300 s, 360 s and 420 s), GR-B outperforms the rest of the MO pairs, and this performance variation is statistically significant with p-values less than 0.05. Regardless of the given time limit, all methods produce a high μ_{norm} over 0.99. The μ_{norm}s produced by GR-B increase slightly from 0.9954 to 0.9997 even if the time limit is increased by a factor of 1.75.

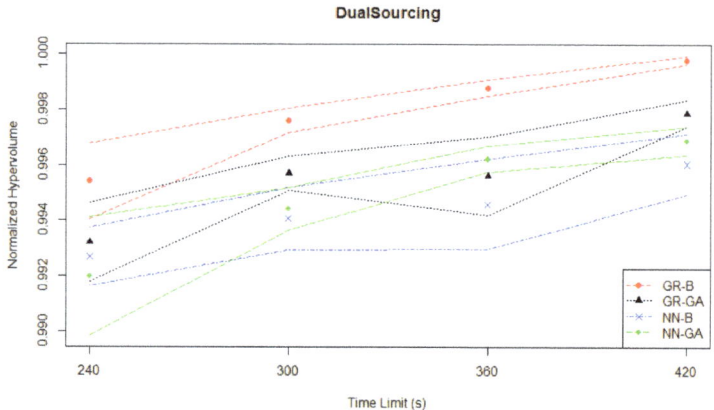

Figure 18. Dual Sourcing experiments—hypervolume evaluation—time series.

Table 4. Dual Sourcing experiments—normalized hypervolume performance comparison of each MO pair with the best-performing one at each time limit.

Time Limit (s)	MO Pair	μ_{norm}	σ	p-Value
240	GR-B	0.995415	6.93×10^{-4}	Best
	GR-GA	0.993214	7.18×10^{-4}	1.10×10^{-4}
	NN-B	0.992700	5.32×10^{-4}	3.49×10^{-4}
	NN-GA	0.991999	1.08×10^{-3}	6.89×10^{-5}
300	GR-B	0.997616	2.22×10^{-4}	Best
	GR-GA	0.995695	3.17×10^{-4}	8.17×10^{-5}
	NN-B	0.994081	5.68×10^{-4}	8.71×10^{-7}
	NN-GA	0.994431	3.89×10^{-4}	2.18×10^{-7}
360	GR-B	0.998792	1.51×10^{-4}	Best
	GR-GA	0.995610	7.16×10^{-4}	6.25×10^{-8}
	NN-B	0.994595	8.22×10^{-4}	9.88×10^{-8}
	NN-GA	0.996224	2.34×10^{-4}	1.82×10^{-8}
420	GR-B	0.999778	7.88×10^{-5}	Best
	GR-GA	0.997865	2.35×10^{-4}	8.83×10^{-10}
	NN-B	0.996043	5.52×10^{-4}	9.75×10^{-9}
	NN-GA	0.996886	2.57×10^{-4}	7.44×10^{-9}

However, the Hausdorff distance evaluation plotted in Figure 19 suggests a large relative separation of solution qualities, which is not observed when considering the normalized hypervolumes. As the Hausdorff distances are normalized, an outlier with a high pre-normalized value will compress the distribution of normalized values towards 0. In fact, the Student Services experiments may exhibit the compression of normalized values issue the most, as the highest plotted point in the Hausdorff distance evaluation plot in Figure 5 which corresponds to the upper confidence interval for NN-GA at the 50 s time limit is close to 0.3, in contrast to the highest plotted point in the Hausdorff distance evaluation for the Dual Sourcing case which is 0.8. The definition of the Hausdorff distance can lead to it being very sensitive to the possibility of a "very bad" solution that is part of a solution Pareto front leading to a very high distance, even though the corresponding point in objective space would not greatly affect the front's measured hypervolume.

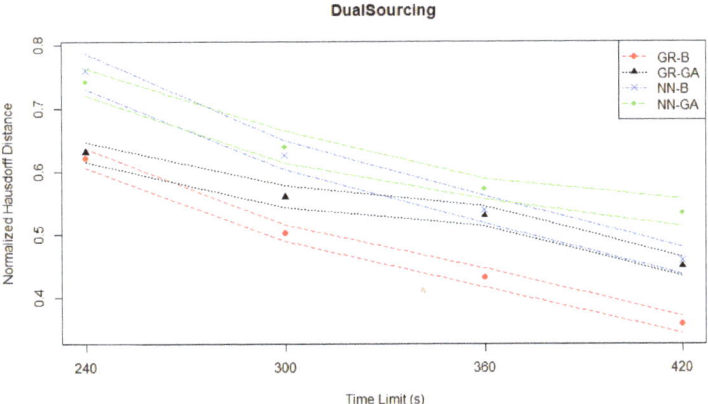

Figure 19. Dual sourcing experiments—Hausdorff distance evaluation—time series.

However, the normalized crowding distances plotted in Figure 20 not only support a significant improvement in Pareto front quality in terms of density, but the patterns of relative performance differ between the Hausdorff distance and crowding distance measures. Taken together, these two suggest that a high level of density is not required to properly characterize the Pareto front.

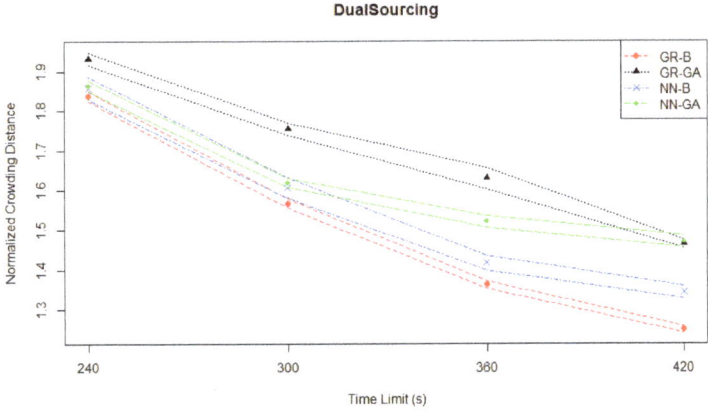

Figure 20. Dual sourcing experiments—crowding distance evaluation—time series.

We can further investigate these features by plotting the best Pareto front obtained from a 420 s time limit in Figure 21 which has a normalized hypervolume above 0.999 despite showing a large section of red points that were missed but do not result in significant loss.

Viewing the Pareto front from another angle, as in the plot Figure 22 shows clearly that the large amount of red points seen previously are very close to (many are exactly on) the plane of minimum average penalty. In this case study, it is entirely plausible to have exactly 0 average penalty, as this corresponds to the stock never running out in all the simulation runs done for the FE. There are also a number of points with very small average penalties as well for the same reason. Not only does this follow the general pattern of corners or boundary edges having the majority of "misses" by MO pairs, but in this case, the hypervolume loss is so extremely small because only a couple of points already capture all the relevant space.

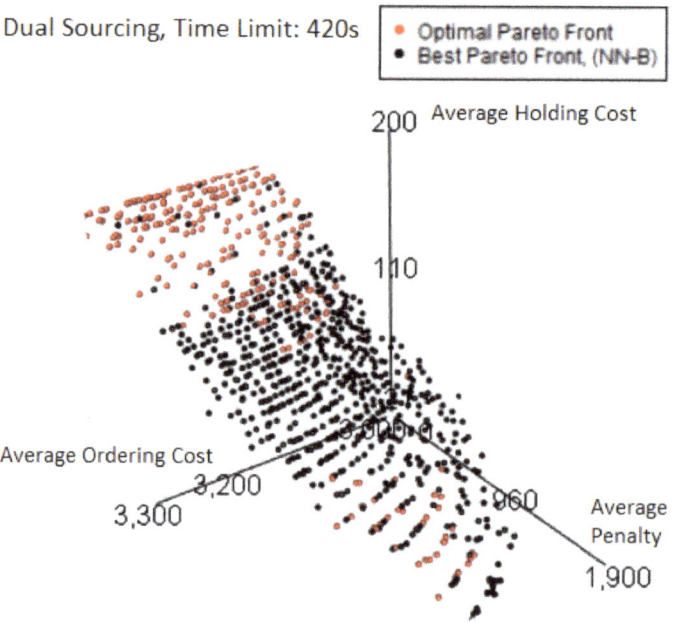

Figure 21. Dual Sourcing experiments—optimal and best Pareto front.

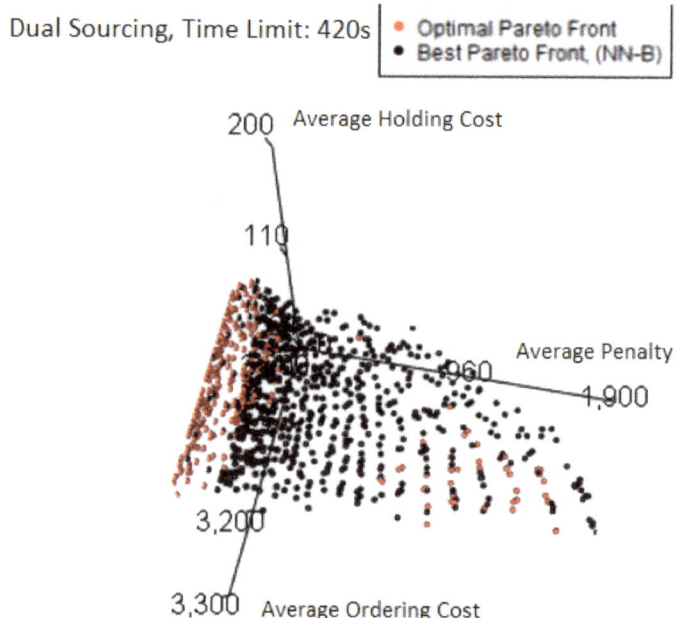

Figure 22. Dual sourcing experiments—optimal and best Pareto front (alternative angle of view).

4.5. Best-Performing MO Pair

In Table 5, we provide the n_{best} value which is the number of times that an MO pair performs the best along with the other top-ranking MO pairs delivering a similar performance to the best (if there are any) considering all four time limits per case study.

Table 5. Best-performing MO pairs per case study.

Case Study	Best MO Pair (s)	n_{best}
Student Services	NN-B & NN-GA	3
Telecom	GR-B & NN-B	3
Continuous News Vendor	GR-B	4
Dual Sourcing	GR-B	4

The GR-B pair is the best overall option in three of the four case studies with a total n_{best} value of 11. The Basic optimization method (B) is the winner when compared to the genetic algorithm metaheuristic, as this method appears as part of the top-ranking MO pairs in almost all cases.

4.6. Experimental Computational Costs

Table 6 shows the MO Time which is the real-world time taken to run the experiments on each simulation problem. While this does not include the time taken for the associated FEs (as these are looked up from the record) the FE times are recorded and "paid for" with the allowed time limit. As a result, an experiment that is given a time limit of 60 s may run for 15 s of the user time, and end with 15 s of MO time and 45 s of FE time. The "FE Record Time" is the time taken to generate the full list of FEs, and helps demonstrate the savings when many experiments are run. For example, the Student Services experiments took under 6 h, but were able to save an additional 11 h by using the FE records. The gains are largest in the Dual Sourcing case where a higher proportion of the allowed time limit is spent on FEs, such that even though time limits are higher for the Dual Sourcing experiments, the real-world time spent does not increase proportionally.

Table 6. Experimental computational costs.

Simulation	MO Time (min)	FE Time (min)	FE Record Time (min)	FE Record Size (KB)
Student Services	352	672	3.6	13
Telecom	205	557	3.7	21
Continuous News Vendor	462	1541	24.2	13
Dual Sourcing	337	3981	10.7	40

5. Discussion

In the experimental investigation of four simulation optimization problems, it turned out that two of them (Student Services and Dual Sourcing) can be considered straightforward in that all the MO pairs evaluated performed similarly and produced high-quality Pareto fronts. In the other two (Telecom and Continuous News Vendor), there was more of a separation of quality with different patterns between the MO pairs evaluated, which comes from the way in which the metamodels estimate objective values for the inputs being explored by the optimizers. One can form more intuitive relationships from MO pair performance patterns to response surface properties than starting from the simulation components or domains, as there are only a limited number of MO pair performance patterns.

Ideally, even a problem with a computationally intensive simulation model of interest would have well-behaved response surfaces, allowing a metamodel to identify areas of interest quickly and with confidence. This would enable the use of expensive FEs more sparingly, focusing on those areas of interest identified by the metamodel to maximize the precision of the optimization. However, being "well-behaved" is not necessarily a simple property that would hold for all MO pairs that might be employed. As seen, some MO pairs may perform better than others for certain problems of interest. Additionally, multi-domain problems may or may not behave similarly to the problems of any particular component domain [40].

The application of metamodeling to ABS is currently a topic of great interest and ongoing research. In the Student Services case study, we showed that despite the agent-based behavior of the model, it was still able to be solved to a high standard across all evaluated MO pairs. In fact, for this problem, the agents' decision-making did not lead to a complex response surface. In contrast, a more challenging problem like the one investigated in the Continuous News Vendor case study has a simple simulation model but a response surface that is not equally responsive to different MO pairs.

It is important to note that the FE times are based on a fixed record. However, the time limit stopping condition treats a second of FE time as equivalent to a second of metamodel or optimizer time. Therefore, if one runs experiments on problems where records were generated on a slower system, the faster system will always obtain better quality solutions within the same time limit, as the faster system has more computational resources. It will be possible to replicate previous results by creating a different version of the record with scaled decreased FE times. This will better match what the faster system is experiencing. Additionally, a smaller time limit can be used in the same proportion. This approach still allows the user to use records, but avoids having to set up numerous simulation models.

While handy for experimental work like that detailed here, the downside of using an FE recording approach is that it does introduce an issue if there is a desire to create records for simulation models with a large input space due to memory constraints. Furthermore, referencing the records will take longer as they grow in size. This can lead to a memory-computation cost tradeoff. However, for the simulation models presented in this paper, the records are small enough so that they do not require a lot of memory to load. The ability to use records without having to run the underlying simulation model is also a form of experiment enabler, especially if the associated model would otherwise be simply inaccessible.

6. Conclusions

In this paper, we have presented and tested a comprehensive methodology designed to facilitate the systematic application and evaluation of metamodeling and optimization heuristics in the form of MO pairs. Our methodology enables researchers to compare setups experimentally, in a way that allows drawing general conclusions about the optimal MO pairs. Hence, the aim detailed in Section 1.4 has been fulfilled. The methodology has been tested with the help of a test environment that allows algorithmic testing and evaluation of MO pair performance for different types of problems. We have demonstrated its use with the help of four illustrative case studies. The performance of the different four MO pairings we tested suggests that patterns of relative performance (and thus the ideal choice) may differ between different models that they are asked to solve.

By critically assessing our work, we have identified several limitations that will need further research: (1) Our methodology has not been tested on highly complex models. (2) Our test cases are limited to the OR domain. (3) Instead of conducting experiments with different time limits, it may be more efficient to run experiments up to the highest time limit and use vertical slicing to directly investigate the evolution of Pareto front quality over time. (4) To evaluate Pareto front quality, we can incorporate additional metrics from the multiple objective literature to gain further insights into the performance of MO pairs. (5) The field of metamodeling and optimization offers numerous other metamodels and optimizers that have not yet been tested.

This presents several opportunities for future work. The most straightforward would be to increase the number of simulation models, metamodels and optimizers available for experimentation and performance comparisons. Since simulation models are represented in the environment by records of their input-objective outcomes (including time taken), additional simulation models from other domains and implemented in various simulation platforms can be integrated into the environment and made accessible for comparison purposes. Better domain coverage from this can enable testing of generalizability across a number of domains and problems without having to manage data links to external simulators for each one.

Additionally, where there are parameters for these components that are currently treated as fixed across all uses in these case studies, it may be possible to improve a component by augmenting them with algorithmic hyper-parameter optimization, although this is a non-trivial addition when keeping to the design goal of allowing generalizability to future models. The possibility exists that having a larger variety of less individually optimized metamodel or optimizer options is more efficient in terms of component-possibility coverage.

Another important aspect that requires further investigation is the question of when and why simulation models behave similarly in terms of the performance of MO pairs. While models with similar response surface properties will show similar patterns of MO pair performance, the question remains of identifying the more abstract properties that lead to these similarities in the performance of MO pairs. Alternatively, the possibility of building a selection-type hyperheuristic that explores the space of metamodel and optimizer selection within the optimization process and selects an optimal pair on the fly could potentially be more beneficial for practical applications. This approach could also be generalizable if performance patterns can be detected early enough in the optimization process to justify allocating computational resources to the hyperheuristic layer, rather than a simple initial MO pair selection.

Supplementary Materials: The following supporting information can be downloaded at: https://www.mdpi.com/article/10.3390/a17010041/s1.

Author Contributions: Conceptualization, K.J.H. and P.-O.S.; methodology, K.J.H., E.Ö. and P.-O.S.; software, K.J.H.; validation, K.J.H. and P.-O.S.; formal analysis, K.J.H.; writing—original draft preparation, K.J.H.; writing—review and editing, K.J.H., E.Ö. and P.-O.S.; supervision, E.Ö. and P.-O.S. All authors have read and agreed to the published version of the manuscript.

Funding: This research received no external funding.

Institutional Review Board Statement: Not applicable.

Informed Consent Statement: Not applicable.

Data Availability Statement: Data are contained within the article and Supplementary Materials.

Acknowledgments: The authors would like to acknowledge the valuable advice provided by Russell R. Barton (Pennsylvania State University) regarding this work.

Conflicts of Interest: The authors declare no conflicts of interest.

Abbreviations

The following abbreviations are used in this manuscript:

MO	Metamodel Optimizer
ABS	Agent-Based Simulation
OR	Operations Research
FE	Full Evaluation
QE	Quick Evaluation
GR	Gaussian Regression
NN	Neural Network
B	Basic
GA	Genetic Algorithm

References

1. Kleijnen, J.P. *Design and Analysis of Simulation Experiments*; Springer: Berlin/Heidelberg, Germany, 2018.
2. Alizadeh, R.; Allen, J.K.; Mistree, F. Managing computational complexity using surrogate models: A critical review. *Res. Eng. Des.* **2020**, *31*, 275–298.
3. Cui, Y.; Geng, Z.; Zhu, Q.; Han, Y. Multi-objective optimization methods and application in energy saving. *Energy* **2017**, *125*, 681–704.
4. Lotov, A.V.; Miettinen, K. Visualizing the Pareto Frontier. *Multiobject. Optim.* **2008**, *5252*, 213–243.
5. Gunantara, N. A review of multi-objective optimization: Methods and its applications. *Cogent Eng.* **2018**, *5*, 1502242. [CrossRef]
6. Afshari, H.; Hare, W.; Tesfamariam, S. Constrained multi-objective optimization algorithms: Review and comparison with application in reinforced concrete structures. *Appl. Soft Comput.* **2019**, *83*, 105631.
7. Barton, R.R. Metamodelling: Power, pitfalls, and model-free interpretation. In Proceedings of the 11th Operational Research Society Simulation Workshop, SW 2023, Southampton, UK, 27–29 March 2023; Operational Research Society: Birmingham, UK, 2023; pp. 48–62.
8. Westermann, P.; Evins, R. Surrogate modelling for sustainable building design—A review. *Energy Build.* **2019**, *198*, 170–186. [CrossRef]
9. Wang, C.; Duan, Q.; Gong, W.; Ye, A.; Di, Z.; Miao, C. An evaluation of adaptive surrogate modeling based optimization with two benchmark problems. *Environ. Model. Softw.* **2014**, *60*, 167–179. [CrossRef]
10. Serra, P.; Stanton, A.F.; Kais, S. Pivot method for global optimization. *Phys. Rev. E* **1997**, *55*, 1162–1165. [CrossRef]
11. Kandris, K.; Romas, E.; Tzimas, A. Benchmarking the efficiency of a metamodeling-enabled algorithm for the calibration of surface water quality models. *J. Hydroinform.* **2020**, *22*, 1718–1726.
12. Lejeune, J. Mechanical MNIST: A benchmark dataset for mechanical metamodels. *Extrem. Mech. Lett.* **2020**, *36*, 100659.
13. Swan, J.; Adriaensen, S.; Brownlee, A.E.; Hammond, K.; Johnson, C.G.; Kheiri, A.; Krawiec, F.; Merelo, J.J.; Minku, L.L.; Özcan, E.; et al. Metaheuristics "in the large". *Eur. J. Oper. Res.* **2022**, *297*, 393–406. [CrossRef]
14. Pamparà, G.; Engelbrecht, A.P. Towards a generic computational intelligence library: Preventing insanity. In Proceedings of the 2015 IEEE Symposium Series on Computational Intelligence, Cape Town, South Africa, 7–10 December 2015; IEEE: Piscataway, NJ, USA, 2015; pp. 1460–1467.
15. Muravev, D.; Hu, H.; Rakhmangulov, A.; Mishkurov, P. Multi-agent optimization of the intermodal terminal main parameters by using AnyLogic simulation platform: Case study on the Ningbo-Zhoushan Port. *Int. J. Inf. Manag.* **2021**, *57*, 102133. [CrossRef]
16. Ivanov, D. *Operations and Supply Chain Simulation with AnyLogic*; Berlin School of Economics and Law: Berlin, Germany, 2017.
17. Railsback, S.F.; Lytinen, S.L.; Jackson, S.K. Agent-based simulation platforms: Review and development recommendations. *Simulation* **2006**, *82*, 609–623. [CrossRef]
18. Soetaert, K.; Herman, P.M. *A Practical Guide to Ecological Modelling: Using R as a Simulation Platform*; Springer: Berlin/Heidelberg, Germany, 2009; Volume 7.
19. Juan, A.A.; Faulin, J.; Grasman, S.E.; Rabe, M.; Figueira, G. A review of simheuristics: Extending metaheuristics to deal with stochastic combinatorial optimization problems. *Oper. Res. Perspect.* **2015**, *2*, 62–72. [CrossRef]
20. Eskandari, H.; Mahmoodi, E.; Fallah, H.; Geiger, C.D. Performance analysis of comercial simulation-based optimization packages: OptQuest and Witness Optimizer. In Proceedings of the 2011 Winter Simulation Conference (WSC), Phoenix, AZ, USA, 11–14 December 2011; IEEE: Piscataway, NJ, USA, 2011; pp. 2358–2368.
21. Eckman, D.J.; Henderson, S.G.; Shashaani, S. SimOpt: A testbed for simulation-optimization experiments. *INFORMS J. Comput.* **2023**, *35*, 495–508. [CrossRef]
22. Sóbester, A.; Forrester, A.I.; Toal, D.J.; Tresidder, E.; Tucker, S. Engineering design applications of surrogate-assisted optimization techniques. *Optim. Eng.* **2014**, *15*, 243–265. [CrossRef]
23. Viana, F.A.; Gogu, C.; Goel, T. Surrogate modeling: Tricks that endured the test of time and some recent developments. *Struct. Multidiscip. Optim.* **2021**, *64*, 2881–2908. [CrossRef]
24. do Amaral, J.V.S.; Montevechi, J.A.B.; de Carvalho Miranda, R.; de Sousa Junior, W.T. Metamodel-based simulation optimization: A systematic literature review. *Simul. Model. Pract. Theory* **2022**, *114*, 102403. [CrossRef]
25. Hey, J.; Siebers, P.O.; Nathanail, P.; Ozcan, E.; Robinson, D. Surrogate optimization of energy retrofits in domestic building stocks using household carbon valuations. *J. Build. Perform. Simul.* **2022**, 1–22. [CrossRef]
26. Beck, J.; Friedrich, D.; Brandani, S.; Fraga, E.S. Multi-objective optimisation using surrogate models for the design of VPSA systems. *Comput. Chem. Eng.* **2015**, *82*, 318–329. [CrossRef]
27. Wu, J.; Luo, Z.; Zheng, J.; Jiang, C. Incremental modeling of a new high-order polynomial surrogate model. *Appl. Math. Model.* **2016**, *40*, 4681–4699. [CrossRef]
28. Prada, A.; Gasparella, A.; Baggio, P. On the performance of meta-models in building design optimization. *Appl. Energy* **2018**, *225*, 814–826. [CrossRef]
29. Razavi, S.; Tolson, B.A.; Burn, D.H. Review of surrogate modeling in water resources. *Water Resour. Res.* **2012**, *48*. [CrossRef]
30. Garzón, A.; Kapelan, Z.; Langeveld, J.; Taormina, R. Machine Learning-Based Surrogate Modeling for Urban Water Networks: Review and Future Research Directions. *Water Resour. Res.* **2022**, *58*, e2021WR031808. [CrossRef]

31. Alzubaidi, L.; Zhang, J.; Humaidi, A.J.; Al-Dujaili, A.; Duan, Y.; Al-Shamma, O.; Santamaría, J.; Fadhel, M.A.; Al-Amidie, M.; Farhan, L. Review of deep learning: Concepts, CNN architectures, challenges, applications, future directions. *J. Big Data* **2021**, *8*, 53.
32. Emmerich, M.T.; Deutz, A.H. A tutorial on multiobjective optimization: Fundamentals and evolutionary methods. *Nat. Comput.* **2018**, *17*, 585–609. [PubMed]
33. Ng, A.; Grimm, H.; Lezama, T.; Persson, A.; Andersson, M.; Jägstam, M. OPTIMISE: An internet-based platform for metamodel-assisted simulation optimization. *Adv. Commun. Syst. Electr. Eng.* **2008**, *4*, 281–296.
34. Konzen, E.; Cheng, Y.; Shi, J.Q. Gaussian process for functional data analysis: The GPFDA package for R. *arXiv* **2021**, arXiv:2102.00249.
35. Günther, F.; Fritsch, S. Neuralnet: Training of neural networks. *R J.* **2010**, *2*, 30.
36. Riedmiller, M. Advanced supervised learning in multi-layer perceptrons—from backpropagation to adaptive learning algorithms. *Comput. Stand. Interfaces* **1994**, *16*, 265–278. [CrossRef]
37. Bogoya, J.M.; Vargas, A.; Schütze, O. The averaged hausdorff distances in multi-objective optimization: A review. *Mathematics* **2019**, *7*, 894. [CrossRef]
38. Deb, K.; Pratap, A.; Agarwal, S.; Meyarivan, T. A fast and elitist multiobjective genetic algorithm: NSGA-II. *IEEE Trans. Evol. Comput.* **2002**, *6*, 182–197.
39. AnyLogic. Cell Telecom Market. 2019. Available online: https://cloud.anylogic.com/model/11e1d402-1fb9-4f6f-8a6b-7f7e91f4c6e3?mode=SETTINGS (accessed on 23 May 2023).
40. Viana, F.A.; Simpson, T.W.; Balabanov, V.; Toropov, V. Special section on multidisciplinary design optimization: Metamodeling in multidisciplinary design optimization: How far have we really come? *AIAA J.* **2014**, *52*, 670–690.

Disclaimer/Publisher's Note: The statements, opinions and data contained in all publications are solely those of the individual author(s) and contributor(s) and not of MDPI and/or the editor(s). MDPI and/or the editor(s) disclaim responsibility for any injury to people or property resulting from any ideas, methods, instructions or products referred to in the content.

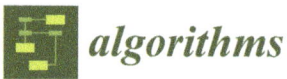 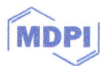

Article

Exploring the Use of Artificial Intelligence in Agent-Based Modeling Applications: A Bibliometric Study

Ștefan Ionescu, Camelia Delcea *, Nora Chiriță and Ionuț Nica

Department of Economic Informatics and Cybernetics, Bucharest University of Economic Studies, 0105552 Bucharest, Romania; stefion09@gmail.com (Ș.I.); nora.chirita@csie.ase.ro (N.C.); ionut.nica@csie.ase.ro (I.N.)
* Correspondence: camelia.delcea@csie.ase.ro

Abstract: This research provides a comprehensive analysis of the dynamic interplay between agent-based modeling (ABM) and artificial intelligence (AI) through a meticulous bibliometric study. This study reveals a substantial increase in scholarly interest, particularly post-2006, peaking in 2021 and 2022, indicating a contemporary surge in research on the synergy between AI and ABM. Temporal trends and fluctuations prompt questions about influencing factors, potentially linked to technological advancements or shifts in research focus. The sustained increase in citations per document per year underscores the field's impact, with the 2021 peak suggesting cumulative influence. Reference Publication Year Spectroscopy (RPYS) reveals historical patterns, and the recent decline prompts exploration into shifts in research focus. Lotka's law is reflected in the author's contributions, supported by Pareto analysis. Journal diversity signals extensive exploration of AI applications in ABM. Identifying impactful journals and clustering them per Bradford's Law provides insights for researchers. Global scientific production dominance and regional collaboration maps emphasize the worldwide landscape. Despite acknowledging limitations, such as citation lag and interdisciplinary challenges, our study offers a global perspective with implications for future research and as a resource in the evolving AI and ABM landscape.

Keywords: bibliometric analysis; agent-based modelling; artificial intelligence; complex systems; RStudio; VOSviewer; Bibliometrix

Citation: Ionescu, Ș.; Delcea, C.; Chiriță, N.; Nica, I. Exploring the Use of Artificial Intelligence in Agent-Based Modeling Applications: A Bibliometric Study. *Algorithms* **2024**, *17*, 21. https://doi.org/10.3390/a17010021

Academic Editors: Nuno Fachada and Nuno David

Received: 6 December 2023
Revised: 29 December 2023
Accepted: 31 December 2023
Published: 3 January 2024

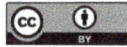

Copyright: © 2024 by the authors. Licensee MDPI, Basel, Switzerland. This article is an open access article distributed under the terms and conditions of the Creative Commons Attribution (CC BY) license (https://creativecommons.org/licenses/by/4.0/).

1. Introduction

In the current era of technology, artificial intelligence (AI) has become a central research field, significantly influencing numerous scientific disciplines. Simultaneously, agent-based modeling (ABM) has captured researchers' attention as a promising framework for simulating and understanding complex phenomena. In this context, this study proposes a detailed exploration of the synergies between AI and ABM, conducting an extensive analysis of the existing scientific literature.

ABM is a powerful simulation technique that characterizes a complex dynamic system through its interacting entities [1–3]. While ABM provides extensive flexibility for various applications, the complexity of real-world models necessitates the intensive use of computing resources and significant computational time. However, to mitigate computational costs, a metamodel can be constructed to provide insights at a less computationally demanding level. ABM has a range of applications that can be modeled, such as simulating emergency evacuation processes [4,5], specific transportation applications [6], modeling Grey economic systems [7], financial process modeling [8], analyzing financial contagion effects [9], medicine [10,11], etc.

Although ABM and AI are two distinct fields, they can interconnect through collaboration and complement each other in various ways. Thus, a series of interconnected features can be identified, such as simulating intelligent behavior [2,12,13], flexibility and adaptability [2,14], interconnection with AI technology [15], decision-making and collective intelligence [16], analysis and visualization of complexity [5,17], as well as innovation and exploration of emergent behaviors in complex systems. Firstly, ABM is considered a modeling method specific to economic cybernetics and complex adaptive systems [17,18]. On the other hand, the complexity of systems, given their dynamic and sometimes unpredictable nature, and the fact that a complex system is composed of a multitude of entities and agents that interact, result in a large volume of data. The most useful tools for analyzing this large volume of data [19], given the current technological and digital era, are provided by AI algorithms and techniques. The combination of these actions can be achieved through modeling applications offered by ABM and AI algorithms. In this case, ABM focuses on simulating the individual behavior of agents or individual entities and their interactions within the complex system, while AI develops algorithms and models that mimic and reproduce intelligent behavior through machine learning techniques. AI, especially in machine learning, focuses on developing models capable of learning and adapting to new data. By completing this process with ABM, its characteristic flexibility in modeling complex systems and adaptability to real-time changes are recognized. In essence, ABM and AI can complement each other in addressing complex problems, bringing together the advantages of simulating agent-level details and those of automated learning in an integrated and synergistic manner.

ABM is a simulation and modeling method that is specific to cybernetics [20]. Cybernetics is an interdisciplinary science that provides a framework for understanding various processes and systems in different fields. AI, as a field of study, offers machine learning algorithms that can be used in managing and analyzing large volumes of data and information, complementing and seamlessly integrating with the methods and frameworks provided by cybernetics. Integrating ABM with AI provides new perspectives for study and applicability in various fields such as sustainable agriculture [21], marketing [22], education [23], biomedical systems [24], agent behavior [25], management [26], etc.

ABM has the capacity to simulate agent behavior, while the AI approach analyzes and understands complex patterns, learning from real-time data. Thus, the interconnection between the two bridges the gap with the aim of contributing to more informed and efficient decision-making, leading to the development of more flexible and resilient systems/models. Additionally, AI is employed to analyze large volumes of data, and in conjunction with modeling individual and collective behavior through ABM, it enables more accurate forecasting and rapid identification of specific trends [27–29].

Turgut and Bozdag [25], in their study, provided a detailed presentation of the relationship between ML technology and agent-based approaches. Based on their analysis, they concluded that the main framework researchers can employ to address specific challenges identified individually in both methods is to use ML models to simulate agent behavior in their ABMs.

Hu et al. [30] conducted a study in which they examined challenges arising from agent behavior governed by rules derived from their bounded rationality and data scarcity. The authors addressed this challenge by incorporating domain expert knowledge with machine learning techniques.

Other investigations focus on the applicability and interconnection between ABM and AI in the medical field. For example, in their research, Sivakumar et al. [24] provided examples of how ABM and ML are integrated into various contexts covering spatial scales, including multicellular biology. The primary aim of their research was to use published studies as a guide to identify suitable approaches to machine learning based on specific types of ABM applications, considering the scale of the biological system and the characteristics of the available data.

Another study combines ABM with AI by constructing a metamodel that integrates ABM with random forest regression and neural networks. This approach has highlighted the benefit of reducing the number of required ABM simulations to validate a model [1].

Models and agent-based simulations are commonly encountered in various fields, providing a means to study systemic patterns resulting from individual behavior and interactions. Achieving the behavioral accuracy required for predictive models represents one of the significant challenges of ABM, and the use of learning algorithms can contribute to enhancing this accuracy in behavioral modeling [31].

The primary purpose of this study is to conduct a comprehensive bibliometric analysis of the utilization of AI in ABM applications. By exploring the existing scholarly literature, the aim is to identify patterns, trends, and the interconnected landscape between these two dynamic fields. This investigation seeks to provide insights into the evolution, challenges, and opportunities at the intersection of AI and ABM, offering a foundation for future research directions in this interdisciplinary domain. Additionally, our study can make a significant contribution by highlighting novelties in the field, identifying key research directions, and providing a comprehensive perspective on the relationship between AI and ABM. As Donthu et al. [32] suggest, the bibliometric analysis best fits the situations in which one aims to present the state of intellectual structure and emerging trends in a research field. The methodology involves a meticulous bibliometric approach, leveraging a well-established database, namely WoS [33]. Selection criteria include articles related to ABM and AI, with a focus on titles, abstracts, and keywords. The chosen data set is then refined through language and document type filters, ensuring a targeted and relevant sample. The bibliometric analysis utilizes the Bibliometrix platform in RStudio [34] and VOSviewer software (version 1.6.20) [35], employing techniques such as keyword co-occurrence clustering and network visualization to unveil patterns and connections within the literature.

This study innovatively combines bibliometric analysis with the exploration of AI and ABM, shedding light on the dynamics of these fields through a quantitative lens. The use of VOSviewer facilitates the visualization of co-occurrences, enabling a more nuanced interpretation of the relationships and interdependencies present in the literature. This approach adds a novel dimension to the examination of AI in ABM applications, offering a systematic and data-driven perspective on the evolution and interconnectedness of these domains. The value of this study lies in its contribution to the scholarly understanding of the synergies between AI and ABM. By offering a comprehensive bibliometric overview, the research provides a valuable resource for scholars, practitioners, and policymakers interested in the evolving landscape of these interconnected fields. The insights gained from this analysis can inform future research directions, guide strategic decision-making, and foster collaboration within the dynamic intersection of AI and ABM.

In addition, the above-mentioned aim, the present study tries to answer the following research questions:

- RQ1: What are the most influential articles in the field of AI utilization in ABM?
- RQ2: Who are the most notable authors in the realm of AI utilization in ABM?
- RQ3: Which journals have been preferred for papers on AI utilization in ABM?
- RQ4: What are the most impactful journals in the field of AI utilization in ABM?
- RQ5: Which universities are at the forefront of AI research based on papers published in ABM?
- RQ6: How has scientific production related to AI in ABM evolved over time?
- RQ7: What are the characteristics of the collaboration network among authors who have published in the field of AI in ABM?

This paper is structured into several sections, as follows, aiming to provide a holistic overview of the utilization of AI in specific applications of ABM. Section 2 presents the materials and methods underlying the bibliometric analysis. RStudio software, the Bibliometrix platform, and VOSviewer will be employed for the stated purpose. Section 3 is dedicated to the analysis of the dataset, covering articles, sources, authors, and knowledge status in the field. Section 4 introduces in-depth discussions based on the results obtained in Section 3, as well as the exploration of potential research limitations. Our study concludes with Section 5, presenting key findings and outlining future research directions.

2. Materials and Methods

Bibliometric analysis relies on statistical methodologies and specialized software tools to extract, process, and interpret data pertaining to scientific output. The primary aim of this approach is to present an unbiased overview of the progression within a research field, delineate the contributions made by authors or institutions, and pinpoint potential directions for future research. In our bibliometric analysis, we utilized the R Studio software, incorporating the bibliometrix package and the "biblioshiny()" function [34]. The "biblioshiny()" function, as outlined in [34,36,37], furnishes a diverse set of functionalities for our intended bibliometric analysis. It enables the extraction of bibliometric data from various sources like Scopus and WoS, generates key bibliometric indicators (e.g., publication count, H-index, citation count), facilitates comparative analyses, and supports the visualization of results through interactive graphics such as network maps, diagrams, and geographic maps. Additionally, it provides the capability to export these results for further use and dissemination. To guarantee transparency and structure in implementing the research [38], we delineated the stages of the methodological process following the guidelines put forth by Zupic and Čarter [39]. The authors have outlined a procedural workflow for executing scientific mapping studies within the realms of management and organization. From this point of view, the process we will follow in conducting the bibliometric analysis will be as presented below, adapted from Torres Silva et al. [38] and Zupic and Čarter [39].

Step 1. Study design: The data selection process is a crucial step in refining the dataset for further exploration. Each stage aims to obtain a set of articles relevant to our study on ABM applications and AI. The keywords used in Table 1 were chosen to cover key aspects of this study domain, ensuring precise and specific coverage. Our study explores the interaction between two distinct research fields: AI and agent-based models, and the chosen keywords reflect the interdisciplinary complexity of our topic. Additionally, the selected keywords stem from our main research question: How can AI be utilized in ABM applications?

Step 2. Synthesis of Bibliometric Data: Regarding this step in the process, the bibliometric database WoS was chosen, and various queries were conducted based on the following keywords: "agent-based modeling", "agent-based modelling", "agent-based model", "agent-based models", "artificial intelligence", "machine learning", and "deep learning". These key concepts were searched in the title, abstract, and keywords of articles, covering the period from 2000 to 2022. The 22-year period chosen for our study acknowledges the swift and substantial evolution witnessed in the field of AI during the past two decades. Our selected time frame encapsulates the era when AI emerged as a prominent domain for research and development [40]. Additionally, significant technological progress, changes in research methodologies, and the advent of new paradigms have prominently characterized recent decades [41]. These factors, which have influenced our decision regarding the time frame, are also underscored in the 2020 technical report issued by the European Commission [42]. Subsequently, only article-type queries written in English as an internationally recognized language were retained. This stage will be extensively described in the interpretation of Table 1.

Regarding the dataset extraction, it shall be stated that the WoS platform offers, based on subscription, personalized access to data. As a result, as Liu [43] and Liu [44] observed, the results of the bibliometric analysis are highly dependent on the user's access to the ten indexes offered by the WoS. In this context, the authors recommend that the bibliometric papers clearly state the access the users had to the index offered by WoS [43,44].

Furthermore, the choice for the WoS platform has been substantiated by the fact—also highlighted in the scientific literature—that it offers extensive coverage of a broad array of disciplines while being recognized as a platform with a strong reputation by the scientific community [45–47]. Nevertheless, WoS is one of the few platforms on which both Bibliometrix and VOSviewer offer a data reading option for the datasets extracted based on the search criteria [34,48,49].

Table 1. Data selection steps.

Exploration Steps	Applied Filters	Description	Query	Query Number	Count
1	Title	Contains one of the agent-based modeling-specific keywords	(((TI = ("agent-based modeling")) OR TI = ("agent-based modelling")) OR TI = ("agent-based model")) OR TI = ("agent-based models")	#1	5135
		Contains one of the artificial intelligence-specific keywords	((TI = (artificial_intelligence)) OR TI = (machine_learning)) OR TI = (deep_learning)	#2	211,005
		Contains the agent-based modeling and artificial intelligence-specific keywords	#1 AND #2	#3	25
2	Abstract	Contains one of the agent-based modeling-specific keywords	(((AB = ("agent-based modeling")) OR AB = ("agent-based modelling")) OR AB = ("agent-based model")) OR AB = ("agent-based models")	#4	11,173
		Contains one of the artificial intelligence-specific keywords	((AB = (artificial_intelligence)) OR AB = (machine_learning)) OR AB = (deep_learning)	#5	470,238
		Contains the agent-based modeling and artificial intelligence-specific keywords	#4 AND #5	#6	257
3	Keywords	Contains one of the agent-based modeling-specific keywords	(((AK = ("agent-based modeling")) OR AK = ("agent-based modelling")) OR AK = ("agent-based model")) OR AK = ("agent-based models")	#7	8868
		Contains one of the artificial intelligence-specific keywords	((AK = (artificial_intelligence)) OR AK = (machine_learning)) OR AK = (deep_learning)	#8	305,228
		Contains the agent-based modeling and artificial intelligence-specific keywords	#7 AND #8	#9	134
4	Title/Abstract/Keywords	Contains one of the artificial intelligence-specific keywords	#3 OR #6 OR #9	#10	344
5	Language	Limit to English	(#10) AND LA = (English)	#11	340
6	Document Type	Limit to Article	(#11) AND DT = (Article)	#12	226
7	Year published	Exclude 2023	(#12) NOT PY = (2023)	#13	180
		Exclude 2024	(#13) NOT PY = (2024)	#14	180

Moreover, it should be stated that the classification of the papers into the "article" category by the WoS platform follows the description provided by Donner [50]. The author states that an article is considered a report of original research with no predefined length, which features the use of meta-analysis. Following the description provided by WoS regarding the inclusion of scientific papers in the article category, it should be noted that the platform mentions that research papers, brief communications, technical notes, chronologies, full papers, and case reports that were published in a journal and/or presented at a symposium/conference are included in this category, explicitly stating that proceedings papers are included in both the article and the proceedings papers category [51]. Also, Donner [50] highlights that, in the field of scientometrics, it is important to clearly differentiate among various types of documents when conducting the analysis, as each type of document generates a specific citation distribution that is highly connected to the purpose and content of the document type.

Step 3. Analysis: The third stage involved using the bibliometric software Biblioshiny from RStudio's Bibliometrix package. The data extracted from WoS was downloaded in BibTeX format, and the cleaning stage was verified in RStudio v2023.09.1+494.pro2, Bibliometrix R (version 4.3.2). No additional exclusions were necessary at this stage.

Step 4. Visualization: In the visualization stage, graphical methods were used to prepare the analysis of sources, authors, and the literature.

Step 5. Interpretation: In the final stage, we utilize the graphical representations from step 4 and describe and interpret the results.

Table 1 summarizes the queries and steps we conducted to build the database. We utilized the WoS [33] platform to retrieve papers related to ABM and AI. The analysis unfolds in several stages, emphasizing a meticulous process for identifying pertinent works. Titles, abstracts, and keywords are employed to encompass diverse aspects of each paper. The initial step defines the keywords identified in the titles.

Table 1 delineates the methodological steps taken in the data selection process during the exploration phase on the WoS. This systematic approach aims to refine the dataset progressively, ensuring relevance to our study on applications of ABM and AI.

- Step 1. Title exploration: This stage focuses on identifying articles with titles relevant to ABM and AI, providing an initial delimitation of the dataset. Queries #1 and #2 focus on titles containing keywords related to ABM and AI, respectively. Following these queries, 5135 articles with terms specific to ABM in the title and 211,005 articles with terms specific to AI in the title were identified. Query #3 combines these aspects, refining the search.
- Step 2. Abstract exploration: This stage adds relevance by identifying articles with key terms in the abstract and amplifying details about their content. Queries #4 and #5 target abstracts with specific keywords. A total of 11,173 articles with terms specific to ABM in the abstract were obtained, along with a substantial number of 470,238 articles with terms specific to AI in the abstract. Query #6 combines ABM and AI criteria from the abstracts.
- Step 3. Keyword exploration: Identifying keyword-based articles consolidates the selection of papers that specifically address the key concepts of the research. Queries #7 and #8 concentrate on keywords associated with ABM and AI. Query #9 combines these keyword criteria. This query focuses on articles that contain both ABM and AI-specific keywords in the keywords section. A total of 134 articles were identified based on this query, providing insights into publications that simultaneously address both ABM and AI in their keyword content. This step further refines the dataset, capturing articles that explicitly mention both key aspects in their keywords.
- Step 4. Title/Abstract/Keywords exploration: This stage combines relevant selection criteria to obtain a narrower and more focused subset of articles. Query #10 consolidates the AI-specific keywords from previous queries. A total of 344 articles with specific terms related to AI were identified, consolidating the criteria from previous steps.
- Step 5. Language restriction: By limiting it to the English language, we ensure that the included articles are accessible and easily comparable, having a broader international circulation. Query #11 limits results to English publications from the refined set. The results were narrowed down to 340 articles written in English.
- Step 6. Document type restriction: This restriction ensures that the analysis focuses on articles, excluding other types of documents that may contain irrelevant information for this study's purpose. Query #12 narrows down the dataset to articles. A total of 226 articles were selected to be consistent with the scope of our study.
- Step 7. Year published restriction: This stage ensures a focus on articles published during the relevant period for this study, preemptively eliminating materials that could negatively influence the results. Queries #13 and #14 exclude publications from

the years 2023 and 2024, respectively. A total of 46 articles were removed, leaving our final database with 180 articles that will be used in the analysis.

This methodical process ensures that the dataset used for our bibliometric analysis is both comprehensive and relevant to the intersection of ABM and AI. The sequential queries help filter articles based on titles, abstracts, keywords, language, document type, and publication years, contributing to the robustness and specificity of our bibliometric study.

The resulting dataset, comprising 180 articles related to AI utilization in ABM, is close to the recommendations from the field related to the size of the data sample [52]. Furthermore, as the purpose of the dataset collection step was to extract all the papers indexed in WoS pertaining to AI utilization in ABM, no further actions were needed to be taken for expanding the dataset as, in this paper, we are not working with small or fractional parts of research output. As Rogers et al. [52] suggested, in cases where the bibliometric analysis uses an approach that relies on small or fractional parts of the researcher's output, one should pay more attention to the size of the dataset, as there might be cases in which the extracted dataset does not accurately represent the average.

To ensure understanding and clarity of the methodological steps undertaken, Figure 1 describes each step that we will apply in our study. Considering the research questions outlined in this study's introduction, the initial step in constructing the methodological flow involves outlining the research framework. Subsequently, the queries from Table 1 are employed to extract the database, and the RStudio software is utilized to generate the graphs that will be visualized and interpreted.

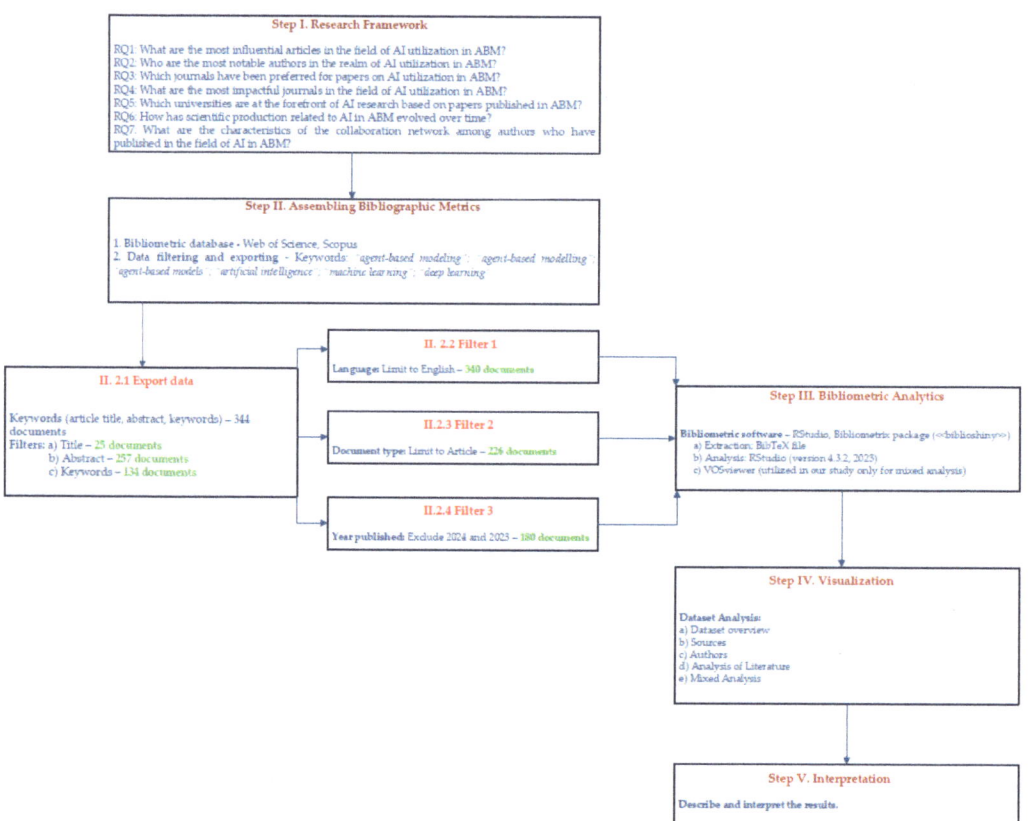

Figure 1. Methodological flow.

3.2. Sources

Regarding the bibliometric analysis of sources, Bibliometrix offers the possibility to conduct analyses based on the most relevant sources, most locally cited sources, Bradford's Law, sources' local impact, and sources' production over time. Figure 6 presents the analysis of the top 20 most relevant journals.

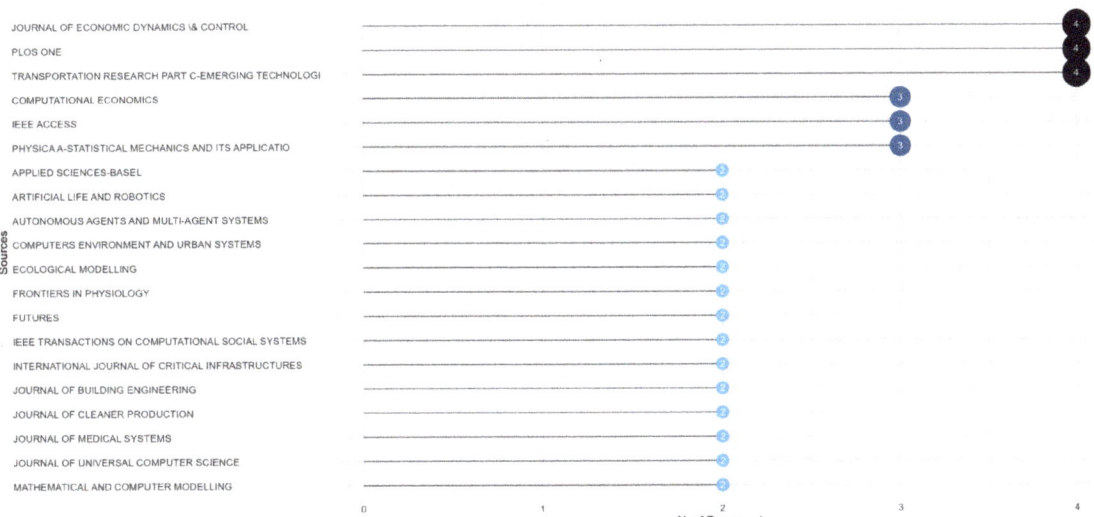

Figure 6. Top 20 most relevant journals.

The analysis of the top 20 most relevant journals in the context of our research provides insights into the key journals contributing to the field, indicating the diversity and significance of research across various platforms. The top 20 most relevant journals span a diverse range of disciplines, indicating the interdisciplinary nature of research in AI and ABM applications. Journals such as *Journal of Economic Dynamics & Control*, *PLOS ONE*, and *Transportation Research Part C-Emerging Technologies* appear to be prominent contributors. The variety of journals with multiple articles suggests a broad exploration of AI applications in ABM, covering economic dynamics, control, emerging technologies, computational economics, and more. This diversity signifies a comprehensive examination of the subject matter. Journals like *Journal of Economic Dynamics & Control* and *PLOS ONE* are notable for having a higher number of articles, indicating a sustained interest and significant contributions in these outlets. Journals such as *IEEE Transactions on Computational Social Systems* highlight engagement with cutting-edge platforms, showcasing an awareness of emerging technologies and social aspects in computational systems. The presence of journals like *Ecological Modelling* and *Frontiers in Physiology* indicates a cross-disciplinary exploration, showcasing the broader impact of AI and ABM beyond traditional domains.

Bradford's Law on Source Clustering categorizes journals into different zones based on the distribution of articles (Figure 7).

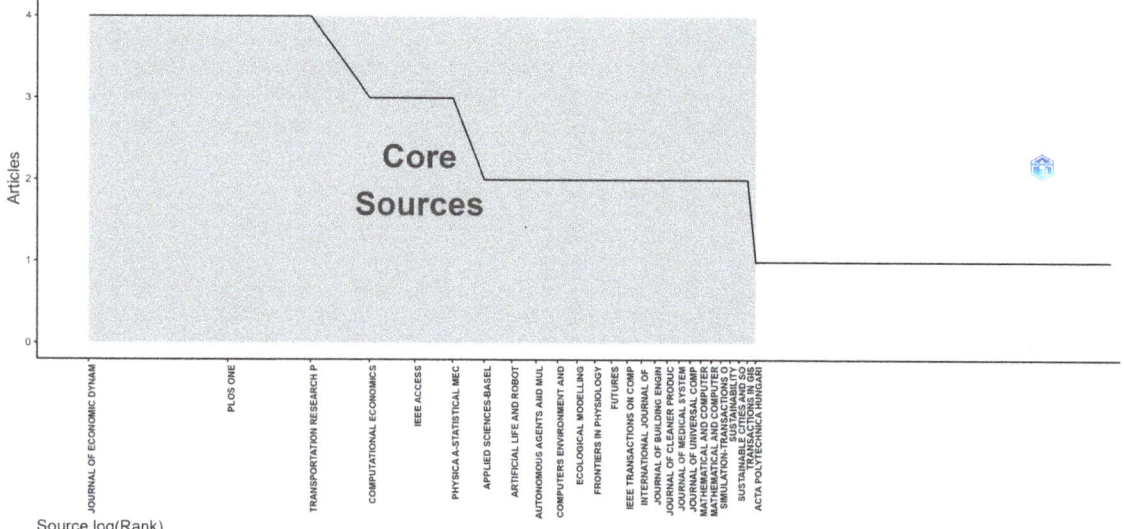

Figure 7. Bradford's law on source clustering.

Journals in Zone 1 have the highest productivity and contribute significantly to the research field. Notable journals include "Journal of Economic Dynamics and Control", "PLOS ONE", and "Transportation Research Part C-Emerging Technologies". These journals have a high frequency of articles, indicating a concentrated focus on the chosen research topic. Journals in Zone 2 have moderate productivity, contributing less than the top journals but still making a substantial impact. Examples include "Administrative Sciences", "Advances in Complex Systems", and "Applied Energy". This zone represents a middle ground in terms of research output. Journals in zone 3 have lower productivity compared to zones 1 and 2. They cover a wide range of topics and may not be as central to the core research focus. Examples include *International Journal of Health Geographics*, *Sensors*, and *SoftwareX*.

Source Local Impact, based on the H-index, highlights the relative impact of various sources (journals) based on the H-index. The H-index represents the number of articles from a source that have at least H citations each. As seen in Figure 8, for example, the journal *Transportation Research Part C-Emerging Technologies* has an H-index of 4, meaning there are 4 articles with at least 4 citations each. *PLOS ONE* has an H-index of 3, indicating there are 3 articles with at least 3 citations each. This analysis provides a quick overview of the relative impact of each source, considering both the number of articles and citations. A higher H-index suggests a more significant influence in the scientific community.

The Sources' Production over Time analyzes the evolution of the number of articles published in various journals over the years. In this context, we can focus on several notable observations (Figure 9):

- *Journal of Economic Dynamics & Control, PLOS ONE*, and *Transportation Research Part C-Emerging Technologies* have shown consistent growth in production since 2008 and have maintained a significant level in recent years;
- The year 2012 marked a significant increase in article production for many of the listed sources, such as *Physica A-Statistical Mechanics and its Applications, Applied Sciences-Based*, and *IEEE Transactions on Computational Social Systems*;
- A significant number of sources have recorded steady growth in recent years, including *Sustainability, Sustainable Cities and Society*, and the *Journal of Building Engineering*;
- After 2020, most sources seem to maintain a high level of production, suggesting a continued interest in the fields covered by these journals.

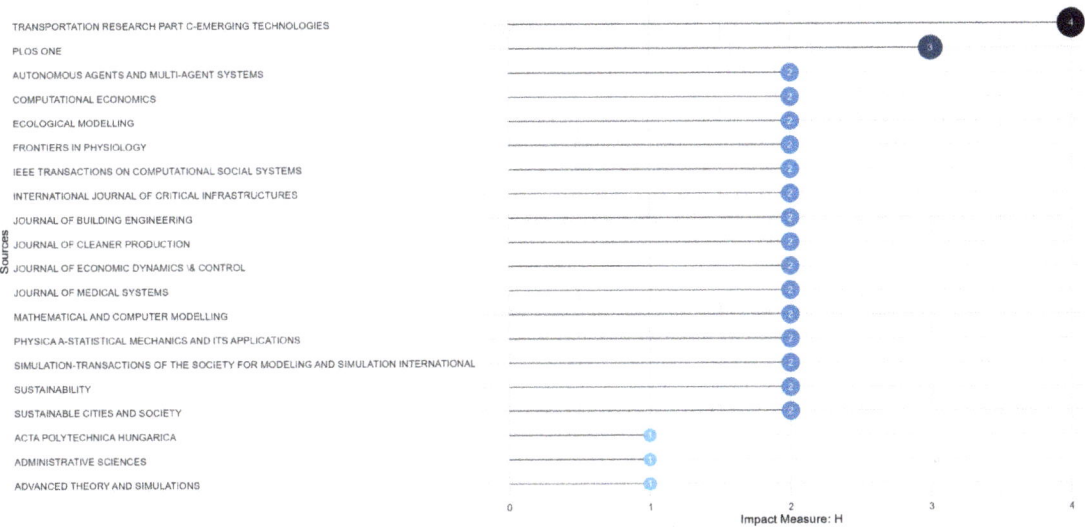

Figure 8. Journals' impact based on H-index.

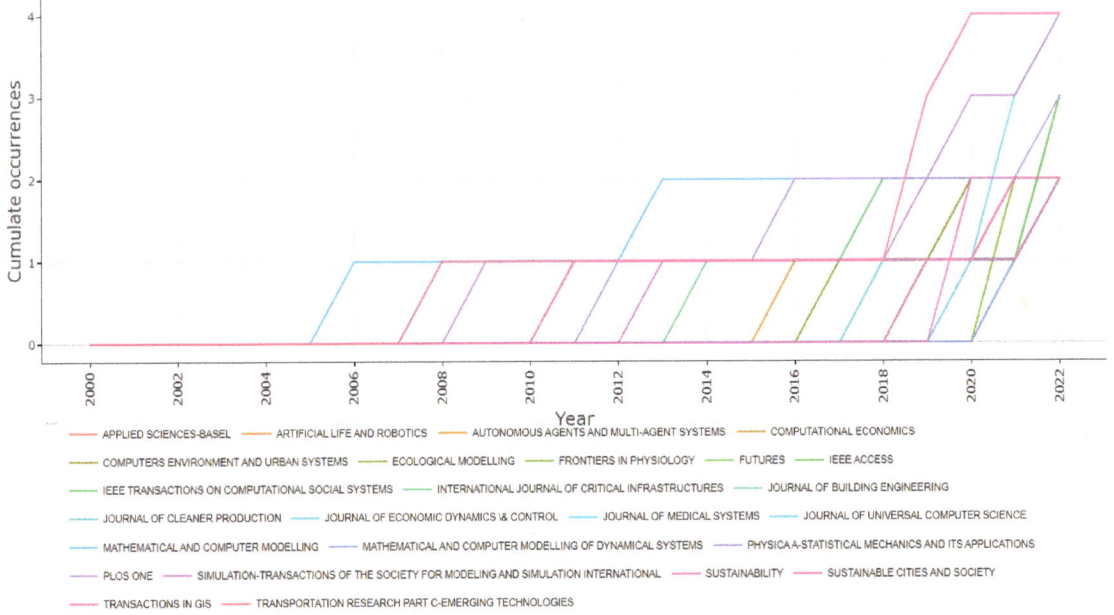

Figure 9. Journals' growth (cumulative) based on the number of papers.

3.3. Authors

When it comes to author analysis, the most relevant authors will be examined, including the top 20 authors' production over time, the top 20 most relevant affiliations, and the top 20 most relevant corresponding author's countries.

Regarding the top 20 relevant authors, according to Figure 10, An G. stands out with 8 articles, followed by Filatova T., Li X., and Malleson N. with 4 articles each.

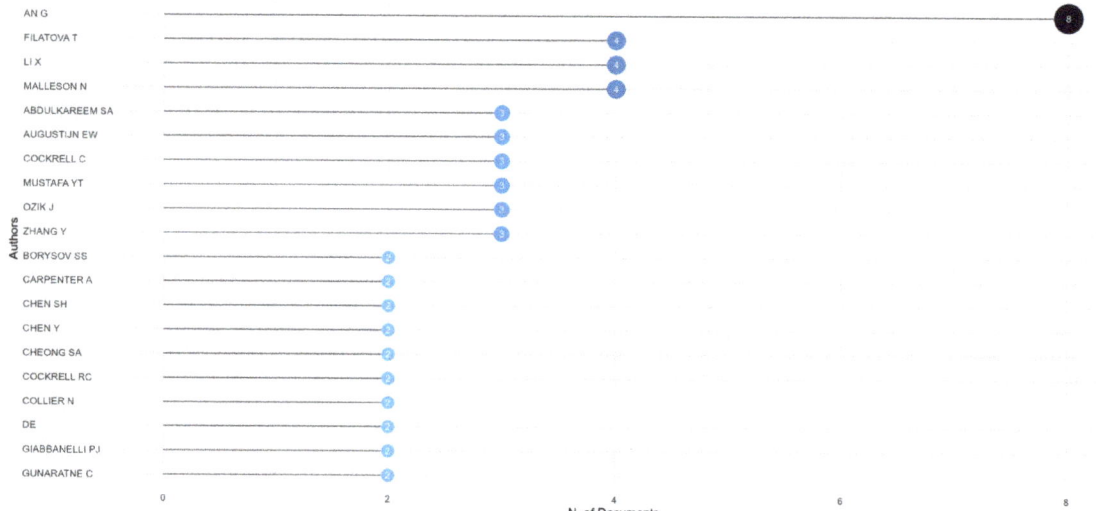

Figure 10. Top-20 authors based on number of documents.

In Figure 11, we display the publication frequency of various authors across different years. For example, Abdulkareem S.A. has published three articles, one in each of the years 2018, 2019, and 2020. The author has received 13 citations, with a yearly citation average of 2.16. Additionally, author An G. has published 8 articles, one of which was cited in 2019 a total of 30 times, averaging 2 citations per year. In 2017, there was an article with 20 citations, and in 2018, there was another article with 19 citations. Similarly, in 2019, another article had a total of 13 citations. In 2021, An G. published 4 articles, accumulating a total of 16 citations, with an average yearly citation of 5.33.

In the context of our study, the most relevant affiliations, based on the number of articles, are represented in Figure 12. These affiliations have shown significant productivity in the fields of AI and ABM, contributing to the breadth and depth of research on the subject.

In the context of our research, focusing on the use of AI in ABM applications, the most relevant countries, based on the number of articles and various metrics, are represented in Figure 13.

These countries, particularly the USA, China, UK, Canada, and Germany, have demonstrated notable contributions to research in the fields of AI and ABM. The SCP (single country publications) and MCP (multiple country publications) metrics provide insights into the collaborative nature of publications, and the frequency and MCP ratio offer additional perspectives on the distribution and collaboration patterns.

The map in Figure 14 illustrates the distribution of scientific production across various countries. The intensity of the blue color on the map corresponds to the volume of scientific production for each country. A darker shade of blue indicates a higher number of publications, while a lighter shade represents a lower number of publications. In this visual representation, the color gradient serves as a quick reference to assess the relative research output across different countries. It is evident that certain countries dominate the research landscape, while others make more modest contributions. Additionally, regional trends and relationships between regions can be observed based on the frequency of scientific production. Furthermore, it is notable that the USA dominates scientific production, indicating a significant contribution to global research.

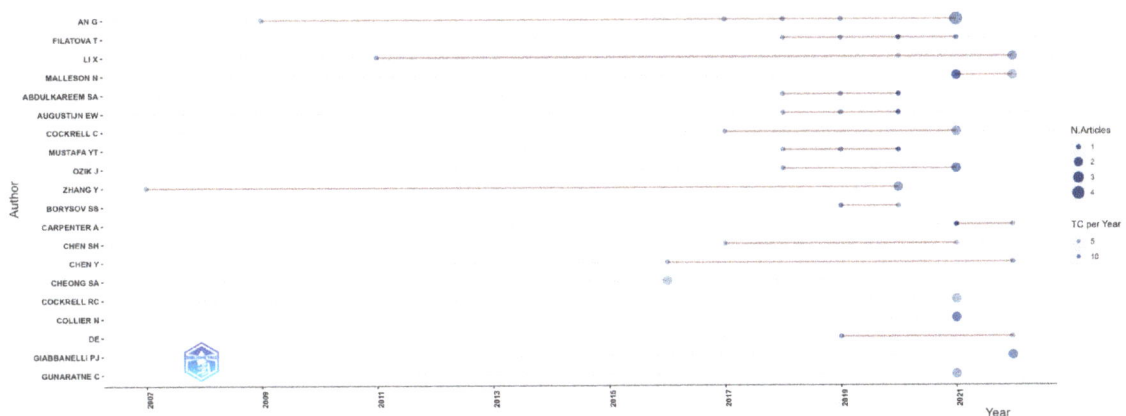

Figure 11. Top-20 authors' production over time.

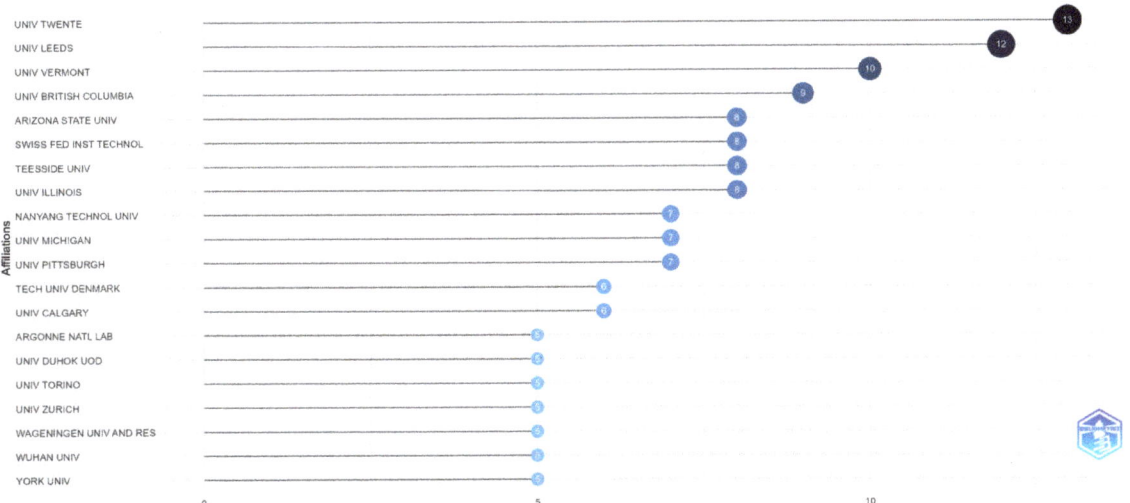

Figure 12. Top 20 most relevant affiliations.

In order to analyze and classify the data underlying Figure 13, a Pareto ABC Diagram was created. This method is based on Pareto's Principle, which states that, in many situations, approximately 80% of results come from 20% of causes [63]. In the context of Pareto ABC analysis, this means that a small number of elements contribute significantly to the total, while the majority of elements contribute less. The primary objective of ABC analysis is to prioritize stringent control for class A items, implement less rigorous control for class B items, and exert minimal control for class C items [64]. According to the representation in Figure 15, class A represents 81% of the contribution to global scientific production. This category includes countries such as the USA, UK, China, Canada, Germany, and Saudi Arabia, and they are the most important countries in this field. Special attention should be given to collaborations, resource exchange, and partnerships to maintain and enhance their impact. Class B contributes 15%, including countries like Poland, Singapore, Spain, Belgium, and Mexico. Although these countries do not have as significant a contribution as those in class A, they remain important for the diversity and amplification of scientific research. Collaborations and information exchange with these countries can bring substantial benefits, even if not as substantial as those in class A. Class C has a contribution of approximately 4% and includes countries such as Bulgaria, Norway, or Portugal. These countries have a smaller contribution to global scientific production but can still play an important role regionally or in specific research areas. Cooperation with these countries could bring benefits in developing more specialized research fields or improving regional collaborations.

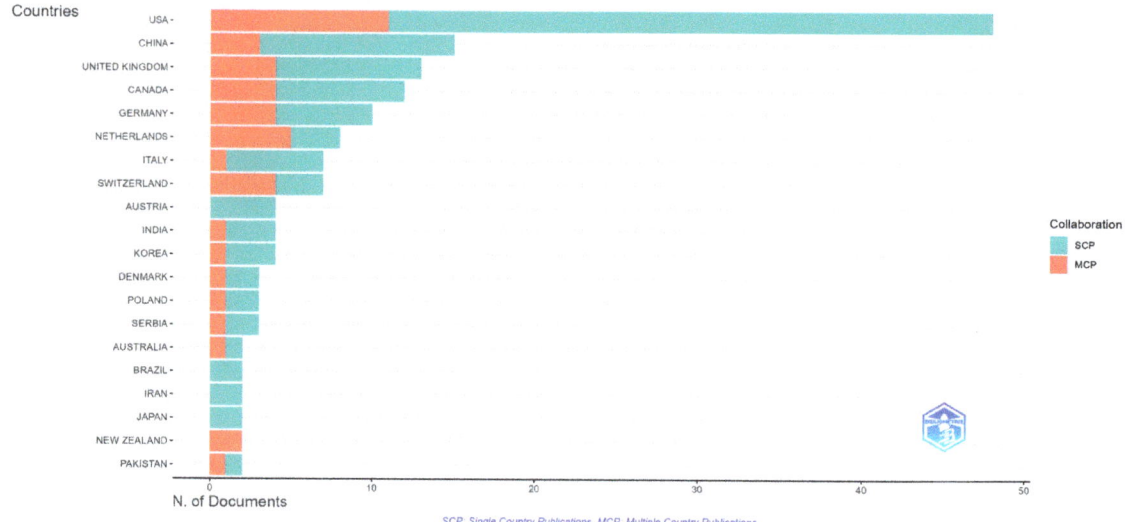

Figure 13. Top-20 most relevant corresponding author's country.

In Figure 16, the top 20 countries are represented based on the total number of citations. Thus, it is observed that the USA has the highest total number of citations (1153) and the highest average citations per article (24.00), indicating a robust and impactful scientific production. The United Kingdom follows with a total of 266 citations and an average of 20.50 citations per article. Switzerland has fewer total citations (181) but a higher average (25.90) compared to other countries, suggesting a high impact per article. Countries like Serbia and Senegal have a relatively small number of articles but a high average number of citations per article, indicating that their research has a significant impact despite the smaller volume.

The map of collaborations between countries can be interpreted by analyzing the frequency of collaborations between different pairs of countries. Specifically, it is important to observe which countries collaborate most frequently and in what contexts. According to Figure 17, the following observations can be made:

- Collaborations between European countries are evident, with multiple connections between Belgium, Finland, France, Germany, the Netherlands, Spain, and Switzerland;
- The USA has frequent collaborations with Canada, the United Kingdom, and Switzerland;
- Asian countries, such as China and Korea, have connections among themselves and with European countries;
- Regarding region-to-region collaborations, countries from a specific region collaborate with each other, such as Finland with Sweden and Denmark or China with Japan and Korea;
- From the perspective of interspecific collaboration, there are collaborations between countries with different geographical and cultural perspectives, such as Australia and Iraq or Brazil and China;

- Intense collaborations are represented by higher frequencies. For example, the USA collaborates frequently with the United Kingdom and Switzerland.

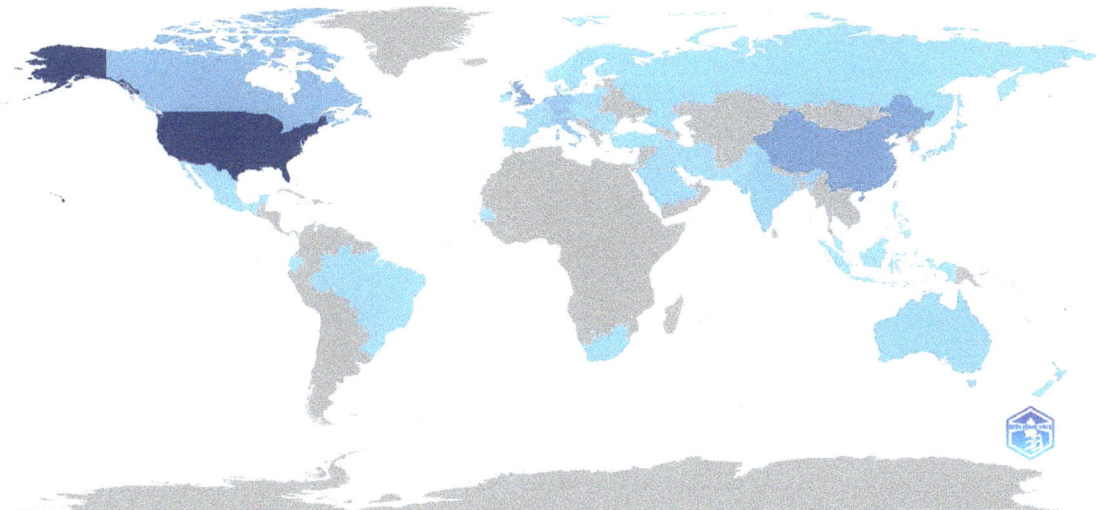

Figure 14. Scientific production based on country.

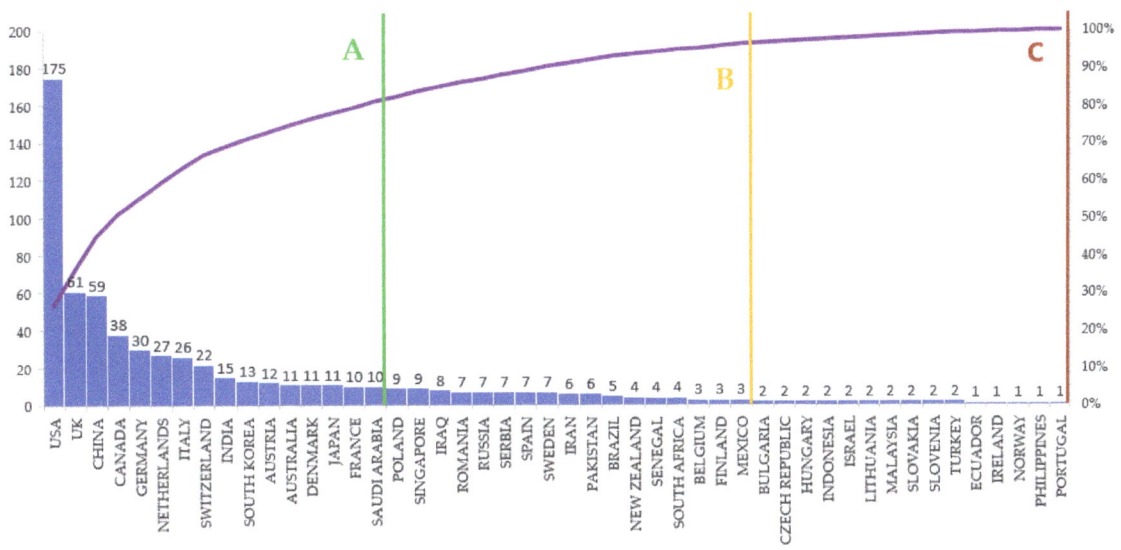

Figure 15. Global Scientific Production represented based on the Pareto distribution.

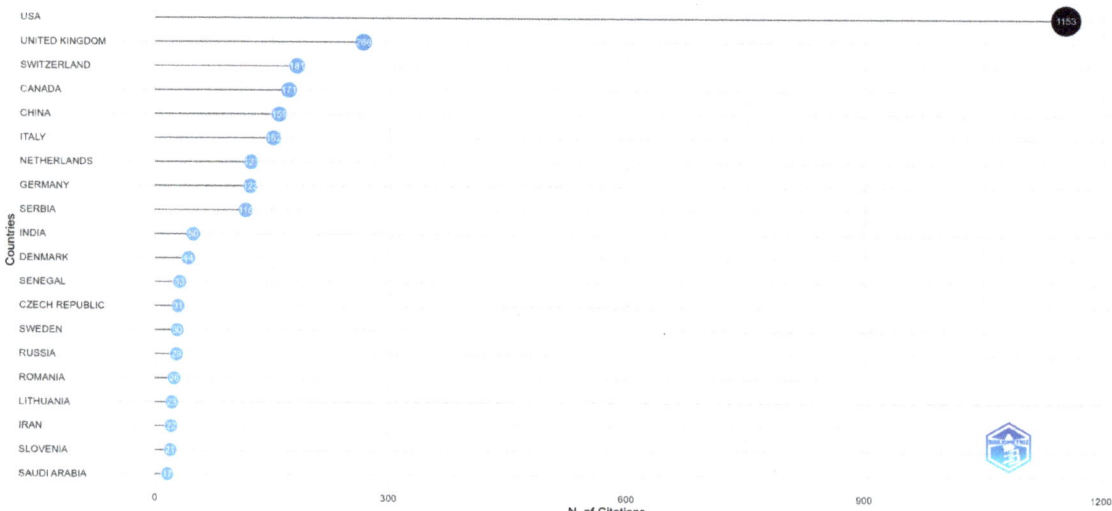

Figure 16. Top 20 countries with the most citations.

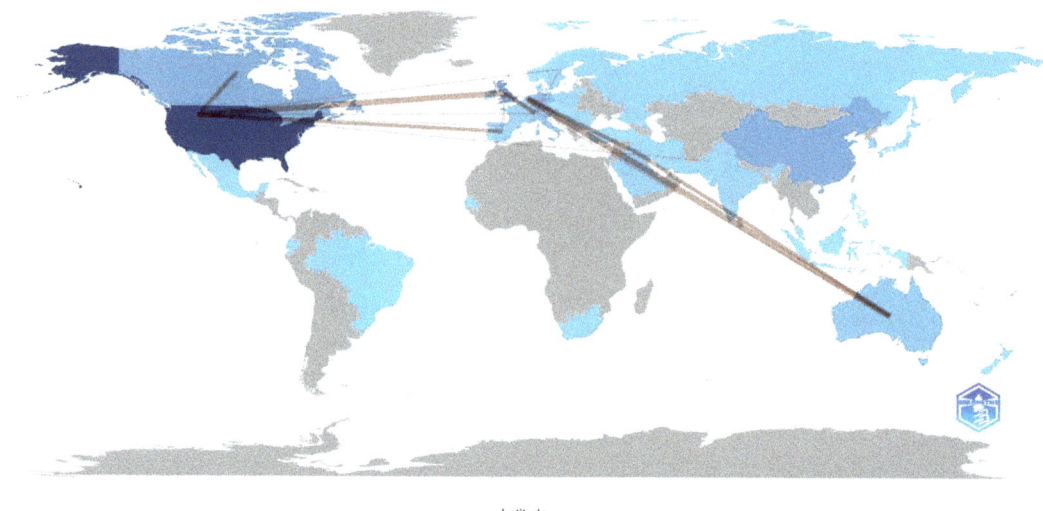

Figure 17. Country collaboration map.

This collaboration map can suggest common research areas or interests between countries, highlighting networks of researchers and international partnerships.

Regarding the author collaboration network, Figure 18 represents the network with the top 50 authors who have collaborated. The lines or connections between nodes represent collaborations, and the more internal the collaboration, the more connections there are between two authors. Larger nodes represent authors who have made a more significant contribution. Our network has been divided into 11 clusters, each of them having a different color, indicating intensive collaborations within these groups.

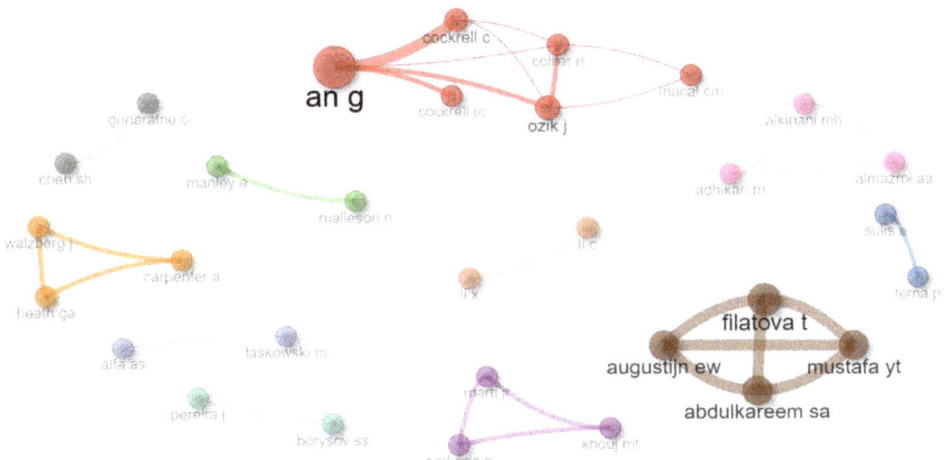

Figure 18. Top 50 authors' collaboration networks.

3.4. Analysis of Literature

Regarding the state of knowledge in the field, the following analyses provide an overview of the scientific landscape and previous contributions in the analyzed domain. In the context of our research, the current state of knowledge indicates a dynamic intersection between two evolving domains: AI and ABM. This exploration reflects a contemporary interest in leveraging advanced AI techniques within ABM, opening up potential new directions for modeling and simulation across various fields. This convergence marks a frontier where traditional ABM methodologies meet advanced AI technologies, promising a more realistic, adaptable model with enhanced predictive capabilities. The synergy between AI and ABM holds the potential to address complex systems with greater fidelity, enabling researchers to simulate and understand intricate real-world scenarios with increased precision. As researchers delve into this interdisciplinary realm, challenges and opportunities emerge. Original contributions in this direction may involve refining existing AI algorithms for ABM contexts, adapting ABM paradigms to harness the learning capabilities of AI, and identifying novel applications that can benefit from this amalgamation. For instance, Taghikhah et al. [28] address the challenges associated with explaining the structure and performance of agent-based models (ABM) in the quantitative social sciences. The authors propose an innovative approach that utilizes AI for both constructing models from data and enhancing the way we communicate these models to stakeholders. While machine learning is actively employed for data preprocessing, this study introduces, for the first time, its use to facilitate the direct development of a simulation model from data. The proposed framework, ML-ABM, is designed to capture causality and feedback loops in complex and nonlinear systems while maintaining transparency for stakeholders [28]. The authors argue that their approach not only leads to the creation of a behavioral ABM but also unveils the internal workings of empirical models, traditionally considered "black boxes". They suggest that integrating AI into simulation practices can bring a new dimension to modeling and provide valuable insights for future applications.

Platas-López et al. [65] explore the integration of Machine Learning (ML) techniques into ABM to enhance the design and analysis of models. The authors propose an extension of the Overview, Design Concepts, and Details (ODD) protocol to standardize the description of ML applications within ABM. The extension categorizes the use of ML based on various factors, facilitating transparent communication of ML workflows in ABM. The proposed approach is exemplified through a tax evasion model, highlighting improved precision with statistical significance.

On the other hand, the role of ABM can be an innovative approach in various fields. For instance, in transportation studies, it can provide an alternative to traditional equation-based models. Delcea and Chirita [6] highlight that specific applications of ABM in transportation, including the aviation, maritime, road, and rail sectors, involve the study of airport operations, maritime efficiency, traffic congestion, evacuation scenarios, and public transportation systems.

3.4.1. Top 10 Most Cited Papers—Overview

In Figure 19, the top 10 most globally cited documents are depicted. The highest number of global citations is observed for the author Bagstad, with 349, followed by Hare with 130 citations. These will be detailed further on.

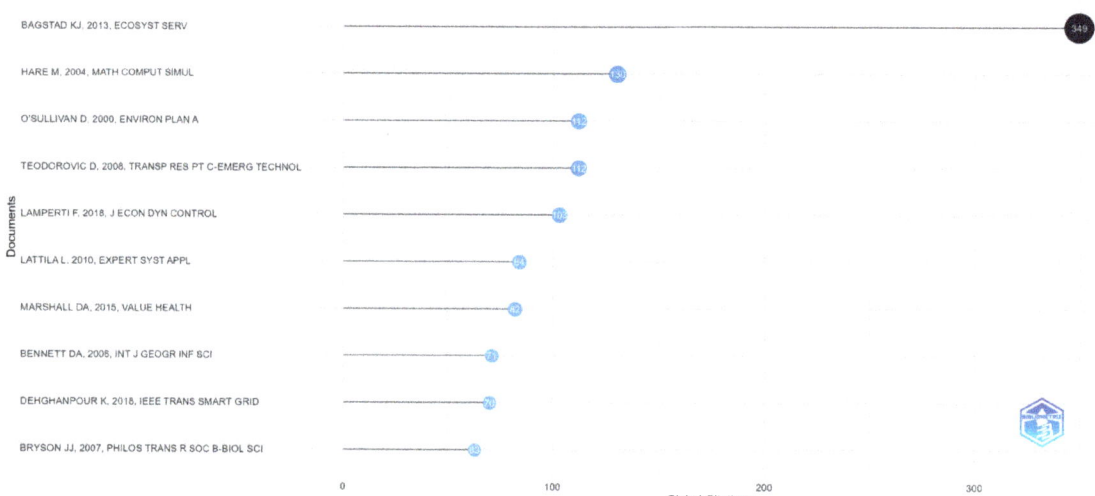

Figure 19. Highly cited documents worldwide.

In Table 6, centralized information provides an overview of the impact and geographic distribution of research documents. Various metrics, such as the total citations per year and normalized citations, offer insights into the ongoing impact and relevance of these documents within the scientific community. For instance, Bagstad et al. [66], the author with the highest citations for their study, have a total of 349 citations, with a TCY (Total Citations per Year) of 31.73 and a value of 8.19 for normalized total citations (NTC). Similarly, Hare and Deadman [26] have a total of 130 citations for their study, with a value of 6.5 citations per year (TCY), but with a relatively small value for the NCT, namely 1.

While the TC and TCY indicators are easy to read and understand, we should further explain the calculus rules for the NTC metric in order to better understand the values listed on the right-column of Table 6. The key point in determining the NTC is the year in which the paper has been published, as the NTC value is obtained by dividing the TC value by the average citations per document recorded in the extracted dataset for the year in which the paper has been published [37]. Thus, for the year 2013 in which the paper authored by Bagstad et al. [66] was published, the average citations per document were equal to 42.61. By dividing the value of TC obtained by Bagstad et al. [66], namely 349 citations, by 42.61, the 8.19 value for the NTC is obtained. Thus, it can be stated that the paper authored by Bagstad et al. [66] has gained approximately 8.19 times more citations than the average of the citations received in the same year by the other papers included in the dataset. As for the papers authored by Hare and Deadman [26] and O'Sullivan and Haklay [67], as both papers have been published in years (2004, respectively, 2000), for which in the database the mentioned papers are the only published papers, the value they have received for the TC equals the average value of the citations obtained by all the papers in the database published in the same year, making the NTC equal to 1.

Table 6. Top 10 most globally cited documents.

No.	Paper (First Author, Year, Journal, Reference)	Number of Authors	Region	Total Citations (TC)	Total Citations per Year (TCY)	Normalized TC (NTC)
1	Bagstad, K.J. (2013), Ecosystem Services [66]	4	Denver, USA	349	31.73	8.19
2	Hare, M. (2004), Mathematics and Computers in Simulation [26]	2	Canberra, Australia	130	6.5	1
3	O'Sullivan, D. 2000, Environment and Planning: A-Economy and Space [67]	2	London, England	112	4.67	1
4	Teodorovic, D. (2008), Transportation Research Part C-Emerging Technologies [68]	1	Belgrade, Serbia	112	7	3.97
5	Lamperti, F. (2018), Journal of Economic Dynamics & Control [69]	3	Pisa, Italy	103	17.17	4.59
6	Lättilä, L. (2010), Expert Systems with Applications [70]	3	Shreveport, USA	84	6	2.63
7	Marshall, D.A. (2015), Value in Health [71]	9	Calgary, Canada	82	9.11	2.67
8	Bennett, D.A. (2006), International Journal of Geographical Information Science [72]	2	Southampton, England	71	3.94	1.37
9	Dehghanpour, K. (2018), IEEE Transactions on Smart Grid [73]	4	Bozeman, Montana	70	11.67	3.12
10	Bryson, J.J, (2007), Philosophical Transactions of the Royal Society B-Biological Sciences [74]	3	Avon, England	63	3.71	1.48

3.4.2. Top 10 Most Cited Papers—Review

In order to build an overview of the impact and ongoing relevance of research in the global scientific community, Table 7 has been compiled. Centralization provides a comprehensive view of the impact and geographic distribution of the most globally cited research documents. Relevant information about each document is provided, including the total number of citations, citations per year, and normalized citations. Additionally, the authors' region of origin and the total number of authors for each document are highlighted.

3.4.3. Words Analysis

The analysis of keywords used in scientific articles provides an efficient way to investigate the language and content of scientific documents, yielding valuable insights in the field of research. This analysis can offer significant information about trends and characteristics within a specific domain or subdomain. The study of keywords can assist in understanding key concepts and the terminology employed in the field, proving helpful when clarification or definition of specific terms is needed. Furthermore, by examining groups of keywords that frequently appear together in documents, thematic clusters or groups of terms often associated with each other can be identified. This can provide an overview of subdomains or main themes within a field. Additionally, keywords associated with a high number of citations may indicate topics of great relevance and impact in the scientific community. This can aid in identifying works and subjects that have had a significant impact in the field.

Table 7. Brief summary of the content of top 10 most global cited documents.

No.	Paper (First Author, Year, Journal, Reference)	Title	Main Elements	Purpose	Qualitative Analysis
1	Bagstad, K.J. (2013), Ecosystem Services [66]	Spatial dynamics of ecosystem service flows: A comprehensive approach to quantifying actual services	Ecosystem services; Spatial flows; Artificial Intelligence for Ecosystem Services (ARIES)	This study introduces "Service Path Attribution Networks" (SPANs), a class of agent-based models, to systematically quantify ecosystem service flows, emphasizing spatial connectivity between ecosystems and beneficiaries. Developed as part of the ARIES project, SPANs extend the existing ecosystem services classification, providing a comprehensive approach to modeling flow dynamics and supporting decision-making for conservation and resource management.	The qualitative analysis highlights the innovative nature of SPANs and their potential impact on decision-making for conservation and resource management.
2	Hare, M. (2004), Mathematics and Computers in Simulation [26]	Further towards a taxonomy of agent-based simulation models in environmental management	Agent-based simulation; Multi-agent systems; Agent-based modeling	This study addresses the challenges in the efficient use of Agent-Based Simulation (ABS) for environmental modeling due to the lack of a fixed definition for ABS and ambiguity regarding the concept of agents. The authors provide an overview of ABS in environmental modeling, clarifying and simplifying terminology to two key terms: agent-based modeling and multi-agent simulation. By reviewing representative case studies, the paper develops a classification scheme as a foundation for a taxonomy, aiming to assist modelers in identifying and implementing ABS techniques aligned with their specific requirements.	Qualitative insights discuss the significance of ABS in addressing challenges and offer practical guidance for environmental modelers.
3	O'Sullivan D. (2000), Environment and Planning A-Economy and Space [67]	Agent-based models and individualism: Is the world agent-based?	Bounded rationality; Increasing returns; economics; Agent-based models (ABMs)	This study discusses the growing popularity of Agent-Based Models (ABMs) in the social sciences, projecting their continued rise in fields like geography, urban planning, and regional planning. The overview spans applications in life sciences, economics, planning, sociology, and archaeology, highlighting a prevailing individualist perspective in ABMs. The discussion emphasizes the need for explicit inclusion or justified omission of institutions and social structures in ABMs. The paper suggests that the individualist bias in ABMs may stem from early research in AI and distributed AI. It urges critical examination of underlying assumptions and advocates engagement with social theory for ABMs to realize their full potential.	The qualitative analysis underlines the importance of addressing individualist biases in ABMs and advocates for engagement with social theory.

Table 7. Cont.

No.	Paper (First Author, Year, Journal, Reference)	Title	Main Elements	Purpose	Qualitative Analysis
4	Teodorovic, D. (2008), Transportation Research Part C-Emerging Technologies [68]	Swarm intelligence systems for transportation engineering; Principles and applications	Swarm intelligence; Transportation modeling; Nature-inspired algorithms; Metaheuristics	Agent-based modeling is an approach that views a system as comprised of decentralized individual "agents", each interacting with others based on localized knowledge. Inspired by social insects like bees and ants, artificial agents mimic their autonomy, distributed functioning, and self-organizing capacities. Social insect colonies demonstrate that simple organisms can achieve complex tasks through dynamic interactions. Swarm intelligence, a branch of AI, studies the behavior of individuals in decentralized systems. The paper classifies and analyzes results obtained using swarm intelligence to model complex traffic and transportation processes, introducing readers to the principles and potential applications of swarm intelligence in this context.	The qualitative analysis focuses on the application and potential impact of swarm intelligence in addressing transportation challenges.
5	Lamperti, F. (2018), Journal of Economic Dynamics & Control [69]	Agent-based model calibration using machine learning surrogates	Agent-based model; Calibration; Machine learning; Meta-model	This paper addresses the challenge of efficiently calibrating agent-based models (ABMs) to real data by employing a novel approach that combines machine learning and intelligent iterative sampling. The method involves the creation of a fast surrogate meta-model through machine learning, capturing the nonlinear relationship between ABM inputs (initial conditions and parameters) and outputs. The effectiveness of this approach is demonstrated in two models: the Brock and Hommes (1998) [75] asset pricing model and the "Islands" endogenous growth model by Fagiolo and Dosi (2003) [76]. Results indicate that the machine learning surrogates obtained through the iterative learning procedure serve as accurate proxies for the true model, significantly reducing computation time for large-scale parameter space exploration and calibration.	The qualitative analysis emphasizes the effectiveness of the proposed approach in calibrating ABMs and its potential implications for modeling complex systems.

Table 7. Cont.

No.	Paper (First Author, Year, Journal, Reference)	Title	Main Elements	Purpose	Qualitative Analysis
6	Lättilä, L. (2010), Expert Systems with Applications [70]	Hybrid simulation models—When; Why; How?	System dynamics; Agent-based modeling and simulation; Hybrid simulation models; Artificial intelligence; Expert Systems; Complex Adaptive Systems;	Agent-Based Modeling and Simulation (ABMS) and System Dynamics (SD) are distinct simulation paradigms, rarely combined despite their shared objectives. This research explores possible ways to integrate these methods, identifying five situations where their combination proves beneficial. Previous studies have successfully employed these approaches, suggesting modelers use them as potential interfaces for merging methodologies. Hybrid simulation models, formed through this integration, offer the potential to enhance the accuracy and reliability of Expert Systems (ES).	Qualitative insights highlight the potential of hybrid simulation models to enhance the accuracy and reliability of Expert Systems (ES).
7	Marshall, D.A. (2015), Value in Health [71]	Selecting a Dynamic Simulation Modeling Method for Health Care Delivery Research, Part 2: Report of the ISPOR Dynamic Simulation Modeling Emerging Good Practices Task Force	Decision-making; dynamic simulation modeling; validation; discrete-event simulation	This report builds on prior work by the ISPOR Task Force, comparing the three main dynamic simulation modeling methods—system dynamics; discrete-event simulation; and agent-based modeling. It provides criteria for method selection based on the problem, model scope, and approach. Emerging good practices for dynamic simulation modeling in healthcare are outlined, emphasizing stakeholder engagement and offering recommendations for informed decision-making. The report aims to assist readers in determining the appropriateness of dynamic simulation modeling for specific health systems problems, providing a concise overview, and directing them to further educational resources.	The qualitative analysis focuses on the recommendations provided for stakeholders and their potential impact on decision-making in healthcare.
8	Bennett, D.A. (2006), International Journal of Geographical Information Science [72]	Modelling adaptive, spatially aware, and mobile agents: Elk migration in Yellowstone	Agent-based modeling; machine learning; simulation; behavior; systems	This paper explores the potential utility of agent-based models (ABMs) featuring adaptive, spatially aware, and mobile entities in geographic and ecological research. Addressing challenges in geographic information science, the study introduces a framework for representing these agents. The framework aims to capture the spatio-temporal behavior of individuals, emphasizing the need for novel representational forms and procedures that simulate experiential learning, adaptation to dynamic environments, and spatial decision-making. To contextualize the research, a multiagent model simulates the migratory behavior of elk on Yellowstone's northern range, showcasing how intelligent agents learn and adapt within a simulated environment.	The qualitative analysis discusses the implications of using adaptive agents in modeling geographic and ecological phenomena and emphasizes the need for novel representational forms.

Table 7. Cont.

No.	Paper (First Author, Year, Journal, Reference)	Title	Main Elements	Purpose	Qualitative Analysis
9	Dehghanpour, K. (2018), IEEE Transactions on Smart Grid [73]	Agent-Based Modeling of Retail Electrical Energy Markets with Demand Response	Agent-based modeling; machine learning; demand response; networks	This paper explores a day-ahead retail electrical energy market with price-based demand response from air conditioning loads using a hierarchical multiagent framework and machine learning. The retailer aims to maximize profit by setting optimal retail prices, while AC agents optimize consumption patterns based on temperature set-points. The retailer relies on machine learning to model aggregate load behavior due to data privacy constraints. Simulation results demonstrate simultaneous optimization of agent behavior, leading to reduced power consumption costs and increased retailer profit. The proposed architecture is also effective in reducing peak loads, offering potential for deferring/avoiding distribution system upgrades in high photovoltaic power penetration scenarios.	The qualitative analysis focuses on the effectiveness of the proposed architecture in reducing power consumption costs and increasing retailer profit.
10	Bryson, J.J. (2007), Philosophical Transactions of the Royal Society B-Biological Sciences [74]	Agent-based modeling as scientific method: a case study analyzing primate social behavior	Agent-based modelling; validation, emergence; evolution; ecology; organization;	This study advocates for the application of agent-based modeling (ABM) as a scientific methodology in the biological sciences, providing a means of explanation and improving explanations through exploration of the collective effects of individual action selection. The article emphasizes the testing, critiquing, generalizing, and specifying capabilities of ABM. A case study is presented, focusing on Hemelrijk's DomWorld, the most widely published agent-based model in the biological sciences, specifically modeling primate social behavior. The analysis reveals discrepancies between the model and observed macaque behavior but highlights the model's robustness, allowing for valid results and extensions to compensate for identified problems. This robustness is presented as a standard advantage of experiment-based AI modeling techniques over analytic modeling.	The qualitative analysis discusses the case study's insights into primate social behavior, highlighting the robustness of experiment-based AI modeling techniques.

Table 8 presents the top 10 most frequently occurring words in the "keywords plus" section of the analyzed documents. We can observe that the term "simulation" appears most frequently, suggesting a prevalent focus on simulated scenarios, experiments, or models in the research. The term "model" is also highly recurrent, indicating a substantial emphasis on the creation and analysis of various models within the documents. The term "systems" is frequently used, suggesting that research often involves the study, development, or analysis of complex systems. The most frequently occurring words in the keywords plus section reflect a strong emphasis on simulation, modeling, system analysis, and the study of dynamic behaviors within various frameworks. The inclusion of terms like networks, optimization, and evolution indicates additional specific areas of interest in the analyzed research.

Table 8. Top-10 most frequent words in keywords plus.

Words	Occurrences
Simulation	23
Model	20
Systems	19
Behavior	13
Framework	12
dynamics	10
System	10
Networks	9
Optimization	9
Evolution	6

Also, Table 9 provides an overview of the top 10 most frequently used words in the authors' keywords across the analyzed documents. The recurring terms reflect the prevalent themes and focuses within the research. The list includes words such as "Machine learning", "Agent-based modeling", "Artificial intelligence", and "Simulation", indicating a strong emphasis on these concepts in the scholarly work. These keywords collectively suggest a significant interest in the application of machine learning and AI techniques, particularly within the context of ABM and simulation. The repetition of terms like "Deep learning" and "Learning" further underscores the importance of advanced learning methodologies in the studies. Overall, the word frequency analysis provides a consolidated view of the key themes and areas of focus within the body of research, offering insights into the prevalent topics and methodologies in the field.

Table 9. Top-10 most frequent words in authors' keywords.

Words	Occurrences
Machine learning	43
Agent-based modeling	31
Agent-based model	25
Artificial intelligence	20
Agent-based modelling	18
Simulation	15
Agent-based models	10
Deep learning	9
Learning	9
Agent-based	8

Additionally, a word cloud for the top 50 words based on keywords plus the author's keywords was generated in Figure 20.

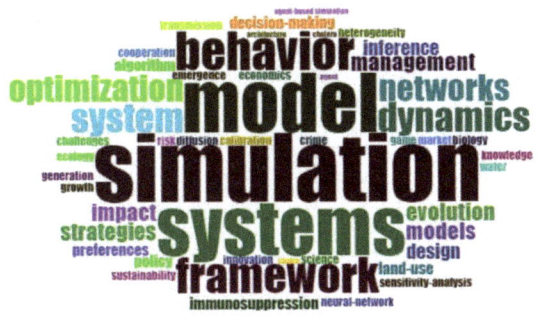 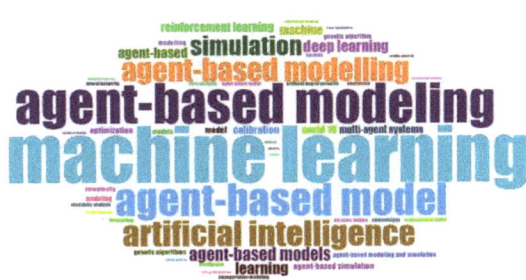

(**A**) Top 50 words based on keywords plus (**B**) Top 50 words based on authors' keywords

Figure 20. Top 50 words based on keywords plus (**A**) and authors' keywords (**B**).

The word cloud based on keywords plus reveals prominent terms within the research landscape. The most frequently occurring terms include "simulation", "model", "systems" "behavior", and "framework", indicating a focus on simulation modeling and system behavior in the research. Additionally, terms like "optimization", "evolution" and "impact" suggest an interest in optimizing systems and understanding their evolutionary impact. The presence of terms such as "management", "strategies", and "design" highlights a concern for effective management strategies and design considerations. The word cloud also reflects a diverse range of topics, including "immunosuppression", "land-use", "policy", and "preferences", indicating a multidisciplinary approach. Terms like "calibration", "inference", and "algorithm" suggest a methodological focus on refining models and making informed inferences. Furthermore, the inclusion of terms like "crime", "diffusion" and "ecology" suggests an application of simulation modeling in various domains, including social sciences and environmental studies. The word cloud provides a snapshot of the key thematic areas and methodological approaches prevalent in the research, offering insights into the diversity and depth of the studies covered.

The word cloud generated from the author's keywords provides insights into the key themes and methodologies prevalent in the research landscape. The most frequently occurring terms include "machine learning", "agent-based modeling", "artificial intelligence", and "simulation", indicating a strong emphasis on these areas in the scholarly work. The prominence of terms such as "deep learning", "reinforcement learning", and "calibration" suggests a focus on advanced learning techniques and refining models for accuracy. The presence of terms like "COVID-19", "epidemiology", and "forecasting" highlights a significant focus on applying these methodologies to address contemporary challenges. Additionally, terms like "multi-agent systems", "genetic algorithms", and "transportation modeling" reflect a diverse set of research areas, demonstrating the interdisciplinary nature of the studies covered. The word "cloud" also reveals a strong emphasis on specific modeling techniques, including "agent-based simulation", "complexity", and "genetic algorithm", underscoring the importance of these methods in the research community. Terms such as "sensitivity analysis", "neural networks", and "mathematical model" indicate a methodological focus on assessing model sensitivity and employing mathematical approaches in the research. Overall, the word cloud based on the author's keywords provides a comprehensive overview of the major themes, methodologies, and application areas within the academic research covered by the analyzed documents.

To analyze the relationships between categorical variables, such as the keywords in our analysis, the Multiple Correspondences Analysis (MCA) technique was employed to conduct a Factorial Analysis of Mixed Data (FAMD) [77]. This technique identifies associations between categories and provides a visual representation of these associations. In Figure 21, we observe that in the first quadrant, keywords such as "agent-based modeling", "decision making", "software agents", and "decision support systems" are prominent. Articles associated with this quadrant are characterized by involvement in ABM, decision-making, and the use of decision support systems. In this quadrant, research could explore the use of agent-based models in decision-making processes and the development of decision support systems. In the second quadrant, keywords like "deep learning", "reinforcement learning", "multi-agent systems", "sensitivity analysis", "economics", and "forecasting" are prevalent. Studies in this quadrant may address ways to improve system performance through technologies such as deep learning and reinforcement learning, with implications for economics and forecasting. Articles in the third quadrant focus on "machine learning", "computer models", "risk assessment", and "algorithms". Articles in this quadrant may delve into the development and application of computer models, the use of machine learning in various contexts, risk assessment, and algorithm development. Finally, the fourth quadrant encompasses articles addressing "decision support systems", "computer modeling", and "AI". Research in this quadrant could explore the implementation and enhancement of decision support systems, the utilization of computerized models, and advancements in the field of AI.

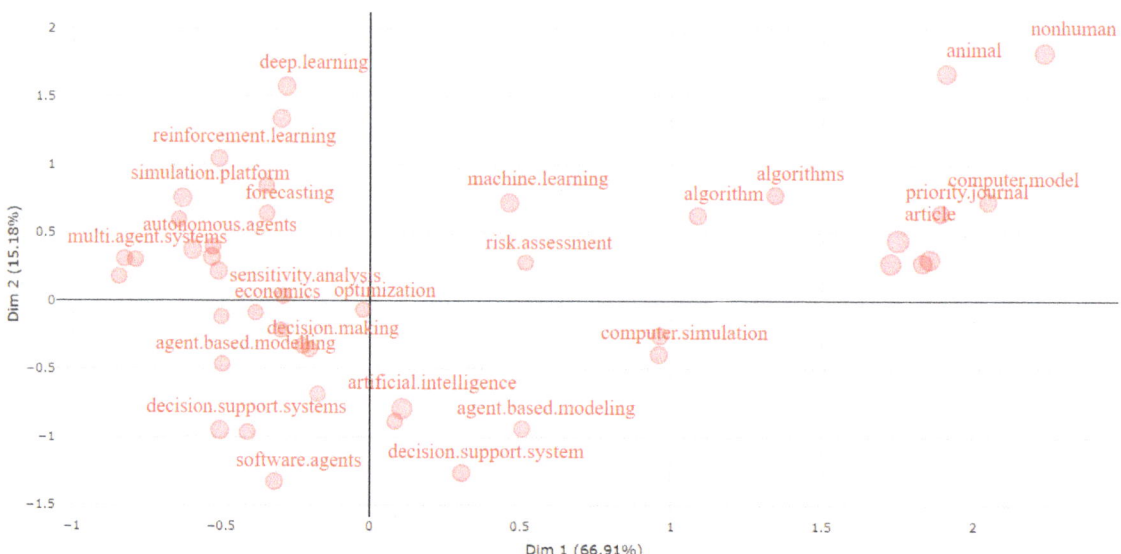

Figure 21. Keyword Plus—Factorial Analysis.

Table 10 represents the results of a dimensionality reduction analysis (factor analysis technique) for a set of words. The values in the "Dim.1" and "Dim.2" columns represent the coordinates of each word in a two-dimensional space, while the "cluster" column indicates the assigned cluster for each word. The words are grouped into a single cluster (cluster 1), suggesting a commonality or similarity among them in the analyzed context. Words with similar coordinates in this space are likely to have similar associations or patterns in the analyzed data. The positive or negative values in each dimension indicate the direction of the association. For instance, words like "networks", "algorithm", "machine learning", and "risk assessment" have positive coordinates in both dimensions, suggesting they share common associations.

Table 10. Factorial Analysis of 15 words by Cluster.

Word	Dim.1	Dim.2	Cluster
Simulation	−0.37	−0.38	1
Model	−0.15	0.09	1
Systems	0.25	−1.09	1
Behavior	0.72	−0.22	1
Framework	−0.34	−0.94	1
dynamics	−0.26	0.49	1
System	−0.33	−0.56	1
Networks	1.68	0.19	1
Optimization	−0.37	−0.21	1
Evolution	−0.57	0.86	1
Algorithm	1.34	0.78	1
Risk assessment	0.52	0.29	1
Artificial Intelligence	0.11	−0.79	1
Machine Learning	0.46	0.72	1
Deep Learning	−0.28	1.58	1

3.5. Mixed Analysis

In this section, we will conduct a mixed analysis by integrating information from multiple perspectives with the aim of providing a comprehensive view of the scientific landscape in our research field.

To achieve this, we employed the Three-fields plot from Bibliometrix. In Figure 22, we generated a Three-fields plot (countries, authors, journals). The first part of the plot illustrates how scientific contributions are distributed based on the countries of origin. This allows us to observe whether certain countries dominate in a specific field or if there is a balanced distribution. The second part of the plot focuses on the authors involved in research, providing insights into collaborations among authors and their influence in a given field. The third section highlights the distribution of results across scientific journals, potentially revealing the top journals where most works in the analyzed field are published.

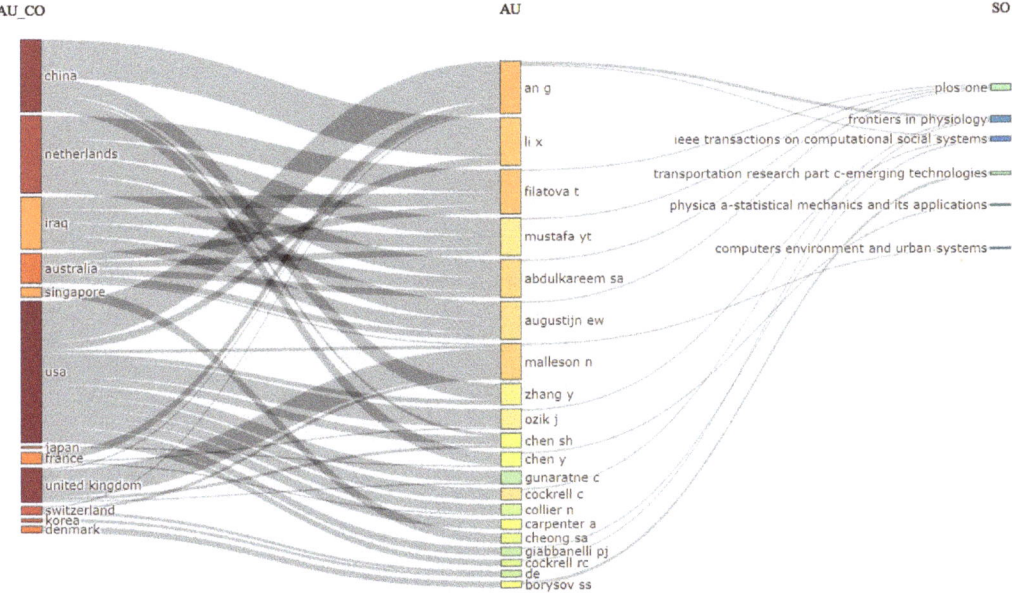

Figure 22. Three-fields plot: countries (**left**), authors (**middle**), journals (**right**).

Additionally, in Figure 23, a Three-fields plot (affiliations, authors, keywords) was generated.

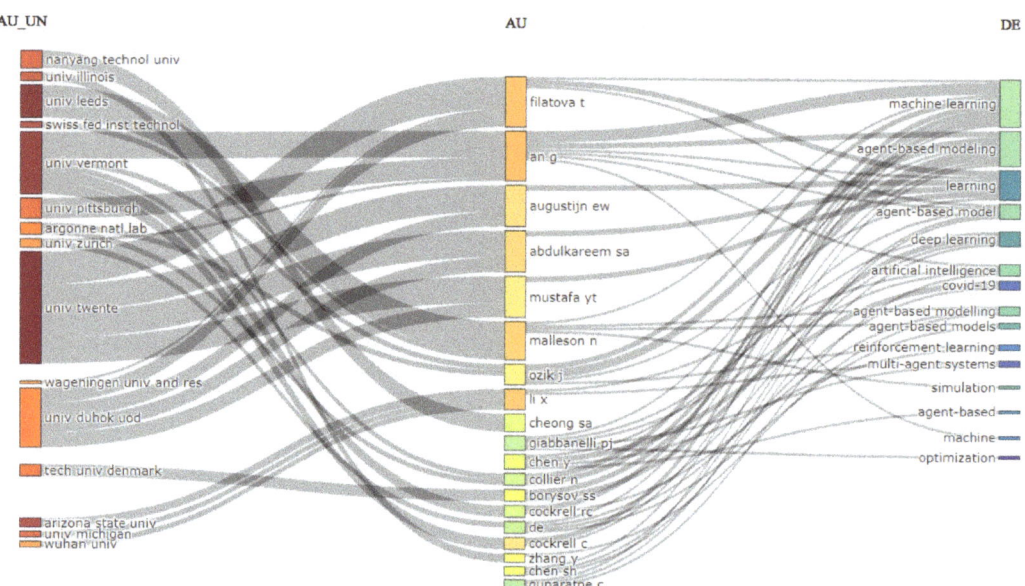

Figure 23. Three-fields plot: affiliations (**left**), authors (**middle**), keywords (**right**).

The first section illustrates how authors' affiliations are distributed in the scientific space, allowing us to observe if certain institutions dominate in specific fields. The second part of the plot focuses on the authors themselves, providing information on how they are connected based on their affiliations. The last section highlights the keywords associated with the research field, offering insights into emerging research trends and directions.

VOSviewer is a powerful tool for visualizing networks in bibliometric data [78,79]. From the analysis conducted in Figure 24, we can observe if there are certain patterns, connections, and relevant trends associated with the specific research field. Each color highlighted in Figure 24 represents a cluster, having their explanation in Table 11.

Table 11. Explanation of the clusters of co-occurrences depicted in Figure 24.

Cluster	Color	Label
1	Red	Agent, algorithm, machine, prediction, population, ability, effect, state, parameter, decision, impact, insight, goal, feature, interest, addition, individual, case study, case.
2	Blue	Artificial intelligence, challenge, modeling, knowledge, development, implementation, article, example, field, information, issue, need, point, problem, research, tool
3	Green	Complexity, ABM, ABMs, performance, number

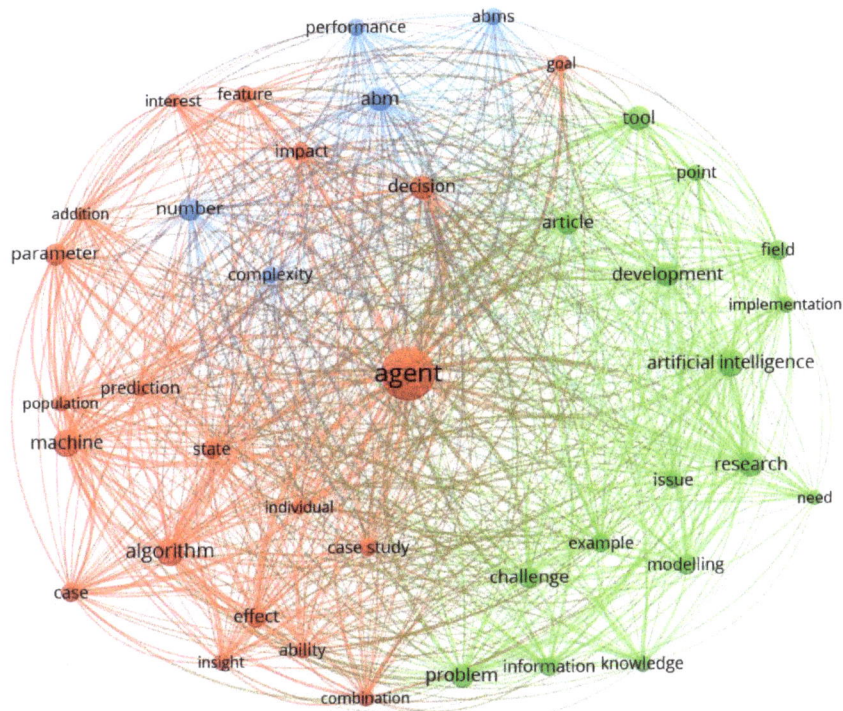

Figure 24. Spatial Patterns of Keyword Co-Occurrences in VOSviewer (LinLog/modularity method)—WoS source.

In Table 11, the formed clusters are described. Regarding Cluster 1 (red), among the representative keywords, we find "agent", "algorithm", "machine", "prediction", "decision", "parameter", "effect", and "case study". Thus, this cluster highlights specific aspects of ABM, such as algorithms, agent abilities, and the effects and impact of predictions on the population or individuals. Special attention is given to "agents", "machines", and "algorithms" in this cluster. Cluster 2 (blue) features representative words such as "AI", "modeling", "development", "knowledge", "issue", "need", etc. This cluster focuses on aspects related to AI in the context of ABM. Cluster 2 addresses the challenges, development, and implementation of AI in this field, highlighting the resolution of needs and associated problems through AI. As for Cluster 3 (green), it includes keywords such as "ABM", "complexity", and "performance". This cluster centers around concepts such as complexity, performance, number, and agent-based models (ABMs). It may also reflect an interest in analyzing how these models behave in complex contexts.

4. Discussion

Our research focuses on constructing a holistic landscape of the interconnections between ABM and artificial intelligence. To create this comprehensive landscape, bibliometric analyses were conducted on the temporal evolution, citations, collaborations, and geographical distribution in the fields of AI and ABM. Thus, we examined the significant growth in interest and activity, the contemporary research explosion, temporal trends and fluctuations, sustainability of impact, diversity, and interdisciplinary nature of journals, as well as the dominance of countries and regional collaborations regarding scientific production.

Regarding the temporal evolution of research, our results reveal a significant increase in scientific production, especially post-2006. The peaks in 2021 and 2022 suggest heightened interest and increased activity, indicating a contemporary surge in exploring AI in ABM. However, fluctuations in the 2000s and stability from 2009 to 2015 raise questions about the influencing factors. Possible causes could include technological advances, global events, or shifts in research focus (RQ6).

From the perspective of citation trends, the consistent growth in citations per year per document signifies sustained impact and recognition. The 2021 peak implies an accumulation of influence, suggesting significant contributions during that period. The continued high level of citations in 2022 underscores the ongoing relevance of recent studies. Understanding the factors behind these citation patterns could provide insights into influential works and emerging trends. Our bibliometric analysis highlights that the study of Bagstad et al. [66] is the most influential article, considering it has the highest number of citations. The authors have developed a systemic approach to quantifying the flow of ecosystem services using a formalized approach in the form of a class of agent-based models developed within the Artificial Intelligence for Ecosystem Services project (RQ1). Thus, we can observe the interest of researchers and specialists in the development of service flows in this area. By using the same criteria regarding the total number of citations globally, the bibliometric analysis has highlighted authors Bagstad et al. [66], Hare and Deadman [26], O'Sullivan and Haklay [67], Teodorović [68], and Lamperti [69], ranking as the top 5 authors based on the total number of citations (RQ2).

The application of Reference Publication Year Spectroscopy (RPYS) to analyze cited references over time reveals historical trends in ABM and AI. The recent decline may indicate a shift in research focus or a reevaluation of seminal works. Further exploration is necessary to understand the implications of these changes and their impact on the current state of the field.

Additionally, Lotka's Law, in line with our article analysis, indicates a small percentage of authors contributing to the majority of research in this field. This is supported by the ABC-Pareto analysis. The diversity of journals and their interdisciplinary nature indicate extensive exploration of AI applications in ABM. According to our analysis of the top 20 most relevant journals in the context of our study, we have identified that these 20 journals cover a diverse range of disciplines, highlighting the interdisciplinary nature of AI and ABM applications. Journals such as the *Journal of Economic Dynamics & Control*, *PLOS ONE*, and *Transportation Research Part C-Emerging Technologies* appear to be prominent contributors. The variety of journals with multiple articles suggests a broad exploration of AI applications in ABM, covering economic dynamics, control, emerging technologies, computational economics, and more. This diversity signifies a comprehensive examination of the subject. The presence of journals such as *Ecological Modelling* and *Frontiers in Physiology* indicates interdisciplinary exploration, highlighting the extended impact of AI and ABM beyond traditional domains (RQ3, RQ4). Identifying key journals and grouping them according to Bradford's Law provides valuable insights into publishing trends and can guide researchers seeking impactful platforms. Furthermore, our analysis highlighted that universities such as Twente, Leeds, Vermont, British Columbia, and Arizona State are at the forefront of research in the field of artificial intelligence, based on articles published in ABM (RQ5).

The dominance of certain countries in scientific production emphasizes the global landscape of AI in ABM research. The collaboration map between countries can be interpreted by analyzing the frequency of collaborations between different pairs of countries. Specifically, it is important to observe which countries collaborate most frequently and in what contexts. Our results have highlighted collaborations among European countries, with multiple connections between Belgium, Finland, France, Germany, the Netherlands, Spain, and Switzerland. Additionally, Asian countries such as China and Korea have connections both among themselves and with European countries. An interesting observation from the perspective of interspecific collaborations is that our results have revealed collaborations between countries with different geographical and cultural perspectives, such as Australia and Iraq or Brazil and China. The most intense collaborations were observed with the USA, which frequently collaborates with the United Kingdom and Switzerland (RQ7). The collaboration map highlights regional, cultural, and interdisciplinary partnerships, offering opportunities for enhanced cooperation and knowledge exchange.

Interpreting the results of cluster analysis for keyword co-occurrences in VOSviewer in connection with the data extracted from WoS, it can be observed that the Red cluster highlights a broad interest in concepts such as "Agent", "Algorithm", "Machine", and "Prediction", suggesting a focus on the technical and technological aspects of AI and algorithms. The Blue cluster reveals terms like "Artificial Intelligence" and "Modelling", reflecting a particular interest in the development and implementation of AI. The Green cluster indicates an interest in "ABMs" and "Performance". This might suggest that the scientific community is united in exploring agent-based models and evaluating their performance. These findings underscore the complexity and diversity of approaches in scientific literature, also highlighting how crucial it is to understand the specific context of each data source in interpreting the results. It is essential to consider these differences when comparing and synthesizing results from different sources.

5. Conclusions

The present research highlights an innovative perspective on the interaction between ABM and AI. Through detailed bibliometric analyses, we have not only emphasized the significant increase in interest and activity in these fields but also the contemporary explosion in their research. This holistic approach has revealed temporal trends, the sustainability of impact, diversity, and interdisciplinarity of the involved journals, as well as the dominance of certain countries and regional collaborations in scientific production.

The results of our study shed light on the interconnections between ABM and AI, with the bibliometric analysis conducted providing a comprehensive view of the temporal evolution, citations, collaborations, and geographical distribution in the fields of AI and ABM. The bibliometric analyses allowed us to examine the significant increase in interest and activity, the contemporary research explosion, temporal trends and fluctuations, sustainability of impact, diversity, and interdisciplinary nature of journals, as well as the dominance of countries and regional collaborations in scientific production.

The utility of this research lies in providing a comprehensive map of the scientific landscape of the interconnections between ABM and AI, offering researchers and professionals a robust framework for understanding the evolution of these domains and identifying relevant research directions.

The significance of this work resides in its ability to synthesize temporal, regional, and thematic perspectives of research, contributing to shaping a comprehensive framework. It not only reflects the current state of the field but also opens doors to new horizons of exploration and development. Our results reinforce the idea that researchers, practitioners, and decision-makers should more extensively implement AI algorithms in ABM, as it can contribute to improving the accuracy and relevance of the results, as demonstrated in their articles and by Turgut et al. [25], Hu et al. [30], Taghikhah et al. [28], Zhang et al. [15], and Sivakumar et al. [24].

Our paper makes a significant contribution to the existing research in the area by highlighting and exploring the complex interactions between ABM and AI. In contrast to previous research, which predominantly focused on specific aspects, our study provides a comprehensive overview of temporal evolution, collaborations, and geographical distribution, bringing forth significant trends and key interconnections. Also, our bibliometric analysis and keyword cluster study offer a detailed perspective on how the scientific community approaches these topics across various data sources, revealing the intricacies and diversity of ABM and AI research.

However, potential limitations of our research include a citation lag that may impact the accuracy of impact assessments, particularly for more recent works. The interdisciplinary nature of AI in ABM may pose challenges in accurately categorizing publications, requiring careful consideration of classification criteria. While the analysis provides a global perspective, regional variations in priorities and research challenges may not be fully captured. A more detailed examination of specific regions could provide additional insights. Additionally, a limitation of our study, which could also serve as a future research direction, is the examination of funding sources and collaborations to provide another perspective on the dynamics of research in the fields of AI and ABM, including the role of industry-academia partnerships and international collaborations.

Future research directions could focus on a deeper analysis of how recent technological advancements influence the evolution of agent-based models and the utilization of artificial intelligence. Evaluating how anticipated technological progress can shape and steer research in ABM and AI is another future objective we have in mind. Additionally, investigating how global events, such as major socio-economic changes or global crises, can impact the research directions in ABM and AI. Furthermore, a more detailed exploration of how ABM and AI interact in specific domains, such as economics, ecology, or medicine, will highlight the unique challenges and opportunities in each field. Moreover, despite the significant contributions made by research in the fields of AI and ABM, it is crucial to be aware of the ethical and societal implications of this integration. Future research should conduct a more in-depth assessment of these aspects, and researchers should pay special attention to ensuring a robust ethical framework in the development and application of agent-based models involving artificial intelligence.

Author Contributions: Conceptualization, Ș.I., C.D., N.C. and I.N.; Data curation, Ș.I., C.D., N.C. and I.N.; Formal analysis, Ș.I., C.D. and I.N.; Investigation, Ș.I., C.D., N.C. and I.N.; Methodology, Ș.I., C.D. and I.N.; Software, Ș.I. and C.D.; Supervision, C.D.; Validation, Ș.I., N.C. and I.N.; Visualization, Ș.I., C.D., N.C. and I.N.; Writing—original draft, Ș.I. and C.D.; Writing—review and editing, N.C. and I.N. All authors have read and agreed to the published version of the manuscript.

Funding: This research received no external funding.

Data Availability Statement: Data are contained within this article.

Acknowledgments: This paper was co-financed by the Bucharest University of Economic Studies during the Ph.D. program.

Conflicts of Interest: The authors declare no conflicts of interest.

References

1. Chen, S.H.; Londoño-Larrea, P.; McGough, A.S.; Bible, A.N.; Gunaratne, C.; Araujo-Granda, P.A.; Morrell-Falvey, J.L.; Bhowmik, D.; Fuentes-Cabrera, M. Application of Machine Learning Techniques to an Agent-Based Model of Pantoea. *Front. Microbiol.* **2021**, *12*, 726409. [CrossRef]
2. Bonabeau, E. Agent-Based Modeling: Methods and Techniques for Simulating Human Systems. *Proc. Natl. Acad. Sci. USA* **2002**, *99*, 7280–7287. [CrossRef]
3. Paudel, R.; Ligmann-Zielinska, A. A Largely Unsupervised Domain-Independent Qualitative Data Extraction Approach for Empirical Agent-Based Model Development. *Algorithms* **2023**, *16*, 338. [CrossRef]
4. Delcea, C.; Cotfas, L.-A.; Craciun, L.; Molanescu, A.G. An Agent-Based Modeling Approach to Collaborative Classrooms Evacuation Process. *Saf. Sci.* **2020**, *121*, 414–429. [CrossRef]
5. Ionescu, Ș.; Nica, I.; Chiriță, N. Cybernetics Approach Using Agent-Based Modeling in the Process of Evacuating Educational Institutions in Case of Disasters. *Sustainability* **2021**, *13*, 10277. [CrossRef]
6. Delcea, C.; Chirita, N. Exploring the Applications of Agent-Based Modeling in Transportation. *Appl. Sci.* **2023**, *13*, 9815. [CrossRef]
7. Delcea, C.; Yang, Y.; Liu, S.; Cotfas, L.-A. Agent-Based Modelling in Grey Economic Systems. In *Emerging Studies and Applications of Grey Systems*; Yang, Y., Liu, S., Eds.; Series on Grey System; Springer Nature: Singapore, 2023; ISBN 978-981-19342-3-0.
8. El Oubani, A.; Lekhal, M. An Agent-Based Model of Financial Market Efficiency Dynamics. *Borsa Istanb. Rev.* **2022**, *22*, 699–710. [CrossRef]
9. Ionescu, Ș.; Chiriță, N.; Nica, I.; Delcea, C. An Analysis of Residual Financial Contagion in Romania's Banking Market for Mortgage Loans. *Sustainability* **2023**, *15*, 12037. [CrossRef]
10. Badham, J.; Chattoe-Brown, E.; Gilbert, N.; Chalabi, Z.; Kee, F.; Hunter, R.F. Developing Agent-Based Models of Complex Health Behaviour. *Health Place.* **2018**, *54*, 170–177. [CrossRef]
11. Hunter, E.; Kelleher, J.D. Validating and Testing an Agent-Based Model for the Spread of COVID-19 in Ireland. *Algorithms* **2022**, *15*, 270. [CrossRef]
12. Zeigler, B.; Muzy, A.; Yilmaz, L. Artificial Intelligence in Modeling and Simulation. In *Encyclopedia of Complexity and Systems Science*; Meyers, R.A., Ed.; Springer: New York, NY, USA, 2009; pp. 344–368, ISBN 978-0-387-75888-6.

13. Brandon, N.; Dionisio, K.L.; Isaacs, K.; Tornero-Velez, R.; Kapraun, D.; Setzer, R.W.; Price, P.S. Simulating Exposure-Related Behaviors Using Agent-Based Models Embedded with Needs-Based Artificial Intelligence. *J. Expo. Sci. Env. Epidemiol.* **2020**, *30*, 184–193. [CrossRef]
14. Murugesan, U.; Subramanian, P.; Srivastava, S.; Dwivedi, A. A Study of Artificial Intelligence Impacts on Human Resource Digitalization in Industry 4.0. *Decis. Anal. J.* **2023**, *7*, 100249. [CrossRef]
15. Zhang, W.; Valencia, A.; Chang, N.-B. Synergistic Integration Between Machine Learning and Agent-Based Modeling: A Multidisciplinary Review. *IEEE Trans. Neural Netw. Learn. Syst.* **2023**, *34*, 2170–2190. [CrossRef]
16. An, L.; Grimm, V.; Bai, Y.; Sullivan, A.; Turner, B.L.; Malleson, N.; Heppenstall, A.; Vincenot, C.; Robinson, D.; Ye, X.; et al. Modeling Agent Decision and Behavior in the Light of Data Science and Artificial Intelligence. *Environ. Model. Softw.* **2023**, *166*, 105713. [CrossRef]
17. Nica, I.; Chirita, N. *Holistic Approach of Complex Adaptive Systems. Theory, Applications and Case Studies.*; LAP Lambert Academic Publishing: Saarbrücken, Germany, 2021; ISBN 978-620-3-30709-2.
18. Bankes, S.C. Tools and Techniques for Developing Policies for Complex and Uncertain Systems. *Proc. Natl. Acad. Sci. USA* **2002**, *99*, 7263–7266. [CrossRef]
19. Xu, Y.; Liu, X.; Cao, X.; Huang, C.; Liu, E.; Qian, S.; Liu, X.; Wu, Y.; Dong, F.; Qiu, C.-W.; et al. Artificial Intelligence: A Powerful Paradigm for Scientific Research. *The Innovation* **2021**, *2*, 100179. [CrossRef]
20. Bae, J.W.; Moon, I.-C. LDEF Formalism for Agent-Based Model Development. *IEEE Trans. Syst. Man. Cybern. Syst.* **2016**, *46*, 793–808. [CrossRef]
21. Sánchez, J.M.; Rodríguez, J.P.; Espitia, H.E. Bibliometric Analysis of Publications Discussing the Use of the Artificial Intelligence Technique Agent-Based Models in Sustainable Agriculture. *Heliyon* **2022**, *8*, e12005. [CrossRef] [PubMed]
22. Romero, E.; Chica, M.; Damas, S.; Rand, W. Two Decades of Agent-Based Modeling in Marketing: A Bibliometric Analysis. *Prog. Artif. Intell.* **2023**, *12*, 213–229. [CrossRef]
23. Chen, X.; Cheng, G.; Zou, D.; Zhong, B.; Xie, H. Artificial Intelligent Robots for Precision Education: A Topic Modeling-Based Bibliometric Analysis. *Educ. Technol. Soc.* **2023**, *26*, 171–186. [CrossRef]
24. Sivakumar, N.; Mura, C.; Peirce, S.M. Innovations in Integrating Machine Learning and Agent-Based Modeling of Biomedical Systems. *Front. Syst. Biol.* **2022**, *2*, 959665. [CrossRef]
25. Turgut, Y.; Bozdag, C.E. A Framework Proposal for Machine Learning-Driven Agent-Based Models through a Case Study Analysis. *Simul. Model. Pract. Theory* **2023**, *123*, 102707. [CrossRef]
26. Hare, M.; Deadman, P. Further towards a Taxonomy of Agent-Based Simulation Models in Environmental Management. *Math. Comput. Simul.* **2004**, *64*, 25–40. [CrossRef]
27. Moret-Bonillo, V. Can Artificial Intelligence Benefit from Quantum Computing? *Prog. Artif. Intell.* **2015**, *3*, 89–105. [CrossRef]
28. Taghikhah, F.; Voinov, A.; Filatova, T.; Polhill, J.G. Machine-Assisted Agent-Based Modeling: Opening the Black Box. *J. Comput. Sci.* **2022**, *64*, 101854. [CrossRef]
29. Helbing, D. Agent-Based Modeling. In *Social Self-Organization*; Helbing, D., Ed.; Understanding Complex Systems; Springer: Berlin/Heidelberg, Germany, 2012; pp. 25–70. ISBN 978-3-642-24003-4.
30. Hu, Y.; Quinn, C.J.; Cai, X.; Garfinkle, N.W. Combining Human and Machine Intelligence to Derive Agents' Behavioral Rules for Groundwater Irrigation. *Adv. Water Resour.* **2017**, *109*, 29–40. [CrossRef]
31. Ale Ebrahim Dehkordi, M.; Lechner, J.; Ghorbani, A.; Nikolic, I.; Chappin, É.; Herder, P. Using Machine Learning for Agent Specifications in Agent-Based Models and Simulations: A Critical Review and Guidelines. *JASSS* **2023**, *26*, 9. [CrossRef]
32. Donthu, N.; Kumar, S.; Mukherjee, D.; Pandey, N.; Lim, W.M. How to Conduct a Bibliometric Analysis: An Overview and Guidelines. *J. Bus. Res.* **2021**, *133*, 285–296. [CrossRef]
33. WoS: Web of Science. Available online: https://webofscience.com/ (accessed on 11 October 2023).
34. Aria, M.; Cuccurullo, C. Bibliometrix: An R-Tool for Comprehensive Science Mapping Analysis. *J. Informetr.* **2017**, *11*, 959–975. [CrossRef]
35. VOSviewer—Visualizing Scientific Landscapes. Available online: https://www.vosviewer.com/ (accessed on 5 December 2023).
36. Kemeç, A.; Altınay, A.T. Sustainable Energy Research Trend: A Bibliometric Analysis Using VOSviewer, RStudio Bibliometrix, and CiteSpace Software Tools. *Sustainability* **2023**, *15*, 3618. [CrossRef]
37. Delcea, C.; Javed, S.A.; Florescu, M.-S.; Ioanas, C.; Cotfas, L.-A. 35 Years of Grey System Theory in Economics and Education. *Kybernetes* **2023**, ahead-of-print. [CrossRef]
38. Silva, M.D.S.T.; Oliveira, V.M.D.; Correia, S.É.N. Scientific Mapping in Scopus with Biblioshiny: A Bibliometric Analysis of Organizational Tensions. *Contextus* **2022**, *20*, 54–71. [CrossRef]
39. Zupic, I.; Čater, T. Bibliometric Methods in Management and Organization. *Organ. Res. Methods* **2015**, *18*, 429–472. [CrossRef]
40. Lu, Y. Artificial Intelligence: A Survey on Evolution, Models, Applications and Future Trends. *J. Manag. Anal.* **2019**, *6*, 1–29. [CrossRef]
41. Goralski, M.A.; Tan, T.K. Artificial Intelligence and Sustainable Development. *Int. J. Manag. Educ.* **2020**, *18*, 100330. [CrossRef]
42. European Commission. *Joint Research Centre. AI Watch, Historical Evolution of Artificial Intelligence: Analysis of the Three Main Paradigm Shifts in AI*; Publications Office: Luxembourg, 2020.
43. Liu, W. The Data Source of This Study Is Web of Science Core Collection? Not Enough. *Scientometrics* **2019**, *121*, 1815–1824. [CrossRef]

44. Liu, F. Retrieval Strategy and Possible Explanations for the Abnormal Growth of Research Publications: Re-Evaluating a Bibliometric Analysis of Climate Change. *Scientometrics* **2023**, *128*, 853–859. [CrossRef] [PubMed]
45. Cobo, M.J.; Martínez, M.A.; Gutiérrez-Salcedo, M.; Fujita, H.; Herrera-Viedma, E. 25 Years at Knowledge-Based Systems: A Bibliometric Analysis. *Knowl. Based Syst.* **2015**, *80*, 3–13. [CrossRef]
46. Modak, N.M.; Merigó, J.M.; Weber, R.; Manzor, F.; Ortúzar, J.D.D. Fifty Years of Transportation Research Journals: A Bibliometric Overview. *Transp. Res. Part. A Policy Pract.* **2019**, *120*, 188–223. [CrossRef]
47. Mulet-Forteza, C.; Martorell-Cunill, O.; Merigó, J.M.; Genovart-Balaguer, J.; Mauleon-Mendez, E. Twenty Five Years of the Journal of Travel & Tourism Marketing: A Bibliometric Ranking. *J. Travel. Tour. Mark.* **2018**, *35*, 1201–1221. [CrossRef]
48. Tay, A. Bibliometric Reviews in Business, Management & Accounting and the Tools Used. Available online: https://library.smu.edu.sg/topics-insights/bibliometric-reviews-business-management-accounting-and-tools-used (accessed on 21 November 2023).
49. Tay, A. Using VOSviewer as a Bibliometric Mapping or Analysis Tool in Business, Management & Accounting. Available online: https://library.smu.edu.sg/topics-insights/using-vosviewer-bibliometric-mapping-or-analysis-tool-business-management (accessed on 22 November 2023).
50. Donner, P. Document Type Assignment Accuracy in the Journal Citation Index Data of Web of Science. *Scientometrics* **2017**, *113*, 219–236. [CrossRef]
51. WoS Document Types. Available online: https://webofscience.help.clarivate.com/en-us/Content/document-types.html (accessed on 3 December 2023).
52. Rogers, G.; Szomszor, M.; Adams, J. Sample Size in Bibliometric Analysis. *Scientometrics* **2020**, *125*, 777–794. [CrossRef]
53. Meng, L.; Wen, K.-H.; Brewin, R.; Wu, Q. Knowledge Atlas on the Relationship between Urban Street Space and Residents' Health—A Bibliometric Analysis Based on VOSviewer and CiteSpace. *Sustainability* **2020**, *12*, 2384. [CrossRef]
54. Waltman, L.; Van Eck, N.J.; Noyons, E.C.M. A Unified Approach to Mapping and Clustering of Bibliometric Networks. *J. Informetr.* **2010**, *4*, 629–635. [CrossRef]
55. Martins, J.; Gonçalves, R.; Branco, F. A Bibliometric Analysis and Visualization of E-Learning Adoption Using VOSviewer. *Univ. Access Inf. Soc.* **2022**. [CrossRef] [PubMed]
56. Yu, Y.; Li, Y.; Zhang, Z.; Gu, Z.; Zhong, H.; Zha, Q.; Yang, L.; Zhu, C.; Chen, E. A Bibliometric Analysis Using VOSviewer of Publications on COVID-19. *Ann. Transl. Med.* **2020**, *8*, 816. [CrossRef] [PubMed]
57. Abdelwahab, S.I.; Taha, M.M.E.; Moni, S.S.; Alsayegh, A.A. Bibliometric Mapping of Solid Lipid Nanoparticles Research (2012–2022) Using VOSviewer. *Med. Nov. Technol. Devices* **2023**, *17*, 100217. [CrossRef]
58. Guleria, D.; Kaur, G. Bibliometric Analysis of Ecopreneurship Using VOSviewer and RStudio Bibliometrix, 1989–2019. *LHT* **2021**, *39*, 1001–1024. [CrossRef]
59. Bornmann, L.; Marx, W. The Proposal of a Broadening of Perspective in Evaluative Bibliometrics by Complementing the Times Cited with a Cited Reference Analysis. *J. Informetr.* **2013**, *7*, 84–88. [CrossRef]
60. Marx, W.; Bornmann, L.; Barth, A.; Leydesdorff, L. Detecting the Historical Roots of Research Fields by Reference Publication Year Spectroscopy (RPYS). *J. Assoc. Inf. Sci. Technol.* **2014**, *65*, 751–764. [CrossRef]
61. Sahu, A.; Jena, P. Lotka's Law and Author Productivity Pattern of Research in Law Discipline. *Collect. Curation* **2022**, *41*, 62–73. [CrossRef]
62. Kawamura, M.; Thomas, C.D.L.; Tsurumoto, A.; Sasahara, H.; Kawaguchi, Y. Lotka's Law and Productivity Index of Authors in a Scientific Journal. *J. Oral. Sci.* **2000**, *42*, 75–78. [CrossRef] [PubMed]
63. Chen, Y.; Li, K.W.; Marc Kilgour, D.; Hipel, K.W. A Case-Based Distance Model for Multiple Criteria ABC Analysis. *Comput. Oper. Res.* **2008**, *35*, 776–796. [CrossRef]
64. Kheybari, S.; Naji, S.A.; Rezaie, F.M.; Salehpour, R. ABC Classification According to Pareto's Principle: A Hybrid Methodology. *Opsearch* **2019**, *56*, 539–562. [CrossRef]
65. Platas-López, A.; Guerra-Hernández, A.; Quiroz-Castellanos, M.; Cruz-Ramírez, N. Agent-Based Models Assisted by Supervised Learning: A Proposal for Model Specification. *Electronics* **2023**, *12*, 495. [CrossRef]
66. Bagstad, K.J.; Johnson, G.W.; Voigt, B.; Villa, F. Spatial Dynamics of Ecosystem Service Flows: A Comprehensive Approach to Quantifying Actual Services. *Ecosyst. Serv.* **2013**, *4*, 117–125. [CrossRef]
67. O'Sullivan, D.; Haklay, M. Agent-Based Models and Individualism: Is the World Agent-Based? *Env. Plan. A* **2000**, *32*, 1409–1425. [CrossRef]
68. Teodorović, D. Swarm Intelligence Systems for Transportation Engineering: Principles and Applications. *Transp. Res. Part. C Emerg. Technol.* **2008**, *16*, 651–667. [CrossRef]
69. Lamperti, F.; Roventini, A.; Sani, A. Agent-Based Model Calibration Using Machine Learning Surrogates. *J. Econ. Dyn. Control* **2018**, *90*, 366–389. [CrossRef]
70. Lättilä, L.; Hilletofth, P.; Lin, B. Hybrid Simulation Models—When, Why, How? *Expert. Syst. Appl.* **2010**, *37*, 7969–7975. [CrossRef]
71. Marshall, D.A.; Burgos-Liz, L.; IJzerman, M.J.; Crown, W.; Padula, W.V.; Wong, P.K.; Pasupathy, K.S.; Higashi, M.K.; Osgood, N.D. Selecting a Dynamic Simulation Modeling Method for Health Care Delivery Research—Part 2: Report of the ISPOR Dynamic Simulation Modeling Emerging Good Practices Task Force. *Value Health* **2015**, *18*, 147–160. [CrossRef]
72. Bennett, D.A.; Tang, W. Modelling Adaptive, Spatially Aware, and Mobile Agents: Elk Migration in Yellowstone. *Int. J. Geogr. Inf. Sci.* **2006**, *20*, 1039–1066. [CrossRef]

73. Dehghanpour, K.; Nehrir, M.H.; Sheppard, J.W.; Kelly, N.C. Agent-Based Modeling of Retail Electrical Energy Markets With Demand Response. *IEEE Trans. Smart Grid* **2018**, *9*, 3465–3475. [CrossRef]
74. Bryson, J.J.; Ando, Y.; Lehmann, H. Agent-Based Modelling as Scientific Method: A Case Study Analysing Primate Social Behaviour. *Phil. Trans. R. Soc. B* **2007**, *362*, 1685–1699. [CrossRef] [PubMed]
75. Brock, W.A.; Hommes, C.H. Heterogeneous Beliefs and Routes to Chaos in a Simple Asset Pricing Model. *J. Econ. Dyn. Control* **1998**, *22*, 1235–1274. [CrossRef]
76. Fagiolo, G.; Dosi, G. Exploitation, Exploration and Innovation in a Model of Endogenous Growth with Locally Interacting Agents. *Struct. Change Econ. Dyn.* **2003**, *14*, 237–273. [CrossRef]
77. Fithian, W.; Josse, J. Multiple Correspondence Analysis and the Multilogit Bilinear Model. *J. Multivar. Anal.* **2017**, *157*, 87–102. [CrossRef]
78. Effendi, D.N.; Anggraini, W.; Jatmiko, A.; Rahmayanti, H.; Ichsan, I.Z.; Mehadi Rahman, M. Bibliometric Analysis of Scientific Literacy Using VOS Viewer: Analysis of Science Education. *J. Phys. Conf. Ser.* **2021**, *1796*, 012096. [CrossRef]
79. Kirby, A. Exploratory Bibliometrics: Using VOSviewer as a Preliminary Research Tool. *Publications* **2023**, *11*, 10. [CrossRef]

Disclaimer/Publisher's Note: The statements, opinions and data contained in all publications are solely those of the individual author(s) and contributor(s) and not of MDPI and/or the editor(s). MDPI and/or the editor(s) disclaim responsibility for any injury to people or property resulting from any ideas, methods, instructions or products referred to in the content.

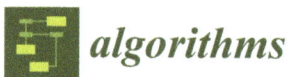 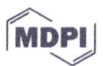

Article

A Largely Unsupervised Domain-Independent Qualitative Data Extraction Approach for Empirical Agent-Based Model Development

Rajiv Paudel [1] and Arika Ligmann-Zielinska [2,*]

[1] Operation Research and Analysis, Idaho National Laboratory, 1955 Fremont Ave., Idaho Falls, ID 83415, USA; rajiv.paudel@inl.gov
[2] Department of Geography, Environment, and Spatial Sciences, Michigan State University, Geography Building, 673 Auditorium Rd, Room 121, East Lansing, MI 48824, USA
* Correspondence: arika@msu.edu

Abstract: Agent-based model (ABM) development needs information on system components and interactions. Qualitative narratives contain contextually rich system information beneficial for ABM conceptualization. Traditional qualitative data extraction is manual, complex, and time- and resource-consuming. Moreover, manual data extraction is often biased and may produce questionable and unreliable models. A possible alternative is to employ automated approaches borrowed from Artificial Intelligence. This study presents a largely unsupervised qualitative data extraction framework for ABM development. Using semantic and syntactic Natural Language Processing tools, our methodology extracts information on system agents, their attributes, and actions and interactions. In addition to expediting information extraction for ABM, the largely unsupervised approach also minimizes biases arising from modelers' preconceptions about target systems. We also introduce automatic and manual noise-reduction stages to make the framework usable on large semi-structured datasets. We demonstrate the approach by developing a conceptual ABM of household food security in rural Mali. The data for the model contain a large set of semi-structured qualitative field interviews. The data extraction is swift, predominantly automatic, and devoid of human manipulation. We contextualize the model manually using the extracted information. We also put the conceptual model to stakeholder evaluation for added credibility and validity.

Keywords: agent-based modeling; natural language processing; unsupervised data extraction; model contextualization

Citation: Paudel, R.; Ligmann-Zielinska, A. A Largely Unsupervised Domain-Independent Qualitative Data Extraction Approach for Empirical Agent-Based Model Development. *Algorithms* **2023**, *16*, 338. https://doi.org/10.3390/a16070338

Academic Editors: Nuno Fachada and Nuno David

Received: 30 May 2023
Revised: 27 June 2023
Accepted: 29 June 2023
Published: 14 July 2023

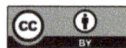

Copyright: © 2023 by the authors. Licensee MDPI, Basel, Switzerland. This article is an open access article distributed under the terms and conditions of the Creative Commons Attribution (CC BY) license (https://creativecommons.org/licenses/by/4.0/).

1. Introduction

Qualitative data provide thick contextual information [1–4] that can support reliable complex system model development. Qualitative data analysis explores systems components, their complex relationships, and behavior [3–5] and provides a structured framework that can guide the formulation of quantitative models [6–10]. However, qualitative research is complex, and time- and resource-consuming [1,4]. Data analysis usually involves keyword-based data extraction and evaluation that requires multiple coders to reduce biases. Moreover, model development using qualitative data requires multiple, lengthy, and expensive stakeholder interactions [11,12], which adds to its inconvenience. Consequently, quantitative modelers often avoid using qualitative data for their model development. Modelers often skip qualitative data analysis or use unorthodox approaches for framework development, which may lead to failed capturing of target systems' complex dynamics and produce inaccurate and unreliable outputs [13].

The development in the information technology sector has substantially increased access to qualitative data over the past few decades. Harvesting extensive credible data is crucial for reliable model development. Increased access to voluminous data presents a challenge and an opportunity for model developers [14]. However, qualitative data analysis has always been a hard nut to crack for complex modelers. Most existing qualitative data analyses are highly supervised (i.e., performed mainly by humans) and hence, bias-prone and inefficient for large datasets.

This study proposes a methodology that uses an efficient, largely unsupervised qualitative data extraction for credible Agent-Based Model (ABM) development using Natural Language Processing (NLP) toolkits. ABM requires information on agents (emulating the target system's decision makers), their attributes, actions, and interactions for its development. The development of a model greatly depends on its intended purpose. Abstract theoretical models concentrate on establishing new relationships and theories with less emphasis on data requirements and structure. In contrast, application-driven models aim to explain specific target systems and tend to be data-intensive. They require a higher degree of adherence to data requirements, validity, feasibility, and transferability [15–17]. Our methodology is particularly applicable to application-driven models rich in empirical data.

ABMs help understand phenomena that emerge from nonlinear interactions of autonomous and heterogeneous constituents of complex systems [18–20]. ABM is a bottom-up approach; interactions at the micro-level produce complex and emergent phenomena at a macro (higher) level. As micro-scale data become more accessible to the research community, modelers increasingly use empirical data for more realistic system representation and simulation [11,21–24].

Quantitative data are primarily useful as inputs for parameterizing and running simulations. Additionally, quantitative model outputs are also used for model verification and validation. Qualitative data, on the other hand, find uses at various stages of the model cycle [25]. Apart from the routine tasks of identifying systems constituents and behaviors for model development, qualitative data support the model structure and output representations [26,27]. Qualitative model representations facilitate communication for learning, model evaluation, and replication.

Various approaches have been proposed to conceptualize computational models. First of all, selected quantitative models have predefined structures for model representation. System dynamics, for instance, uses Causal Loop Diagrams as qualitative tools [28]. Causal Loop Diagrams elucidate systems components, their interrelationships, and feedback that can be used for learning and developing quantitative system dynamics models. ABM, however, does not have a predefined structure for model representation; models are primarily based on either highly theoretical or best-guess ad-hoc structures, which are problematic for model structural validation [16,29].

As a consequence, social and cognitive theories [30–34] often form the basis for translating qualitative data to empirical ABM [35]. Since social behavior is complex and challenging to comprehend, using social and cognition theories helps determine the system's expected behavior. Moreover, using theories streamlines data management and analysis for model development.

Another school of thought bases model development on stakeholder cognition. Rather than relying mainly on social theories, this approach focuses on extracting empirical information about system components and behaviors. Participatory or companion modeling [36], as well as role-playing games [11], are some of the conventional approaches to eliciting stakeholder knowledge for model development [23,24]. Stakeholders usually develop model structures in real time, while some modelers prefer to process stakeholders' information after the discussions. For instance, [37] employs computer technologies to post-process stakeholder responses to develop a rule-induction algorithm for her ABM.

Stakeholders are assumed to be the experts of their systems, and using their knowledge in model building makes the model valid and reliable. However, stakeholder involvement is not always feasible; for instance, when modeling remote places or historical events. In such cases, modelers resort to information elicitation tools for information extraction. In the context of ABM, translating empirical textual data into agent architecture is complex and requires concrete algorithms and structures [25,38]. Therefore, modelers first explore the context of the narratives and then identify potential context-specific scopes. Determining narrative elements becomes straightforward once context and scopes are identified [38].

Many ABM modelers have formulated structures for organizing qualitative data for model development. For instance, [39] used Institutional Analysis and Development framework for managing qualitative data in their Modeling Agent system based on Institutions Analysis (MAIA). MAIA comprises five structures: collective, constitutional, physical, operational, and evaluative. Information on agents is populated in a collective structure, while behavior rules and environment go in constitutional and physical structures. Similar frameworks were introduced by [40,41], to name but a few. However, all these structures use manual, slow, and bias-prone data processing and extraction. A potential solution presented in this paper is to employ AI tools, such as NLP, for unsupervised information extraction for model development [30].

The remainder of the paper is structured as follows: After the introduction, we briefly characterize NPL, focusing on its utility for ABM conceptualization. Next, we describe the proposed methodology. Finally, we demonstrate the framework in a case study of processing narratives from in-depth household interviews on individual food security in Mali, noting the framework's advantages and limitations.

2. Background, Materials, and Methods

Software engineers have been exploring various supervised and unsupervised approaches for information extraction. In supervised approaches, syntactical patterns are defined [42], and text is manually scanned for such patterns. In unsupervised information extraction, the machine does the pattern matching.

Supervised approaches are reliable but slow. Contrarily, the faster, unsupervised approaches are difficult and prone to errors, mainly due to word sense ambiguation [43]. A purely syntactical analysis cannot capture the nuanced meaning of texts, which is often the culprit of the problem. Recently, pattern matching also involves semantic analysis. External databases of hierarchically structured words such as WordNet or VerbNet [44] and machine learning tools are increasingly used for understanding semantics for reduced word sense ambiguity [45,46].

NLP toolkits are increasingly used for unsupervised pattern matching and information extraction [47–52]. Tools such as lemmatizing, tokenizing, stemming, and part-of-speech tagging [53] are helpful for syntactic information extraction. These tools can normalize texts and identify subjects and main verbs from their sentences.

The ability to convert highly unstructured texts to structured information through predominantly unsupervised approaches is one of the main advantages of NLP in qualitative data analysis. NLP efficiently analyzes intertextual relationships using syntactic and semantics algorithms. Approaches such as word co-occurrence statistics and sentiment analysis [54] are beneficial for domain modeling [42] and for exploring contextual and behavioral information from textual data. Similarly, its efficiency in pattern matching for information extraction is essential for model development.

Although present for decades in object-oriented programming and database development [55,56], NLP has a minimal footprint in ABM development. The introduction of NLP in ABM development is very recent. Refs. [14,57] used NLP to model human cognition through word embedding, which is a contextually analyzed vector representation of a text. The procedure places closely related texts next to each other. Specifically, placing agents with similar worldviews together to support theorizing agent decision-making. Although their approach helps develop agent decision-making, it is not well-equipped for developing a comprehensive agent architecture.

Another example is the study by [58], who applied NLP in conjunction with machine learning to create an ABM structure from unstructured textual data. In their framework, texts are translated to the agent–attribute–rule framework. They define agents as nouns (e.g., person and place) that perform some actions and attributes as words that represent some variables. Similarly, sentences containing agents or attributes and action verbs are considered rules. The primary goal of their approach is to create an ABM structure mainly for communicating the model to non-modelers.

As with machine learning approaches in general, Padilla et al.'s approach required a large amount of training data. They used ten highly concise, formally written ABM descriptions from published journals as training datasets. Another limitation, according to the researchers, was the lack of precise distinctions between agents and attributes, attributes could also be nouns, which might confuse the machine. Repeated training with extensive data effectively increased the accuracy of the agent–attribute rule detection. However, the model frequently resulted in underpredictions and overpredictions.

Our work is of significant importance in the context of ABM development, particularly in relation to the utilization of machine learning and artificial intelligence. The recent research papers, refs. [30,59,60], also emphasized the role of these technologies in this domain. Ref. [60] go as far as to argue that natural language processing (NLP) can potentially replace the conventional method of developing ABMs, which heavily relies on field interviews. This perspective highlights the relevance and timeliness of our work, as we effectively incorporated machine learning and artificial intelligence techniques into our ABM development process.

Additionally, we discussed the relevance of prior works such as [14,57,58], and that exhibit similarities to our approach. However, these studies lack certain aspects of model development that our proposed methodology aims to address. For instance, ref. [58] relied on extensive training datasets and struggled to differentiate between agents and attributes effectively, whereas our methodology overcomes these limitations. Furthermore, unlike Runck's approach, which primarily focuses on developing agents' decision-making abilities, our approach strives to create a comprehensive agent architecture.

3. The Proposed Framework

In response to these limitations, our study proposes and tests a largely unsupervised domain-independent approach for developing ABM structures from informal semi-structured interviews using Python-based semantic and syntactic NLP tools (Figure 1). The method primarily uses syntactic NLP approaches for information extraction directly to the object-oriented programming (OOP) framework (i.e., agents, attributes, and actions/interactions) using widely accepted approaches in database design and OOP [61]. Database designers and OOP programmers generally exploit the syntactic structure of sentences for information extraction. Syntactic analysis usually treats the subject of a sentence as a class (an entity for a database) and the main verb as a method (a relationship for a database). Since the approach is not based on machine learning, it does not require large training data. The semantic analysis is limited to external static datasets such as WordNet (https://wordnet.princeton.edu/) (accessed on 8 July 2020) and VerbNet (https://verbs.colorado.edu/verbnet/) (accessed on 21 July 2020).

In the proposed approach, information extraction includes systems agents, their actions, and interactions from qualitative data for model development using syntactic and semantic NLP tools. As our information extraction approach is primarily unsupervised and does not require manual interventions, we argue that, in addition to being efficient, it reduces the potential for subjectivity and biases arising from modelers' preconceptions about target systems.

The extracted information is then represented using Unified Modeling Language (UML) for an object-oriented model development platform. UML is a standardized graphical representation of software development [62]. It has a set of well-defined class and activity diagrams that effectively represent the inner workings of ABMs [63]. UML diagrams represent systems classes, their attributes, and actions. Identified candidate agents, attributes, and actions were manually arranged in the UML structure for supporting model software development. Although there are other forms of graphical ABM representations such as Petri Nets [64], Conceptual Model for Simulation [29], and sequence and activity diagrams [65], UML is natural in representing ABM, named by [66] the default lingua franca of ABM.

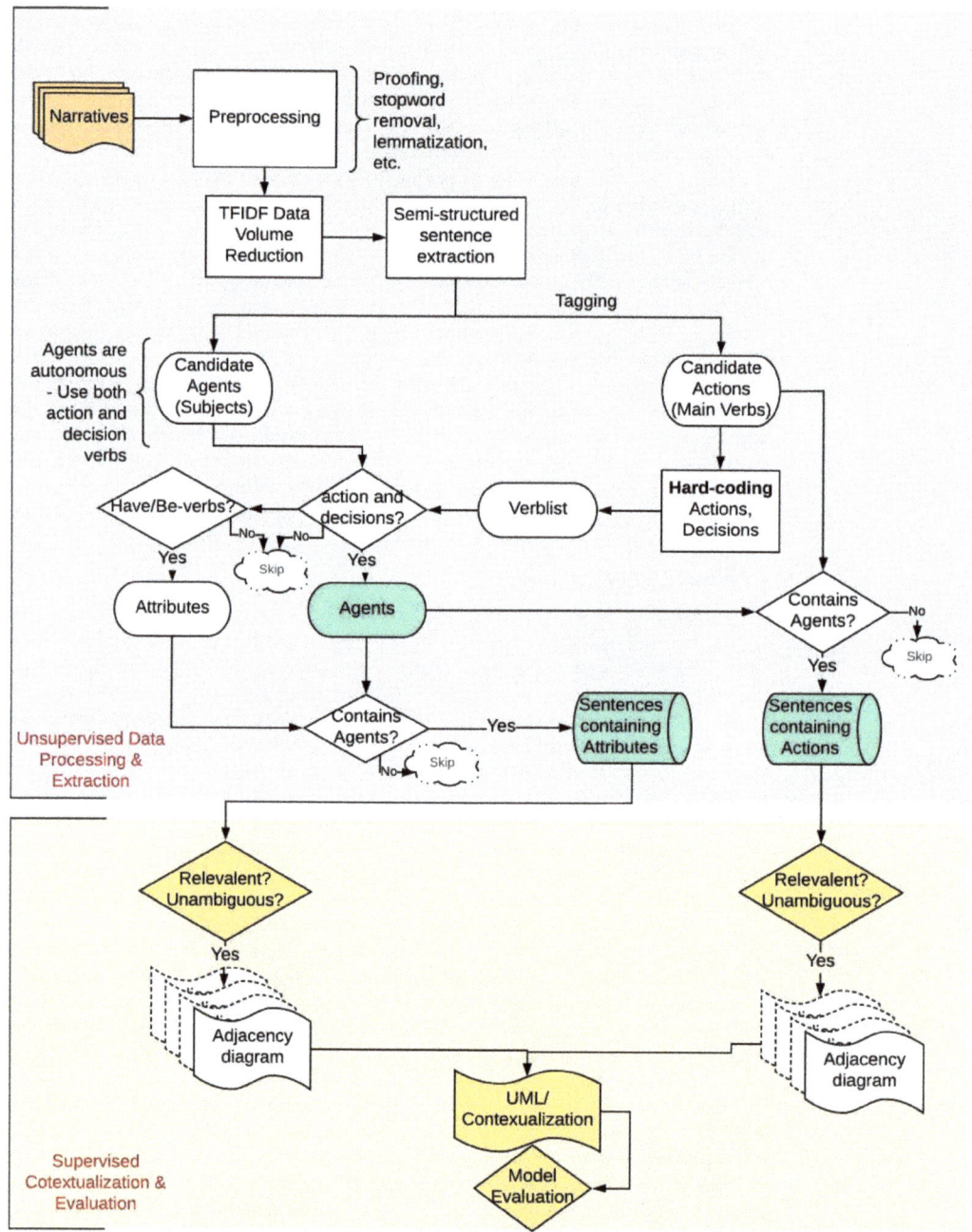

Figure 1. Largely unsupervised information extraction for ABM development. TFIDF: term frequency inverse document frequency.

In our approach, model development is mainly unsupervised and involves the following steps (Figure 1):
1. Unsupervised data processing and extraction;
2. Data preprocessing (cleaning and normalization);
3. Data volume reduction;
4. Tagging and information extraction;
5. Supervised contextualization and evaluation;
6. UML/Model conceptualization;
7. Model evaluation.

Steps one and two are required since semi-structured interviews often contain redundant or inflected texts that can bog down NLP analysis. Hence, removing non-informative contents from large textual data is highly recommended at the start of the analysis. NLP is well-equipped with stop words removal tools that can effectively remove redundant texts. Similarly, tools such as stemming and lemmatizing help normalize texts to their base forms [67].

Step three is data volume reduction, which can tremendously speed up NLP analyses. Traditional volume reduction approaches usually contain highly supervised keyword-based methods. Data analysts use predefined keywords to select and extract sentences perceived to be relevant [68]. Keyword identification generally requires a priori knowledge of the system and is often bias-prone. Consequently, we recommend a domain-independent unsupervised Term Frequency Inverse Document Frequency (TFIDF) approach [69] that eliminates manual keyword identification requirements. The approach provides weightage to individual words based on their uniqueness and machine-perceived importance. The TFIDF differentiates between important and common words by comparing their frequency in individual documents and across entire texts. Sentences that have high cumulative TFIDF scores are perceived to have higher importance. Given a document collection D, a word w, and an individual document $d \varepsilon D$, TFIIDF can be defined as follows:

$$f_{w,d} * log(|D|/f_{w,D}) \qquad (1)$$

where $f_{w,d}$ equals the number of times w appears in d, $|D|$ is the size of the corpus, and $f_{w,D}$ equals the number of documents in which w appears in D [69].

Step four involves tagging and information extraction. Once the preprocessed data are reduced, we move to tagging agents, attributes, and actions/interactions that can occur. We propose the following approaches for tagging agent architecture:

Candidate agents: Following the conventional approaches in database design and OOP [61], we propose identifying the subjects of sentences as candidate agents. For instance, the *farmer* in 'the farmer grows cotton' can be a candidate agent. NLP has well-developed tools such as part-of-speech tagger and named-entity tagger that can be used to detect subjects of sentences.

Candidate actions: The main verbs of sentences can become candidate actions. The main verbs need candidate agents as the subject of the sentences. For example, in the sentence 'the farmer grows cotton,' the *farmer* is a candidate agent, and the subject of the sentence; *grows* is the main verb and, hence, a candidate action.

Candidate attributes: Attributes are properties inherent to the agents. Sentences containing candidate agents as subjects and *be* or *have* as their primary (non-auxiliary) verbs provide attribute information, e.g., 'the farmer *is* a member of a *cooperative*,' and 'the farmer *has 10 ha* of land.' Additionally, the use of possessive words also indicates attributes, e.g., *the cow* in the sentence 'my cow is very small' is an attribute.

Candidate interactions: Main verbs indicating relationships between two candidate agents are identified as interactions. Hence the sentences containing **two or more candidate agents** provide information on *interactions*, e.g., '**The government** *trains* **the farmers**.'

Since the data tagging is strictly unsupervised, false positives are likely to occur. The algorithm can over-predict agents, as the subjects of all the sentences are treated as candidate agents. In ABM, however, agents are defined as autonomous actors, they act and make decisions. Hence, we propose to use a hard-coded list of action verbs (e.g., eat, grow, and walk) and decision verbs (e.g., choose, decide, and think) to filter agents from the list of candidate agents. Only the candidate agents that use both types of verbs qualify as agents. Candidate agents not using both verbs are categorized as *entities* that may be subjected to manual evaluation. Similarly, people use different terminologies that are semantically similar. We recommend using external databases such as WordNet to group semantically similar terminologies.

Step five involves supervised contextualization and evaluation. While the unsupervised analysis reduces data volume and translates semi-structured interviews to the agent–action–attribute structure, noise can percolate to the outputs since the process is unsupervised. Additionally, the outputs need to be contextualized. Consequently, we suggest performing a series of supervised output filtration followed by manual contextualization and validation. The domain-independent unsupervised analysis extracts individual sentences that can sometimes be ambiguous or domain irrelevant. Hence the output should be filtered based on ambiguity and domain relevancy. Once output filtration is performed, contextual structures can be developed and validated with domain experts and stakeholders.

The last two steps (UML/model conceptualization and model evaluation) are described in the following sections.

For this study, we used Python 3.7 programming language (https://www.python.org/) (accessed on 10 May 2020) along with a plethora of NLP libraries (e.g., scikit-learn, NLTK, spaCy, and textacy) to perform data reduction, tagging, extraction, and structuration. Scikit-learn provides a wide range of machine learning algorithms for classification, regression, clustering, and dimensionality reduction tasks. Similarly, NLTK, spaCy, and textacy are useful for analyzing natural language data. We primarily used scikit-learn for dimensionality reduction and NLTK, spaCy, and textacy for tokenization and part of speech tagging.

4. Results and Discussion

We tested the above approach by developing a structural ABM of household food security using semi-structured field interviews, for example, the excerpt in Figure 2. Our qualitative data contain 42 semi-structured interviews from different members (young and old, male and female) of farming households in Koutiala, Southern Mali. The interviews were initially conducted to develop mental models of household food security in the region [70]. Verbal consent was obtained from the participants prior to the interviews. The interviews were originally conducted in the local Bambara dialect and then translated into English for model development. The mental model development followed the lengthy conventional qualitative data analysis approach that used multiple coders and keyword-based sentence extraction. That inspired the research team to develop a more efficient alternative data processing and extraction approach for ABM development, presented here.

First, we grouped the interviews by the member types (i.e., elder male, younger male, elder female, and younger female) and analyzed the grouped narratives collectively. After preprocessing the interviews using NLTK tools, we used the scikit-learn Tfidf Vectorizer to reduce the volume of qualitative data. Textacy was primarily used for identifying candidate agents, actions, and attributes. Additionally, textacy extract (textacy.extract. semi-structured statements) was used in converting sentences to structured outputs. Finally, we manually filtered the unsupervised outputs based on their domain relevancy and ambiguity. The final outputs were then visualized and conceptualized using Gephi (https://gephi.org/) (accessed on 18 May 2020) and Lucid Chart (https://www.lucidchart.com/) (accessed on 21 May 2020) platforms (Figure 3).

Enumerator: When the production reaches home, how do you consume it?

Surveyed: First of all, we are 48 people in my household. After harvesting, we beat and weigh the crops. Then, we pick the quantity of food that is needed to feed the household. That quantity is given to women for cooking. We continue with that quantity until the new crop is harvested. When food is cooked and ready for eating, it is distributed by a plate to five and six persons who eat together. As the daily food consumption is known, we know what quantity we can sell to address household needs. You know, when crops are harvested, we tie them. Then we pick some pieces for beating. After beating, we weigh and stock. Then, we know the existing quantity in the store. If it is maize, for example, we have a cart and beating machine. We take one load of maize in the cart. Then we beat and weigh it and finally stock in the store. Farmers start beating crops and stock them. Because, a researcher like you, **IER** of **Sikasso** and **CMDT** trained us on post-harvest management. By following lessons learned from training, our food won't be over. Even if it happens that our food finishes, we would know what food to buy without any difficulties. With lessons acquired, we can produce and increase our production that will feed all our household over the year. Unless our food is stolen, it will cover for the year.

Enumerator: What are the main crops you are producing?

Surveyed: We produce maize, sorghum, millet, and cowpea in one hand and use the same crops to feed ourselves on the other hand. Some farmers prefer feeding themselves with millet all over the year. Even if they produce maize, they sell it. Although other farmers prefer maize, we consume all the crops we produce. We may consume one crop in one month and shift to another for another month. This is how we shift food consumption.

Enumerator: Who decides to shift from one food to another?

Surveyed: It depends. Some crops are easier to process than others. So, when there is the farm, we decide to consume crop, which is easy and quick to process. But, only one person is responsible for picking the food for daily consumption.

Figure 2. Excerpt from sample interview.

As expected, the unsupervised tagging overpredicted the agents. Subjects that do not make decisions were also identified as candidate agents. To overcome the issue, we created an external database of action/decision verbs (Table 1) that somewhat addressed the problem. Using the external database resulted in more than 60% reduction in the number of agents (e.g., Figure 4). The filtration process discarded the initially identified candidates, such as porridge, food, cereal, or farm. We also obtained multiple similar actions (synonyms). We used an external WordNet database to group semantically similar actions. The process resulted in a highly manageable and structured output for model conceptualization.

Next, we used the extracted information to develop UML class diagrams (Figure 5) and contextual diagrams (Figure 6). The diagrams revealed that different members of households support household food security differently. Male members of the households are generally involved in farming. They grow cereal crops and vegetables and are also into cash cropping, i.e., growing plants for selling on the market rather than subsistence farming to feed their families. Women principally look after household work and assist men in the fields. Households consume the food they produce. During food shortages, households seek help from their fellow villagers or buy food from the market. They use money obtained from cash crops to buy food.

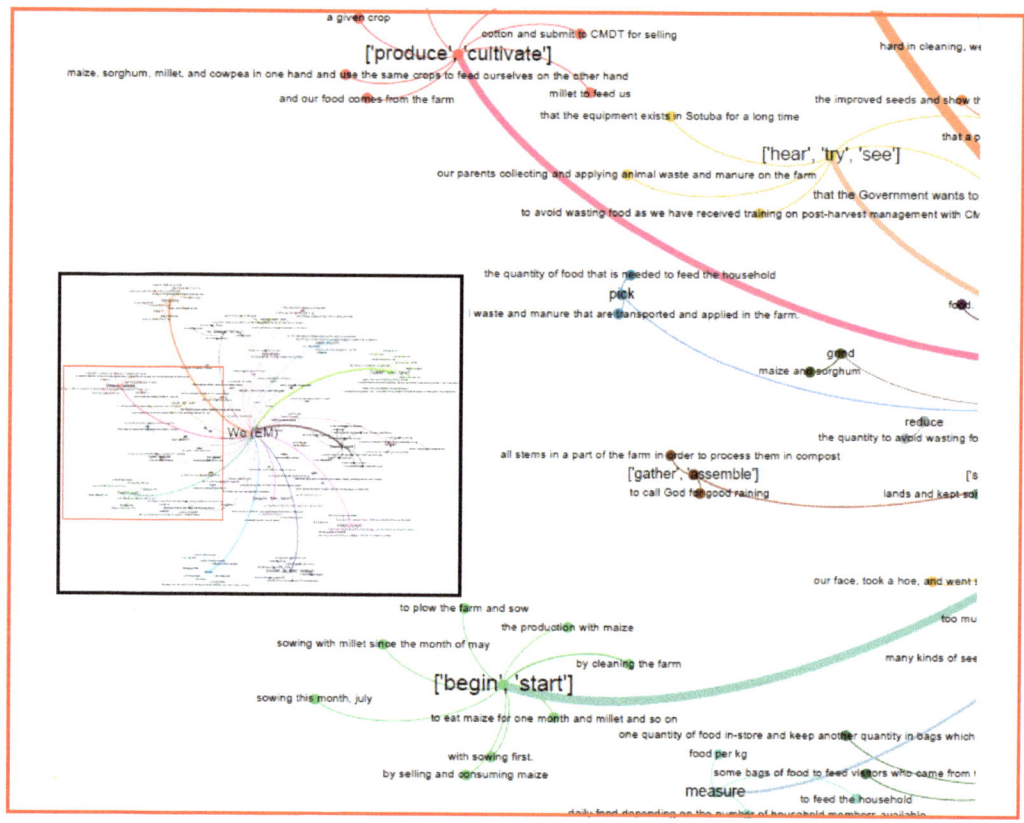

Figure 3. Visual representation of data processing and extraction (fragment).

Table 1. An excerpt of action and decision verbs.

Decision Verbs	Action Verbs
adhere	abandon
advise	accelerate
approve	accept
assess	access
choose	accompany
comply	accord
consult	achieve
decide	acquaint
determine	acquire
discourage	add
educate	adjust
encourage	adopt
expect	advertise
favor	affect
guide	afford
instruct	aim
learn	allow
obey	analyze
oblige	apply
plan	argue

```
candidate agents: {'money', 'woman', 'water', 'porridge', 'household', 'father', 'i', 'food, 'it', 'we', 'they', 'she', 'he', 'cereal', 'farm'}

agents: ['i', 'it', 'we', 'they', 'she']
```

Figure 4. Candidate agents before and after using the external database.

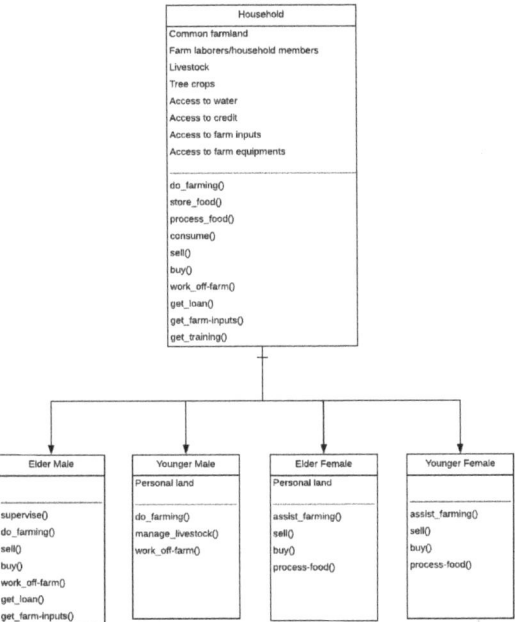

Figure 5. UML class diagram of agents of household food security.

Additionally, household women are involved in small businesses that can support food purchases. For example, some households might need to rely on off-farm jobs or sell their livestock to buy food. Other organizations and credit agencies provide households with credits and support.

Following our framework, the conceptual model required evaluation. We applied model-to-model (M2M) comparison [71,72] and stakeholder validation. M2M involved comparing model output with the mental model of household food security developed using the same dataset, reported by [70]. We found that our approach captured all the essential components of household food security that were identified in the mental model.

Initially, we aimed to develop an efficient, bias-free, completely unsupervised information extraction for conceptualizing an ABM. However, after preliminary algorithm development, we realized that entirely unsupervised data processing and conceptualization is unrealistic with the current NLP capabilities. Therefore, we decided to use manual filtration and contextualization that potentially introduced subjectivity and biases in model development. We performed a stakeholder validation to address this deficiency to check for subjectivity and biases. Consequently, we converted the contextual model to a pictorial representation (Figure 7) and brought it to the stakeholders (interviewees) for validation.

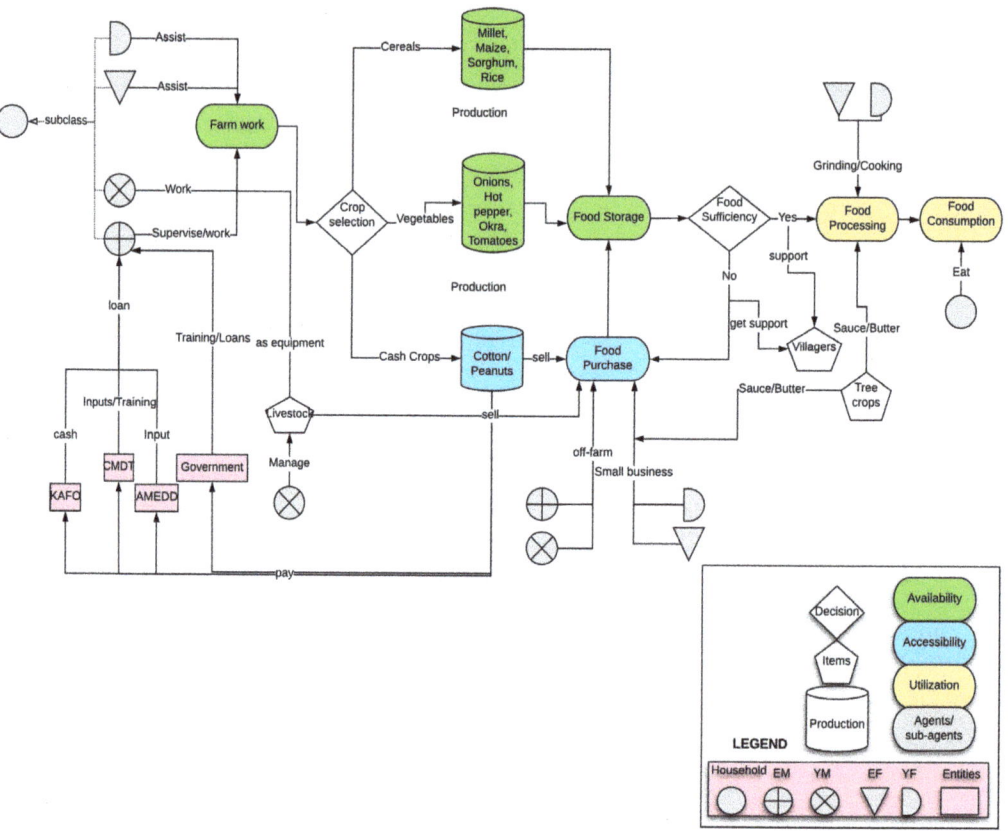

Figure 6. Conceptual model of household food security in Koutiala, Mali (EM: Elderly male; YM:. Younger male; EF: Elderly female; YF: Younger female).

The stakeholders positively evaluated the model and acknowledged that it included all the principal dynamics of the household food system. They, however, pointed out that the contextualized structure did not provide the dynamics of the government and non-government actors. Since the input data only contained interviews from farm households, we failed to capture the dynamics occurring outside of the households. Consequently, the model revealed data gaps where more information needs to be gathered on household food security's government and non-government actors.

The proposed unsupervised information extraction picked individual sentences based on their cumulative TFIDF weights. However, some of the individually extracted sentences lacked contextuality and were ambiguous. To add context and reduce this ambiguity, we used neighboring sentences during the unsupervised data extraction and processing phase (Figure 1). We hypothesized that extracting a tuple of preceding and trailing sentences along with the identified sentence can provide vital contextual information; for example, some of the extracted sentences contained pronouns. These pronouns were impossible to resolve without the information in the preceding sentences. Therefore, extracting the preceding sentence should help in resolving their references.

The NLP also has a coreference resolution tool that automatically replaces pronouns with their referenced nouns. However, the tool is in development. We found that it generated too many errors that would require manual checks. Hence, we proceeded without using the tool, and the pronouns identified as agents were ignored.

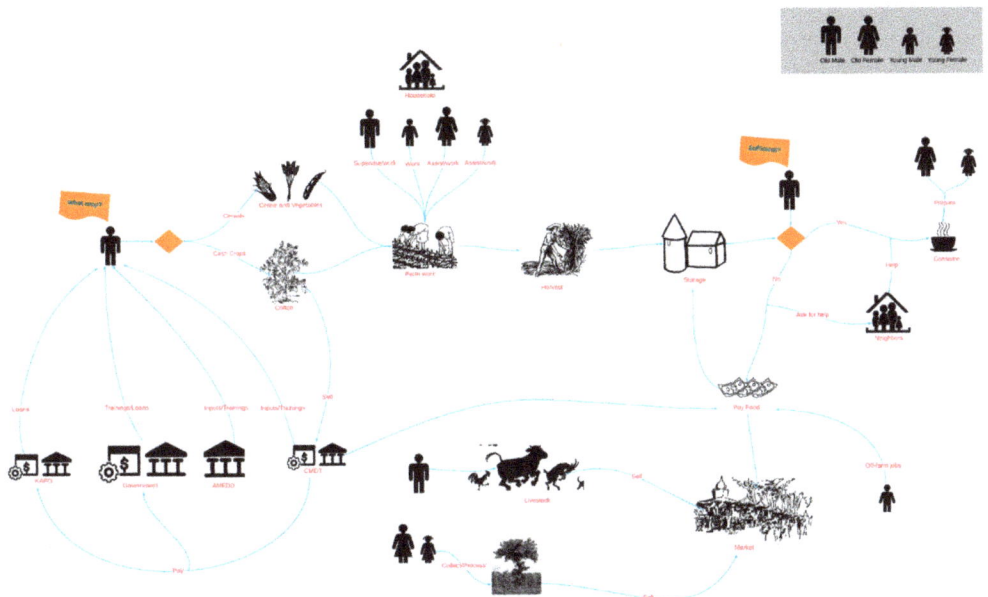

Figure 7. Pictorial representation of the conceptual model presented in Figure 6.

Using our framework, we only collected information on agents, attributes, and actions/interactions. However, ABM also requires information on agent decision-making. Although using social and behavioral theories in defining agent decision-making is predominant, empirically derived decision-making frameworks are context-specific and, therefore, more desirable when ABMs are applied in real-world situations [15,24]. We realize that some sentences are particularly useful in deriving agent decision-making. Specifically, conditional sentences such as 'if it rains, we plant maize' and compound sentences such as 'when production is low, we buy food from the market' can reveal decision-making. Harvesting these sentences with semantics and machine learning approaches can open new avenues for formulating empirically based decision-making rules for ABM.

It is important to note that the derived information is limited by the information contained in the input. For example, we noticed that agent tagging underpredicted agents after using the action and decision verbs. Entities such as 'father' and 'the government' should also be identified as agents of this particular system. However, some information was missed since subjects did not use both types of verbs (action and decision) in the provided interviews. Additionally, stakeholders pointed out that our model structure did not include the dynamics of the governmental and non-governmental actors. It prompts a need for a careful analysis of entities that failed to qualify as agents for data gaps. Furthermore, the interviews went through different translation stages (from local dialects to French and English) that could have corrupted some of their original meanings.

5. Conclusions

Complexities, ambiguities, and difficulties in data processing often discourage ABM developers from using qualitative data for model development, preventing modelers from using rich contextual information about their target systems. ABMs are often developed using ad-hoc approaches, potentially producing models that lack credibility and reliability. We introduced a systematic approach for ABM development from semi-structured qualitative interviews using NLP to address these gaps. The proposed methodology contained a largely unsupervised, domain-independent, efficient, and bias-controlled data processing and extraction approach aimed at ABM conceptualization. We demonstrated its effectiveness by developing an ABM of household food security from large open-ended qualitative field interviews.

Additionally, we outlined some of the significant limitations of the approach and recommended improvements for future development. Our framework is only relevant to data-driven models that focus on applications and address specific geographic regions and localities. It is not aimed at theory-driven modeling, which requires generalizable observations, where other methods, such as metamodeling, are more appropriate. It is also important to note that the proposed framework was developed only to handle information derived from text. Future improvements should focus on algorithms and tools combining text-derived and quantitative information using data analytics tools. Moreover, our framework requires further testing and experimentation, for example, contrasting it with alternative approaches, which is one of the objectives of our future research. Hopefully, since the NLP development community is highly active, these limitations will soon be resolved, making semantic and syntactic NLP more effective for unsupervised information extraction and model conceptualization.

Although we could not fully develop a completely unsupervised approach, we successfully managed to reduce subjectivity and biases by limiting data extraction manipulation. Data processing and extraction were fully unsupervised, and manual inputs were only required towards the end of model conceptualization, limiting the opportunities for introducing human bias in model development. Furthermore, the unsupervised approach was much faster compared with manual coding.

Author Contributions: Conceptualization: R.P. and A.L.-Z.; Methodology: R.P.; Code: R.P.; Formal Analysis: R.P.; Investigation: A.L.-Z.; Writing—Original Draft Preparation: R.P.; Writing—Review and Editing: A.L.-Z.; Manuscript Visualization: R.P.; Graphical Abstract: A.L.-Z.; Supervision, Project Administration and Funding Acquisition: A.L.-Z. All authors have read and agreed to the published version of the manuscript.

Funding: This project was supported by National Science Foundation Grant SMA 1416730, titled IBSS: Participatory-Ensemble Modeling to Study the Multiscale Social and Behavioral Dynamics of Food Security, Ligmann-Zielinska A (PI) et al. The sponsors or funders played no role in the study design, data collection, analysis, decision to publish, or manuscript preparation.

Data Availability Statement: The results presented in this manuscript were extracted from unprocessed (i.e., original) data collected through open-ended interviews from individual households. The interviews contain confidential information such as geographic location, employment, ethnicity, household structure, relationships, and interactions among household members, or number of dependents. The Institutional Review Board (Michigan State University) approval restricted the data access only to the research team. All subjects who provided the interviews provided their informed consent for inclusion before participating in the study. Consequently, the data are protected under the rights of privacy.

Acknowledgments: We want to thank Laura Schmitt-Olabisi from Michigan State University, USA, and Amadou Sidibe' from 4IPR/IFRA de Katibougouand, Koulikoro, Mali, for assistance in data collection and result validation.

Conflicts of Interest: The authors declare no conflict of interest.

References

1. Miles, M.B. Qualitative data as an attractive nuisance: The problem of analysis. *Adm. Sci. Q.* **1979**, *24*, 590–601. [CrossRef]
2. Mortelmans, D. Analyzing qualitative data using NVivo. In *The Palgrave Handbook of Methods for Media Policy Research*; Palgrave Macmillan: London, UK, 2019; pp. 435–450.
3. Rich, M.; Ginsburg, K.R. The reason and rhyme of qualitative research: Why, when, and how to use qualitative methods in the study of adolescent health. *J. Adolesc. Health* **1999**, *25*, 371–378. [CrossRef] [PubMed]
4. Watkins, D.C. Qualitative research: The importance of conducting research that doesn't "count". *Health Promot. Pract.* **2012**, *13*, 153–158. [CrossRef]
5. Kemp-Benedict, E. From Narrative to Number: A Role for Quantitative Models in Scenario analysis. In Proceedings of the International Congress on Environmental Modelling and Software, Osnabrück, Germany, 1 July 2004.

6. Ackermann, F.; Eden, C.; Williams, T. Modeling for litigation: Mixing qualitative and quantitative approaches. *Interfaces* **1997**, *27*, 48–65. [CrossRef]
7. Coyle, G. Qualitative and quantitative modelling in system dynamics: Some research questions. *Syst. Dyn. Rev. J. Syst. Dyn. Soc.* **2000**, *16*, 225–244. [CrossRef]
8. Forbus, K.D.; Falkenhainer, B. Self-Explanatory Simulations: An Integration of Qualitative and Quantitative Knowledge. In Proceedings of the AAAI, Boston, MA, USA, 29 July–3 August 1990; pp. 380–387.
9. Jo, H.I.; Jeon, J.Y. Compatibility of quantitative and qualitative data-collection protocols for urban soundscape evaluation. *Sustain. Cities Soc.* **2021**, *74*, 103259. [CrossRef]
10. Wolstenholme, E.F. Qualitative vs quantitative modelling: The evolving balance. *J. Oper. Res. Soc.* **1999**, *50*, 422–428. [CrossRef]
11. Djenontin, I.N.S.; Zulu, L.C.; Ligmann-Zielinska, A. Improving representation of decision rules in LUCC-ABM: An example with an elicitation of farmers' decision making for landscape restoration in central Malawi. *Sustainability* **2020**, *12*, 5380. [CrossRef]
12. Polhill, J.G.; Sutherland, L.-A.; Gotts, N.M. Using qualitative evidence to enhance an agent-based modelling system for studying land use change. *J. Artif. Soc. Soc. Simul.* **2010**, *13*, 10. [CrossRef]
13. Landrum, B.; Garza, G. Mending fences: Defining the domains and approaches of quantitative and qualitative research. *Qual. Psychol.* **2015**, *2*, 199. [CrossRef]
14. Runck, B. GeoComputational Approaches to Evaluate the Impacts of Communication on Decision-Making in Agriculture. Ph.D. Thesis, University of Minnesota, Minneapolis, MN, USA, 2018.
15. Du, J.; Ligmann-Zielinska, A. The Volatility of Data Space: Topology Oriented Sensitivity Analysis. *PLoS ONE* **2015**, *10*, e0137591. [CrossRef] [PubMed]
16. Grimm, V.; Augusiak, J.; Focks, A.; Frank, B.M.; Gabsi, F.; Johnston, A.S.; Liu, C.; Martin, B.T.; Meli, M.; Radchuk, V. Towards better modelling and decision support: Documenting model development, testing, and analysis using TRACE. *Ecol. Model.* **2014**, *280*, 129–139. [CrossRef]
17. Ligmann-Zielinska, A.; Siebers, P.-O.; Magliocca, N.; Parker, D.C.; Grimm, V.; Du, J.; Cenek, M.; Radchuk, V.; Arbab, N.N.; Li, S. 'One size does not fit all': A roadmap of purpose-driven mixed-method pathways for sensitivity analysis of agent-based models. *J. Artif. Soc. Soc. Simul.* **2020**, *23*. [CrossRef]
18. An, L.; Linderman, M.; Qi, J.; Shortridge, A.; Liu, J. Exploring Complexity in a Human–Environment System: An Agent-Based Spatial Model for Multidisciplinary and Multiscale Integration. *Ann. Assoc. Am. Geogr.* **2005**, *95*, 54–79. [CrossRef]
19. Railsback, S.F.; Grimm, V. *Agent-Based and Individual-Based Modeling: A Practical Introduction*; Princeton University Press: Princeton, NJ, USA, 2019.
20. Wilensky, U.; Rand, W. *An Introduction to Agent-Based Modeling: Modeling Natural, Social, and Engineered Complex Systems with NetLogo*; Mit Press: Cambridge, MA, USA, 2015.
21. Janssen, M.; Ostrom, E. Empirically based, agent-based models. *Ecol. Soc.* **2006**, *11*. [CrossRef]
22. O'Sullivan, D.; Evans, T.; Manson, S.; Metcalf, S.; Ligmann-Zielinska, A.; Bone, C. Strategic directions for agent-based modeling: Avoiding the YAAWN syndrome. *J. Land. Use Sci.* **2016**, *11*, 177–187. [CrossRef] [PubMed]
23. Robinson, D.T.; Brown, D.G.; Parker, D.C.; Schreinemachers, P.; Janssen, M.A.; Huigen, M.; Wittmer, H.; Gotts, N.; Promburom, P.; Irwin, E.; et al. Comparison of empirical methods for building agent-based models in land use science. *J. Land. Use Sci.* **2007**, *2*, 31–55. [CrossRef]
24. Smajgl, A.; Barreteau, O. *Empirical Agent-Based Modelling-Challenges and Solutions*; Springer: Berlin/Heidelberg, Germany, 2014; Volume 1.
25. Seidl, R. Social scientists, qualitative data, and agent-based modeling. In Proceedings of the Social Simulation Conference, Barcelona, Spain, 1–5 September 2014.
26. Grimm, V.; Berger, U.; DeAngelis, D.L.; Polhill, J.G.; Giske, J.; Railsback, S.F. The ODD protocol: A review and first update. *Ecol. Model.* **2010**, *221*, 2760–2768. [CrossRef]
27. Müller, B.; Balbi, S.; Buchmann, C.M.; De Sousa, L.; Dressler, G.; Groeneveld, J.; Klassert, C.J.; Le, Q.B.; Millington, J.D.A.; Nolzen, H. Standardised and transparent model descriptions for agent-based models: Current status and prospects. *Environ. Model. Softw.* **2014**, *55*, 156–163. [CrossRef]
28. Ford, A.; Ford, F.A. *Modeling the Environment: An Introduction to System Dynamics Models of Environmental Systems*; Island press: Washington, DC, USA, 1999.
29. Heath, B.L.; Ciarallo, F.W.; Hill, R.R. Validation in the agent-based modelling paradigm: Problems and a solution. *Int. J. Simul. Process Model.* **2012**, *7*, 229–239. [CrossRef]
30. An, L.; Grimm, V.; Bai, Y.; Sullivan, A.; Turner II, B.; Malleson, N.; Heppenstall, A.; Vincenot, C.; Robinson, D.; Ye, X. Modeling agent decision and behavior in the light of data science and artificial intelligence. *Environ. Model. Softw.* **2023**, *166*, 105713. [CrossRef]
31. Balke, T.; Gilbert, N. How Do Agents Make Decisions? A Survey. *J. Artif. Soc. Soc. Simul.* **2014**, *17*, 13. [CrossRef]
32. Doscher, C.; Moore, K.; Smallman, C.; Wilson, J.; Simmons, D. An Agent-Based Model of Tourist Movements in New Zealand. In *Empirical Agent-Based Modelling-Challenges and Solutions: Volume 1, The Characterisation and Parameterisation of Empirical Agent-Based Models*; Springer: Berlin/Heidelberg, Germany, 2014; pp. 39–51.
33. Edwards-Jones, G. Modelling farmer decision-making: Concepts, progress and challenges. *Anim. Sci.* **2006**, *82*, 783–790. [CrossRef]

34. Janssen, M.; Jager, W. An integrated approach to simulating behavioural processes: A case study of the lock-in of consumption patterns. *J. Artif. Soc. Soc. Simul.* **1999**, *2*, 21–35.
35. Becu, N.; Barreteau, O.; Perez, P.; Saising, J.; Sungted, S. A methodology for identifying and for-malizing farmers' representations of watershed management: A case study from northern Thailand. In *Companion Modeling and Multi-Agent Systems for Integrated Natural Resource Management in Asia*; International Rice Research Institute: Manila, Philippines, 2005; p. 41.
36. Voinov, A.; Bousquet, F. Modelling with stakeholders. *Environ. Model. Softw.* **2010**, *25*, 1268–1281. [CrossRef]
37. Bharwani, S. Understanding complex behavior and decision making using ethnographic knowledge elicitation tools (KnETs). *Soc. Sci. Comput. Rev.* **2006**, *24*, 78–105. [CrossRef]
38. Edmonds, B. A context-and scope-sensitive analysis of narrative data to aid the specification of agent behaviour. *J. Artif. Soc. Soc. Simul.* **2015**, *18*, 17. [CrossRef]
39. Ghorbani, A.; Schrauwen, N.; Dijkema, G.P.J. Using Ethnographic Information to Conceptualize Agent-based Models. In Proceedings of the European Social Simulation Association Conference, Warsaw, Poland, 16–20 September 2013.
40. Gilbert, N.; Terna, P. How to build and use agent-based models in social science. *Mind Soc.* **2000**, *1*, 57–72. [CrossRef]
41. Huigen, M.G. First principles of the MameLuke multi-actor modelling framework for land use change, illustrated with a Philippine case study. *J. Environ. Manag.* **2004**, *72*, 5–21. [CrossRef]
42. Clark, M.; Kim, Y.; Kruschwitz, U.; Song, D.; Albakour, D.; Dignum, S.; Beresi, U.C.; Fasli, M.; De Roeck, A. Automatically structuring domain knowledge from text: An overview of current research. *Inf. Process. Manag.* **2012**, *48*, 552–568. [CrossRef]
43. Al-Safadi, L.A.E. Natural Language Processing for Conceptual Modeling. *JDCTA* **2009**, *3*, 47–59.
44. Navigli, R. Word sense disambiguation: A survey. *ACM Comput. Surv. (CSUR)* **2009**, *41*, 1–69. [CrossRef]
45. Husain, M.S.; Khanum, M.A. Word Sense Disambiguation in Software Requirement Specifications Using WordNet and Association Mining Rule. In Proceedings of the Second International Conference on Information and Communication Technology for Competitive Strategies, Udaipur, India, 4–5 March 2016; pp. 1–4.
46. Orkphol, K.; Yang, W. Word sense disambiguation using cosine similarity collaborates with Word2vec and WordNet. *Future Internet* **2019**, *11*, 114. [CrossRef]
47. Fraga, A.; Moreno, V.; Parra, E.; Garcia, J. Extraction of Patterns Using NLP: Genetic Deafness. In Proceedings of the SEKE, Pittsburgh, PA, USA, 5–7 July 2017; pp. 428–431.
48. Liddy, E.D. Natural Language Processing. 2001. Available online: https://surface.syr.edu/cgi/viewcontent.cgi?article=1043&context=istpub (accessed on 28 June 2023).
49. Loper, E.; Bird, S. NLTK: The natural language toolkit. In Proceedings of the ACL-02 Workshop on Effective Tools and Methodologies for Teaching Natural Language Processing and Computational Linguistics, Philadelphia, PA, USA, 7 July 2002; pp. 63–70.
50. Manning, C.; Surdeanu, M.; Bauer, J.; Finkel, J.; Bethard, S.; McClosky, D. The Stanford CoreNLP natural language processing toolkit. In Proceedings of the 52nd annual meeting of the association for computational linguistics: System demonstrations, Baltimore, MD, USA, 22–27 June 2014; pp. 55–60.
51. Salloum, S.A.; Al-Emran, M.; Monem, A.A.; Shaalan, K. Using text mining techniques for extracting information from research articles. In *Intelligent Natural Language Processing: Trends and Applications*; Springer: Berlin/Heidelberg, Germany, 2018; pp. 373–397.
52. Sun, S.; Luo, C.; Chen, J. A review of natural language processing techniques for opinion mining systems. *Inf. Fusion.* **2017**, *36*, 10–25. [CrossRef]
53. Bird, S.; Klein, E.; Loper, E. *Natural language processing with Python: Analyzing text with the natural language toolkit*; O'Reilly Media Inc.: Sebastopol, CA, USA, 2009.
54. Nasukawa, T.; Yi, J. Sentiment analysis: Capturing favorability using natural language processing. In Proceedings of the 2nd International Conference on Knowledge Capture, Sanibel Island, FL, USA, 23–25 October 2003; pp. 70–77.
55. Harris, L.R. The ROBOT System: Natural language processing applied to data base query. In Proceedings of the 1978 Annual Conference, Washington, DC, USA, 4–6 December 1978; pp. 165–172.
56. Lees, B. Artificial Intelligence Education for Software Engineers. In *WIT Transactions on Information and Communication Technologies*; 1970; Volume 12. Available online: https://www.witpress.com/elibrary/wit-transactions-on-information-and-communication-technologies/12/10537 (accessed on 28 June 2023).
57. Runck, B.C.; Manson, S.; Shook, E.; Gini, M.; Jordan, N. Using word embeddings to generate data-driven human agent decision-making from natural language. *GeoInformatica* **2019**, *23*, 221–242. [CrossRef]
58. Padilla, J.J.; Shuttleworth, D.; O'Brien, K. Agent-Based Model Characterization Using Natural Language Processing. In Proceedings of the 2019 Winter Simulation Conference (WSC), National Harbor, MD, USA, 8–11 December 2019; pp. 560–571.
59. Heppenstall, A.; Crooks, A.; Malleson, N.; Manley, E.; Ge, J.; Batty, M. Future Developments in Geographical Agent-Based Models: Challenges and Opportunities. *Geogr. Anal.* **2021**, *53*, 76–91. [CrossRef] [PubMed]
60. Liang, X.; Luo, L.; Hu, S.; Li, Y. Mapping the knowledge frontiers and evolution of decision making based on agent-based modeling. *Knowl.-Based Syst.* **2022**, *250*, 108982. [CrossRef]
61. Harmain, H.M.; Gaizauskas, R. CM-Builder: An automated NL-based CASE tool. In Proceedings of the ASE 2000 Fifteenth IEEE International Conference on Automated Software Engineering, Grenoble, France, 11–15 September 2000; pp. 45–53.
62. Bersini, H. UML for ABM. *J. Artif. Soc. Soc. Simul.* **2012**, *15*, 9. [CrossRef]

63. Collins, A.; Petty, M.; Vernon-Bido, D.; Sherfey, S. A Call to Arms: Standards for Agent-Based Modeling and Simulation. *J. Artif. Soc. Soc. Simul.* **2015**, *18*, 12. [CrossRef]
64. Bakam, I.; Kordon, F.; Le Page, C.; Bousquet, F. Formalization of a spatialized multiagent model using coloured petri nets for the study of an hunting management system. In Proceedings of the International Workshop on Formal Approaches to Agent-Based Systems, Greenbelt, MD, USA, 5–7 April 2000; pp. 123–132.
65. Gilbert, N. Agent-based social simulation: Dealing with complexity. *Complex. Syst. Netw. Excell.* **2004**, *9*, 1–14.
66. Miller, J.H.; Page, S.E. *Complex Adaptive Systems: An Introduction to Computational Models of Social Life*; Princeton University Press: Princeton, NJ, USA, 2009.
67. Manning, C.; Raghavan, P.; Schütze, H. Introduction to information retrieval. *Nat. Lang. Eng.* **2010**, *16*, 100–103.
68. Namey, E.; Guest, G.; Thairu, L.; Johnson, L. Data reduction techniques for large qualitative data sets. *Handb. Team-Based Qual. Res.* **2008**, *2*, 137–161.
69. Ramos, J. Using tf-idf to determine word relevance in document queries. In Proceedings of the First Instructional Conference on Machine Learning, Piscataway, NJ, USA, 3–8 December 2003; pp. 133–142.
70. Rivers III, L.; Sanga, U.; Sidibe, A.; Wood, A.; Paudel, R.; Marquart-Pyatt, S.T.; Ligmann-Zielinska, A.; Olabisi, L.S.; Du, E.J.; Liverpool-Tasie, S. Mental models of food security in rural Mali. *Environ. Syst. Decis.* **2017**, *38*, 33–51. [CrossRef]
71. Ligmann-Zielinska, A.; Sun, L. Applying time-dependent variance-based global sensitivity analysis to represent the dynamics of an agent-based model of land use change. *Int. J. Geogr. Inf. Sci.* **2010**, *24*, 1829–1850. [CrossRef]
72. Xiang, X.; Kennedy, R.; Madey, G.; Cabaniss, S. Verification and validation of agent-based scientific simulation models. In Proceedings of the Agent-Directed Simulation Conference, San Diego, CA, USA, 3 April 2005; p. 55.

Disclaimer/Publisher's Note: The statements, opinions and data contained in all publications are solely those of the individual author(s) and contributor(s) and not of MDPI and/or the editor(s). MDPI and/or the editor(s) disclaim responsibility for any injury to people or property resulting from any ideas, methods, instructions or products referred to in the content.

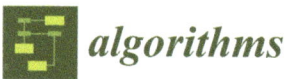 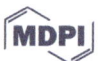

Article

Validating and Testing an Agent-Based Model for the Spread of COVID-19 in Ireland

Elizabeth Hunter * and John D. Kelleher *

ADAPT Centre, Technological University Dublin, Grangegorman, Dublin 7, D07 H6K8 Dublin, Ireland
* Correspondence: elizabeth.hunter@tudublin.ie (E.H.); john.d.kelleher@tudublin.ie (J.D.K.)

Abstract: Agent-based models can be used to better understand the impacts of lifting restrictions or implementing interventions during a pandemic. However, agent-based models are computationally expensive, and running a model of a large population can result in a simulation taking too long to run for the model to be a useful analysis tool during a public health crisis. To reduce computing time and power while running a detailed agent-based model for the spread of COVID-19 in the Republic of Ireland, we introduce a scaling factor that equates 1 agent to 100 people in the population. We present the results from model validation and show that the scaling factor increases the variability in the model output, but the average model results are similar in scaled and un-scaled models of the same population, and the scaled model is able to accurately simulate the number of cases per day in Ireland during the autumn of 2020. We then test the usability of the model by using the model to explore the likely impacts of increasing community mixing when schools reopen after summer holidays.

Keywords: agent-based model; epidemiology; infectious disease; simulation; COVID-19

Citation: Hunter, E.; Kelleher, J.D. Validating and Testing an Agent-Based Model for the Spread of COVID-19 in Ireland. *Algorithms* 2022, 15, 270. https://doi.org/10.3390/a15080270

Academic Editors: Nuno Fachada and Nuno David

Received: 14 July 2022
Accepted: 1 August 2022
Published: 3 August 2022

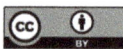

Copyright: © 2022 by the authors. Licensee MDPI, Basel, Switzerland. This article is an open access article distributed under the terms and conditions of the Creative Commons Attribution (CC BY) license (https://creativecommons.org/licenses/by/4.0/).

1. Introduction

During an infectious disease outbreak, modeling can be an essential tool to help understand how a disease might spread and the possible impact of any interventions [1]. Modeling has been used to respond to the UK foot and mouth epidemic in 2001 [2], the H1N1 pandemic in 2009 [3] and more recently during the COVID-19 pandemic. Infectious disease modeling has shown to be an important part of many government responses. For example, models have been used as evidence for lockdowns in the UK and USA [4], models have also been used in the Irish response to the pandemic [5], and Australia has used models to understand the impacts of lifting restrictions [6].

Equation-based models, in particular, compartmental models, are the most common type of model used for infectious disease modeling. A compartmental model is made up of a set of differential equations. The simplest compartmental model is the SIR model that is made up of three compartments: susceptible (S), infected (I) and recovered (R). Variations of the model can include additional compartments, such as the SEIR model, which includes an exposed (E) compartment [7]. The population in a compartmental model is assumed to be homogeneous and well mixed [8].

While the homogeneous SEIR model is often used and is able to accurately predict infectious disease dynamics, in some scenarios, more detail is needed, and the heterogeneity of the population needs to be taken into account. One common method for this is to add additional compartments to the SEIR model that represent different cohorts of the population. This can be done for age groups [9] or vaccination status [10]. These models can play an important role in understanding how an infectious disease will spread when the heterogeneity of the population is important, such as when vaccinations are implemented by age group. Although a cohort SEIR model allows for heterogeneity in the mixing between compartments, there are some drawbacks. Each compartment is still homogeneous, and the model might not be able to capture the individual actions and variations in characteristics that drive a pandemic [8].

Agent-based models (ABMs) can be used when this greater level of detail is necessary. ABMs are a type of computer simulation made up of agents who interact with each other and their environment [11]. Those agents can be created so that they emulate a real population. This synthetic agent population can match the real population on different characteristics and geographic distribution, and agent networks can produce results due to the interactions between these factors [12].

There are a number of situations where there is an advantage to using ABMs compared to equation-based models. They allow us to create a baseline scenario where we can look at what would have happened if a certain intervention had not occurred, for example, if there was no lockdown, or if vaccinations were not introduced. Additionally, as ABMs are stochastic and are driven by agent decisions, each model run is slightly different, and this stochasticity gives a range of outcomes that could occur within the system. Because of these advantages, a number of ABMs have been developed to help respond to and better understand the COVID-19 pandemic [4,6,13–16]. The model we present in this paper was part of a suite of modeling tools developed by the Irish Epidemiological Modeling Advisory Group (IEMAG). IEMAG was a group formed to provide statistical and mathematical modeling support and advice to the chief medical officer and the national public health emergency team during the COVID-19 pandemic.

ABMs, however, can be computationally intensive, which can limit their usefulness when speed of results is necessary [17]. A number of studies have attempted to reduce the computing power while still retaining model fidelity. One method is using a hybrid agent-based and equation-based method designed to save computing power by switching between the two modeling types, depending on the number of infected agents in the simulation [18]. Alternatively, computing power can be saved by only simulating infected agents and modeling healthy agents as a property of the environment [19]. Another method of decreasing the amount of computing power needed to run a model while still increasing the population size is using scaling methods. Dynamic re-scaling is another method that scales agents when certain thresholds of infection are reached [13,16]. In this paper, we present an agent-based model for the Republic of Ireland with a population that has been scaled so that 1 agent represents 100 people. The model can be used to understand how changes in behaviors and movements impact the spread of COVID-19 in Ireland. In the next section, we discuss the different components of the model. We then discuss the validation of the model to show that the model results are trustworthy, and finally we test the scaled model, running an experiment looking at the impacts of different levels of community mixing when schools re-open after summer holidays, and present the result of the experiment to show the model's usability.

2. Materials and Methods

We use an ABM to model the spread of COVID-19 through Ireland. In this section, we provide a brief description of the model that is used in our work and then discuss the experiments run to validate and test the model.

2.1. Model Description

The model presented here is a version of a previous model [20] that has been scaled to simulate the entire population of the Republic of Ireland. It was created and implemented in the modeling environment, Netlogo [21]. The Republic of Ireland is a country in Northwestern Europe. In 2016, when the last Irish census was completed, there were 4,757,976 people in Ireland; in the scaled model, this would equate to approximately 47,580 agents. There are 26 counties that make up the country. Approximately 40% of the population of the country live in the region of the nation's capital city, Dublin. The model is an agent-based model that was created for the spread of measles in an Irish county [20] and has been adapted to simulate the spread of COVID-19 [22]. The model is made up of four main components: environment, transportation, disease, and society [23]. It uses census data from the Irish Central Statistics Office to create a population that matches the demographic characteristics of the county at the small area level (small areas are the smallest geographic area over which census statistics are aggregated in Ireland, and contain between 50 and 200 dwellings) [24] and transportation patterns [25]. The scaled-up model presented here has the same four components and a similar structure. The largest difference between the two models is that the scaled-up model is designed to simulate the entire population and capture the interactions between counties. There are, however, other differences that are mainly meant to reduce the computing power necessary to run a county-level agent-based model. The more complex an agent-based model is and the more agents in the simulated population, the more computing power that is needed [17]. Thus, to simulate at a larger scale while still being able to produce timely results, we reduce the complexity of the environment matching population distributions at the county level instead of the small area level, and we scale the model so that each agent represents 100 similar people in Ireland. The following sections discuss the different model components used in the model in more detail as well as the model schedule, the initial conditions of the model and the interventions that can be implemented in the model. Further details including model parameters can be found in the model ODD [26].

2.1.1. Agents

At its heart, an agent-based model is made up of agents. The agents in this model represent people in Ireland and have a number of characteristics that define them. Agent characteristics fall into different categories. They have demographic information, such as age, sex and employment status; a set of social networks, including a family network and a work network; information on their disease status, such as if they are susceptible, exposed, infected or immune; and information on their location (home, school, work or the community). For more detail and for the full list of variables that define an agent, see the model ODD [26].

2.1.2. Environment Component

The model environment is made up of grid cells or patches in NetLogo. Thirty-one patches in the model are designated as counties (e.g., Leitrim County, and Cork County) or city and city/county areas (e.g., Dublin City, Cork City, Waterford City and County). These county and city labels are defined by the CSO and are referred to as county patches going forward. The number of primary and secondary schools in each actual county in Ireland can be found from the data from the Irish Department of Education. However, because we are scaling the model for 1 agent to represent 100 people, we reduce the number of schools in the counties. We do this by dividing the number of schools in the county by 50 (half the scale for agents to people) and rounding up. This gives us at least one primary and one secondary school in each county and also approximately reproduces the class and school network sizes that are found in the 1 to 1 scaling in the county model.

Agents will only occupy the county patches in the model and can move between them. Although all agents on a county patch will physically be coded in the same location, the agents keep track of their location within the county and will be at either home, work, school, or in the community. Agents will only come into contact with other agents in the same location as them in the same county. For example, an agent in the community will not be in contact with an agent at home. Additionally, all agents in the community on the same patch will not be in contact with every other agent in the community. Instead, a set of parameters derived using the POLYMOD contact matrix data [27] is used to determine the number of community contacts that an agent will have. Agents can move between county patches. Agent movement is discussed in more detail in Section 2.1.4. While on a patch, we can access certain information about the patch, including the number of agents on the patch and the physical distance to the other patches.

2.1.3. Disease

The disease component in the model is set to simulate the dynamics of COVID-19 and follows the dynamics of an SEIR model with the agents moving from susceptible to exposed then infected and finally recovered. In addition to the four stages of infection, we match the disease component of the model to the Irish population-based SEIR model [5]. In the model, individuals start in a susceptible component, then if infected, they move to an exposed component, and from the exposed component, individuals will move to one of two infectious components: asymptomatic or presymptomatic. If the individual is presymptomatic, they will then move to one of the following components: isolating, not isolated, waiting for a test, and tested. Once recovered, individuals will move to a recovered state. Thus in our model, an infectious agent can be in one of the following states: asymptomatic, presymptomatic, isolating, not isolated, waiting for a test and tested. When a susceptible agent comes into contact with an infectious agent, they have a chance of becoming exposed. Once exposed, the agent will stay exposed for a predetermined period of time before becoming infectious. This predetermined period of time is different for each agent. When an agent is exposed, the agent is assigned a length of time for their exposure period, using an exponential distribution with a mean of the exposure period taken from the literature. Agents will remain infectious for a predetermined period of time before recovering. Similar to the exposure period, this predetermined period of time is different for each agent. When an agent becomes infectious, the agent is assigned a length of time for their infectious period using an exponential distribution with a mean of the infectious period taken from the literature. Once recovered, the agents can no longer be infectious and cannot be re-infected. This assumption was made, as the risk of reinfection early in the pandemic was low [28], and the model was initially designed to look at short term outcomes of the pandemic (i.e., during a single wave). When an agent becomes infectious, the agent will either become asymptomatic or symptomatic. If they are symptomatic, they can either be isolating, not isolating, or waiting for a test. If waiting for a test, the agent will be waiting for a test for a predetermined time and then have tested positive. The infectious component that an agent is in (asymptomatic, isolating, etc.) determines how infectious an agent is. The base infectious rate is determined using the basic reproduction number, R_0, the average contacts an agent has, and the infection period [29]. The method for calculating the infectiousness of the agents and all the parameter values are discussed more in the model ODD [26]. Those who are presymptomatic, asymptomatic, and isolated have a reduction in their infectiousness. We implement these reductions to match with those in the SEIR model. The main disease parameters needed to initialize the model are the basic reproduction number, R_0, the length of the exposed period, the length of the pre-symptomatic period, and the length of the infectious period, and are taken from the literature.

Additionally, as there have been multiple variants of COVID-19 during the course of the pandemic, the model allows for agents to pass on specific variants. For example, if an agent is infected with the alpha variant, any agents they infect will also be infected with the alpha variant. As the variants that are widely circulated in the population tend to be more infectious, we also include a variant multiplier that adjusts the infectiousness of an agent for a specific variant.

2.1.4. Transport

The transportation component of the model is not altered compared to the transportation component in [20]. In the model, there are two drivers of agent movement within the model: scheduled movements determined by the time of day and the agent type and community movements determined from a gravity model. The schedule of movements and the parameters that define the community movements are defined further in the model ODD [26], but in this section, we provide a brief description of both, as well as an analysis of the contact patterns that are generated from the model and the process of updating the contact patterns to be more realistic using real contact data.

Scheduled movements define the movement of agents who are students or workers. On weekdays, these agents will move from home to school or home to work at certain times of the day and then will return home after work or school. Additionally, all agents will return home at a certain time of the day and will remain at home until the morning. Commuting patterns are determined using data from the CSO Place of Work, School or College—Census of Anonymity Records (POWSCAR) [25].

On weekdays, the movements of all agents who are not students or working and on the weekends, the movements of all agents are determined using a gravity model. A gravity model uses the characteristics of a location and the distances between locations to determine interactions between location pairs [30]. In the case of our model, the interactions between the location pairs is the probability that an agent at one location will move to the other location in the next time step. The idea behind using a gravity model for movements is that agents are pulled toward areas or counties that are closer to their current location and areas that have a high population density and pushed away from areas that are farther away and areas that have a low population density. Although not a perfect model of human transportation, it is a proxy for human mobility.

When an agent's movements are determined by a gravity model, they can be either at home or in the community. In reality, there are many locations within a community that agents might travel to, such as parks or shops; however, for simplicity, we only include a "community" location. While this makes the model slightly less realistic, the model is built so that not all agents in the community in the same county are in contact. Instead the contacts are determined by agent networks. If two agents in the community in the same county are in the same family network, they are more likely to be in contact than two agents in the community in the same school or work network who are more likely to come into contact than two random agents. The time that agents spend in the community and the likelihood of coming into contact with other agents in their networks was originally determined by parameterizing the model to match contact patterns and infection rates with the [12] model, where the agents moves in steps around a town and only comes into contact with another agent in the community if they are on the same patch. While this was done to preserve model fidelity when scaling up the model, to make the model more realistic, we adjust the parameters in the model so that the contact patterns simulated in the model match those from real-world studies of contact patterns. We use the contact patterns found in the POLYMOD study that examined the social contacts of people in eight European countries. The participants of the study recorded their contacts and locations of the contacts including home, work, school, leisure, transportation or other. As Ireland is not one of the eight countries, we use the data from the Netherlands to estimate the Irish contact rates [27]. The parameters determined from this analysis can be found in the model ODD [26].

2.1.5. Society

As we are simulating the spread of COVID-19 in the Republic of Ireland, we aim to match the characteristics of our agent population to the characteristics of the Irish population at the county level. Thus every county in the model has the correct portion of agents of the following characteristics: age, sex and economic status (student, working, retired, unemployed, etc). The counties also have the correct portion of households by type (single, couple, couple with children, etc.), and by number and ages of children (under 15, over 15 and both under and over 15). To make the contact networks in the model more realistic, we allow for agents to have an extended family network. This network connects two households one with agents over 65 and one with agents under 65. The reasons for creating these extended networks are two-fold. The first is to capture interactions and thus transmission between children and grandparents who act as carers. The second is to capture interactions between families during holiday periods, such as Christmas, when inter-generational mixing typically increases. Further discussion of the creation of these networks can be found in the model ODD [26].

From the 2016 census, the last Irish census collected at the time of model creation, there were 4,757,976 people in Ireland. An agent-based model with that many agents requires a large amount of computing time and power to run such that the results may take days or weeks. Thus we introduce a scaling factor into the model that equates 1 agent to 100 people. This greatly reduces the number of agents needed to simulate the population, from 4,757,976 to 47,580, which allows us to model the social and economic structure of Ireland without decreasing the level of detail in the model or taking an overly large amount of time to run the model.

Although we still keep the same population structure with the scaling factor, we are changing the total number of agents and need to make sure that the reduction in agents does not impact the model results. Section 2.2 discusses the scaling factor in more detail and the tests run to validate the changes introduced when scaling the model.

2.1.6. Schedule

The model is run on discrete time steps. Each time step represents two hours of the day, thus 12 time steps make up a day and 84 time steps make up a week. During "nighttime" hours, agents are not moving around the environment but are instead at home, and transmission can only occur between others in their household network. The model keeps track of the week of the year, as this determines when schools are open or closed for the summer and for winter holidays. From week 26 to week 34, schools are closed for the summer, and agents who are students do not attend school but instead move throughout the community as they would on weekends for the summer. Additionally, schools are closed down for weeks 51 and 52 to simulate the impacts of Christmas holidays. During two days in week 51, agents move to a household within their extended family network for the day and spend time to simulate family gatherings for the holidays.

2.1.7. Initial Conditions

To start the simulation the initial conditions for the disease component need to be set. As the society and environment are set based off of real census data, these do not change between model scenarios. For each scenario of the agent-based model that is run, we determine the number of agents who are vaccinated, exposed, infectious, and recovered. If vaccinations are included in the model, the number of initially vaccinated agents are determined first from the vaccination model discussed in Section 2.1.8. The start week of the model is used to select the number of agents in each age group that have been vaccinated. After vaccinations, the number of infectious, exposed and immune agents are determined. In order to run the model, there needs to be at least one agent who is either exposed or infectious. A given number of agents, determined by the user, who are not fully vaccinated are assigned to be sick. If variants are included, of those agents who are sick, a certain percentage of them are assigned to being infected with each variant. Then a given number, again assigned by the user, of sick agents are assigned to be asymptomatic, isolating, not isolating, or waiting for a test. Following the assignment of the initially infectious agents, we determine the exposed agents. Half of the predetermined number of exposed agents are chosen to be agents in the households of those agents who are sick and infectious. This is to make the distribution of exposed agents more realistic, as it is more likely that an infectious agent will have infected a member of their close contacts versus a random agent outside of their networks. Finally, a certain number of agents are set to be immune. We first ask a number of agents who are infectious to set at least one agent in their networks to be immune and then if the number of desired immune agents is greater than those selected in the infectious agents networks, the additional immune agents are selected from random agents in the model.

2.1.8. Interventions

The above sections describe the agent movements and patterns when the model is not adapting its behaviors to a pandemic situation. This would be a likely scenario for the spread of an endemic disease such as influenza or measles where the population does not greatly adjust their behaviors during an outbreak. However, to better capture the response to the COVID-19 pandemic, the ability to simulate interventions and behavioral adaptations is important. Thus, we have included a number of interventions in the model.

Lockdowns and School Closures

Prior to the introduction of vaccinations, one of the main measures used to reduce the spread of the virus was change in behaviors. The fewer contacts individuals have, the less the virus will spread. In the model, the agents' behaviors are changed in two ways: schools are closed, or lockdowns are introduced.

Primary and/or secondary schools can be closed: this requires all agents in the school to stay at home during school hours instead of attending school. A lockdown can be introduced that restricts agents' movements. During a lockdown, schools can be either opened or closed and the user can determine the percentage of agents who are working from home or no longer working as well as the reduction in movement around the community, compared to "normal" movements.

Contact Tracing

Ireland implemented a comprehensive contact tracing program during the pandemic, where those who tested positive were contacted by contact tracers and their close contacts were identified and referred to a test [31]. The contact tracing program successfully completed contact tracing for 96% of the cases notified in Ireland between 17 March 2020 and 30 April 2021 [31]. However, due to the changing nature of the pandemic, the number of close contacts identified, the length of time to complete calls and the number of calls made varied throughout the pandemic. Additionally, not all contacts who were identified through contact tracing attended testing [32].

In the model, when an agent tests positive, a probability determines if they take part in contact tracing. This probability is estimated using the percent of cases in Ireland where contact tracing has been completed for a given month as a proxy. If the agent participates in contact tracing, then their contacts are identified, and a probability determines for each contact identified if that contact also participates in contact tracing. The probability is estimated using the percent of contacts that receive a test as a proxy. If an agent who is a contact of an infectious agent does participate in contact tracing, the agent isolates for a set number of days. In the first year of the pandemic, this isolation period was set to 14 days, as this was the suggested time to restrict movements when identified as a close contact.

Contact tracing in the model can be turned on and off, and the parameters defining contact tracing (probability of a case participating, probability of a contact isolating and the number of days a contact isolates) can be adjusted to match what occurred at different times during the pandemic or to investigate potential scenarios.

Vaccinations

Vaccinations can also be turned on or off to investigate their impact on the pandemic. We include vaccinations in the model, but allow the user to turn vaccinations on and off. If vaccinations are turned on, then a vaccination spreadsheet is used as input to the model that provides information on the number of individuals by age group who have been vaccinated, who have successfully been protected against severe disease, who have successfully been protected against symptomatic disease and who have successfully been protected against asymptomatic disease. There are also different levels of protection against the two main variant, alpha and delta, that were circulating in Ireland in 2021. Thus an individual could be protected against asymptomatic disease from the alpha variant but only against symptomatic disease from the delta variant. This was calculated based off the supply of COVID-19 vaccines to Ireland and the predicted efficacy of the different vaccines supplied.

2.2. Model Validation

The model presented in the previous sections is a scaled version of the Irish county agent-based model [20]. Although it is based off a previously validated model, we made fundamental changes to the society component of the model with the introduction of the scaling factor and altered the level of detail in the environmental component. Thus, it is necessary to validate the new scaled-up version of the model.

To validate the model, we follow the framework laid out in [33]. Agent-based model validation has three main steps: cross validation, where we compare the model output to a previously validated model, sensitivity analysis, and comparing model output to real data.

2.2.1. Cross Validation

The first step of validating an agent-based model is using cross validation, where the model output is compared to the output from a previously validated model. To show that the scaling factor does not have a major impact on the output of the model, we run tests comparing the output of the scaled model for a single county to the output of the original county model output presented and validated in [20]. The idea is that in the scaled-up model, the output from a single county should not change from the county model if we consider the county in isolation. In this cross-validation experiment, we are not aiming to compare the results to real data, which is done later in the validation, but to show that the assumptions we made to scale the model do not impact the output. Thus, the county model is a good benchmark for cross validation because it serves as the base model that was scaled up to obtain the scaled Irish country model. In the county model, 1 agent equates to 1 person. The model is run for Leitrim in the original county-level model, and also in the scaled version, where we equate 1 agent to 100 people. This means that in the original county model, there will be approximately 36,000 agents and in the scaled model there will only be 360, with each agent representing 100 agents. The initial conditions of the model will be adjusted accordingly. The model is run with no interventions in place. We study three different scenarios with different initial conditions: the first starts with 300 agents infected in the county model and 3 in the scaled model, the second has 1000 agents infected in the county model and 10 in the scaled model, and the third starts with 10,000 agents infected in the county model and 100 agents infected in the scaled model. We do not include any exposed or immune agents in the initial conditions for any of the three scenarios. For both the county model and the scaled model, we run the model 30 times. The reason why we run the model multiple times is that agent-based models are stochastic in nature, with each model run producing different results. The stochasticity is introduced in a number of ways: agents sample from distributions to determine the number of days they are exposed before becoming infectious and the number of days before they recover. Agents will also make decisions that determine their actions, which affect their contacts. Thus, there is a question of how many times should the agent-based model be run to accurately capture the true results of the model. Too few runs and the model results might not be accurate, and too many and it could waste computing time. To determine the number of runs necessary, we use the method outlined in [33]. The method looks at the size of a confidence interval around a statistic produced by the model to determine the number of runs necessary to account for the stochasticity in the model. We choose to look at the R_e statistic as the size of R_e can help to determine the speed at which the outbreak is spreading. We aim to pick the number of runs where the size of the confidence interval around R_e is determined to be stable and small enough. The methodology in [33] does not specify an exact metric to determine when the confidence interval is small enough but leaves it to the modeler to make the decision. Using this method, we determine that 30 runs are enough to capture the variability in the model.

2.2.2. Sensitivity Analysis

A sensitivity analysis is performed to determine if changes in the model inputs impact the model output as expected. In our sensitivity analysis, we look at changes in agent behavior and determine how increased community mixing impacts the number of infectious agents. It is expected that as an agent mixes more in the community, there will be more cases. If we do not see an increase in cases as mixing increases, there is likely something fundamentally wrong with the model.

For the sensitivity analysis, we run four different scenarios, looking at how changes in agent movement impact the model results. In all scenarios, we start with 156 infectious agents, and because of the scaling factor, this equates to 15,600 people. Eighty-eight of those infectious agents are asymptomatic, ten are isolating, nine are not isolating and twenty-one are isolating and have tested positive. There are 92 agents exposed to the virus and 5784 agents who have recovered. These initial conditions are similar to the situation in Ireland prior to the start of the school year in 2020. Vaccinations are included in the model, schools are not open, and there is no contact tracing. Each scenario starts with movement at a 50% reduction from the pre-pandemic movement. In order to account for any model burn-in phenomenon, in this experiment, in each run, we allow two weeks of the simulation to pass before we include any changes in mixing. Four different mixing scenarios are considered: (1) agents stay at a 50% reduction from the pre-pandemic movement, (2) agents reduce their movements by 66% of the pre-pandemic movement, (3) agents increase their movements by 33% of the pre-pandemic movement, and (4) agents return to the pre-pandemic movement.

2.2.3. Comparison to Real Data

After cross validation, the next step to validate an agent-based model is to compare the output of the model to real data. To do this, we simulate the time between February and December 2020 in Ireland and compare the average model output across 30 runs to the real number of cases per day in Ireland. We start the model from 1 February 2020. There were no cases notified in Ireland until 29 February 2020; however, starting the model prior to the initial cases allows for a model burn-in period. At the start of the model runs, there are three infectious agents: one is asymptomatic, and one is presymptomatic. Two agents are exposed but not yet infectious, and all other agents are susceptible. We match all agent movements and intervention strategies to those that were in place in Ireland during that time period. Initially, schools are open and agents are mixing at regular pre-pandemic levels. In the third week of March, schools are closed. In the fourth week of March, a lockdown is introduced; agents reduce their mixing to approximately 50% of pre-pandemic levels and 70% of agents who would normally be working are either working from home or not working. In April,, agents reduce their mixing levels again to about 17% of pre-pandemic mixing. Lockdowns and other restrictions start to lift by June, and thus agents increase their mixing to 33% of pre-pandemic levels in June. In the model, schools reopen in September, and agents remain at the same community mixing level. In the beginning of October, agents increase their mixing back to approximately 60% of pre-pandemic levels; however, movements are reduced to 33% of pre-pandemic levels in the last week of October, as a new lockdown is introduced in Ireland. At the start of December, the lockdown is lifted, and agents increase their movements to near pre-pandemic levels. Table 1, gives a summary of the dates that interventions were implemented and when agent mixing changed.

Vaccinations are not included in the model, as vaccinations did not begin until late December 2020. However, we do include contact tracing, as this was an important part of the response to the pandemic and will impact the case numbers.

The number of new cases per day in Ireland during the summer of 2020 was low, under 100 cases. This can be a problem with the scaling factor of the model. Fewer than 100 cases equates to less than 1 agent. This resulted in a number of runs where COVID-19 would have gone extinct in Ireland. As this did not happen, we included a scenario, where if the number of COVID-19 cases in the model was 0, a new case would be imported into the model. This would represent a case that occurred due to travel.

Table 1. Interventions and changes in agent mixing implemented in the model.

Date	Lockdown	School Closure	Vaccinations	Reduction in Mixing
1 February 2020	No	No	No	Normal
12 March 2020	No	Yes	No	Reduced to 50%
27 March 2020	Yes	Yes	No	Reduced to 33%
20 April 2020	Yes	Yes	No	Reduced to 17%
1 June 2020	Yes	Yes	No	Reduced to 33%
29 June 2020	No	Yes	No	No Change
1 September 2020	No	No	No	No Change
1 October 2020	No	No	No	Increased to 60%
21 October 2020	Yes	No	No	Increased to 33%
1 December 2020	No	No	No	Normal Mixing

2.3. Model Testing

Once a model is validated, it is important to test the model and understand if it can help the user to learn something useful about an infectious disease outbreak or pandemic scenario. Thus, the final step in the validation and testing framework is to test the model and show model usability [33]. Unless the user is able to learn something about the system from the agent-based model, it is not a useful model.

To test our model, we run an experiment to better understand how changes in movements can interact with other interventions or the lifting of measures and impact the pandemic in the short term. We perform 30 runs of two scenarios of the model that focus on the period of time when schools reopen in the autumn: (1) schools re-open and community mixing remains the same at a 50% lower rate of mixing than pre-pandemic levels (2) schools re-open and when schools reopen community mixing returns to pre-pandemic levels. We run the model for the equivalent of 60 days, starting a month before schools open and running for a month after schools open. The model is only run for a month after schools open to determine the immediate and short term impacts of opening schools. These are the impacts that will likely occur before an intervention is put in place. For each set of runs, we compare the total infected agents at a given time step and the number of newly infectious agents per day. As we did in the sensitivity analysis, we expect that increased movement and opening schools will lead to an increase in cases. Understanding the magnitude of the increase is important, and we can learn this from the model; however, simpler infectious disease models, such as the SEIR model, will also be able to model this increase in cases. To emphasize the importance of using an agent-based model and the additional information we can learn from a model that simulates at the individual level, we also look at the location of the infection (home, school, work or the community) and the age groups of those infected, and discuss possible implications from the model output.

The initial conditions for our model testing experiment are the same as those used in the sensitivity analysis.

3. Results

The results we present in this section are from two distinct experiments. The first set of results presented are from a validation experiment designed to show the validity of the model. The second set of results are from an experiment designed to test the model to show its potential usefulness.

3.1. Validation

In the following sections, we discuss the results from the experiments run for each part of the agent-based model validation framework (cross validation, sensitivity analysis, and comparison to data).

3.1.1. Cross Validation

Looking at the cross validation results, we first start with 300 infected agents, and in the scaled version we start with 3 infected agents. Figure 1a,b show the total number of agents infected at a given time point and the number of newly infectious agents each day in both models for individual runs and the average across all runs for the scaled model. Looking at the figures, we can see that the scaled model produces a much greater variation in results than the county level model in both total infectious and newly infectious per day. This is likely due to the scaling factor in the model, which means that only three agents are infected at the start of the scaled up model. When few agents are infected, the individual actions of those agents play a larger part in the course the outbreak takes. It is important to note, however, that even though the scaled-up model produces more variation, the runs from the county level model are within the range of the runs from the scaled-up model and are close to the average across the runs from the scaled-up model.

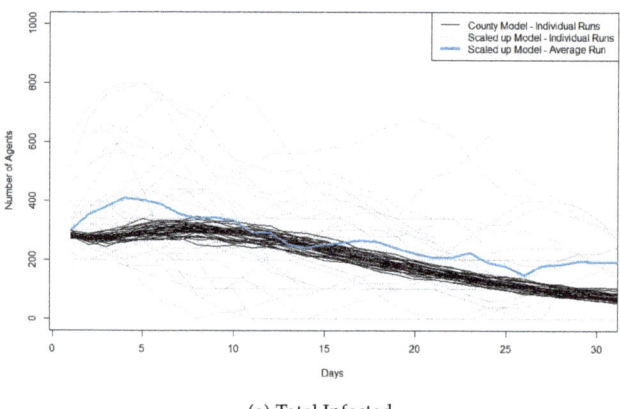

(**a**) Total Infected

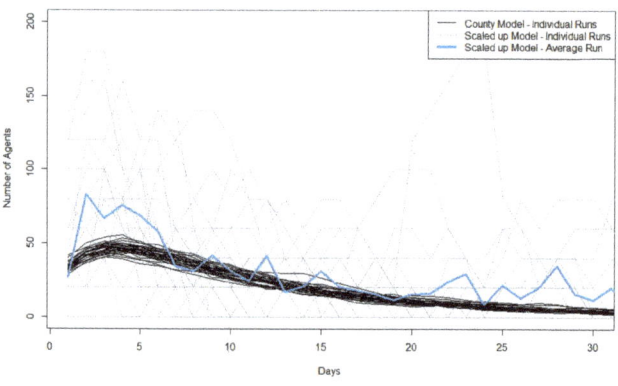

(**b**) Newly Infectious per Day

Figure 1. Plots showing cross validation results when 300 agents are infected at the start of the run in the original model and 3 agents are infected at the start of the run in the scaled model. (**a**) shows the total number of infected agents per day and (**b**) shows the newly infectious agents per day. For the scaled model the y-axis is the number of infected $\times 100$. We also plot the average value across the 30 runs of the scaled model. Best viewed in color.

We then compare runs for scenarios with 1000 agents infected in the county model and 10 agents infected in the scaled up model. Although there is still significant variation in the scaled model compared to the county model, we see less variation in model runs than when we started with only three agents infected. Figure 2a,b plots for this second scenario the total infectious and the new infectious agents per day, respectively. We see that in the first approximately 5 days, the scaled model has higher peaks for new infectious cases compared to the county model and a slightly higher average for total. However, by 10 days, the average curve for the scaled model appears to match well with the runs for the original county model.

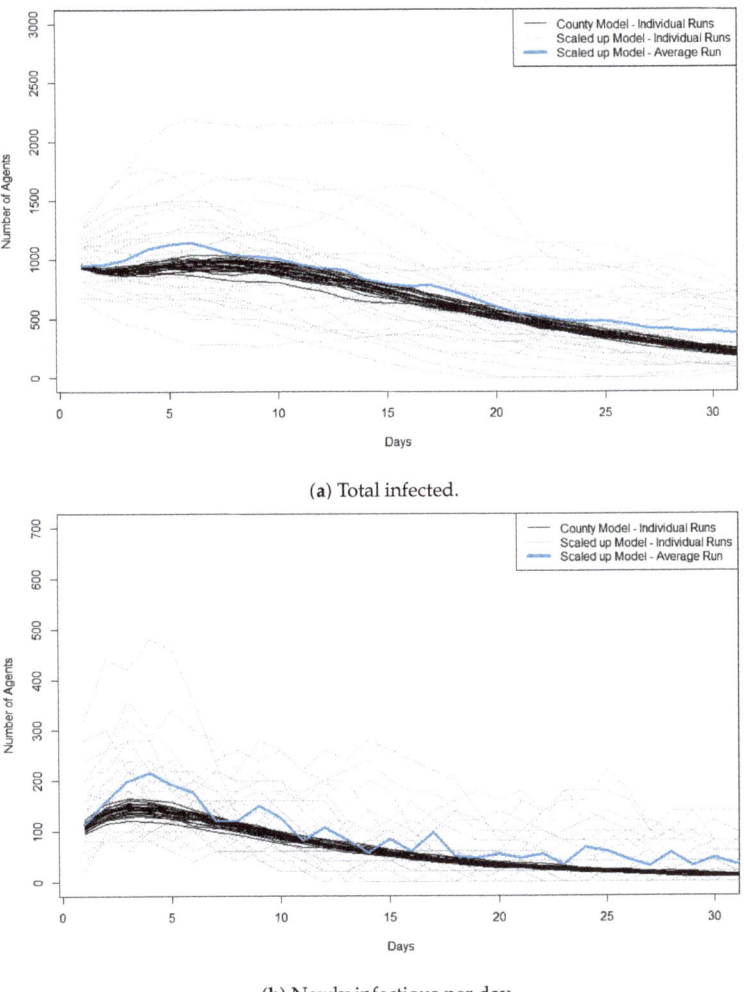

(a) Total infected.

(b) Newly infectious per day.

Figure 2. Plots showing cross validation results when 1000 agents are infected at the start of the run in the original model and 10 agents are infected at the start of the run in the scaled model. (**a**) shows the total number of infected agents per day and (**b**) shows the newly infectious agents per day. For the scaled model the y-axis is the number of infected $\times 100$. We also plot the average value across the 30 runs of the scaled model. Best viewed in color.

Finally, we run scenarios with 10,000 agents infected in the original county model and 100 agents infected in the scaled model. Figure 3a,b plots the total infectious and the new infectious per day for this scenario. Here, we see a much greater match between the two models. Although there is a greater variation in the scaled model, the trajectories for total infected match well across the simulation. Similar to scaling from 10 to 1000 agents, we still see a higher peak of new infectious cases in the scaled model compared to the county model, but by day 10 of the simulation, the average curve for the scaled model is much closer to the runs of the county model.

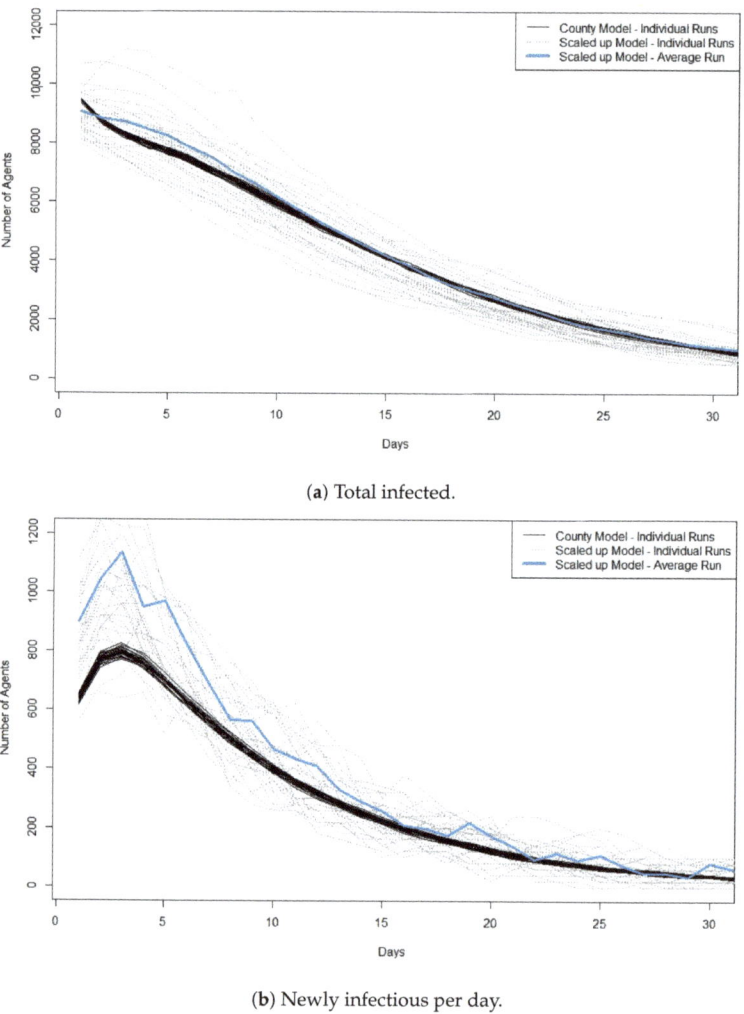

(a) Total infected.

(b) Newly infectious per day.

Figure 3. Plots showing cross validation results when 10,000 agents are infected at the start of the run in the original model and 100 agents are infected at the start of the run in the scaled model. (**a**) shows the total number of infected agents per day and (**b**) shows the newly infectious agents per day. For the scaled model the y-axis is the number of infected $\times 100$. We also plot the average value across the 30 runs of the scaled model. Best viewed in color.

As the average runs for the scaled model appear to match well with the county model, this suggests that even though we see more variation in the scaled model any statistics determined from the model output (total infected, new cases, exposed, recovered, R_f, etc.) will likely tend toward the statistics from the county model, meaning that we do not lose any information when we use the scaling factor. Across the different levels of scaling, we do consistently see that there tends to be a higher peak in newly infected cases in the first 5 days of the simulation. This might signify that there is a burn-in period with the scaled model that should be noted in any analysis of model output.

Our results show that for the first week to two weeks, the scaled model produces similar results for a single county to the original county-level model. However, the scaled model produces more varying output from each run when a smaller number of agents is infected. We think that when the number of infected is close to the number used in scaling (i.e., if the scale is 1 agent to 100 people and the initial conditions are that there are 100 people infected scaled down to 1) then the model will not perform as well.

3.1.2. Sensitivity Analysis

Figure 4 shows the new cases per day for each of the four scenarios.

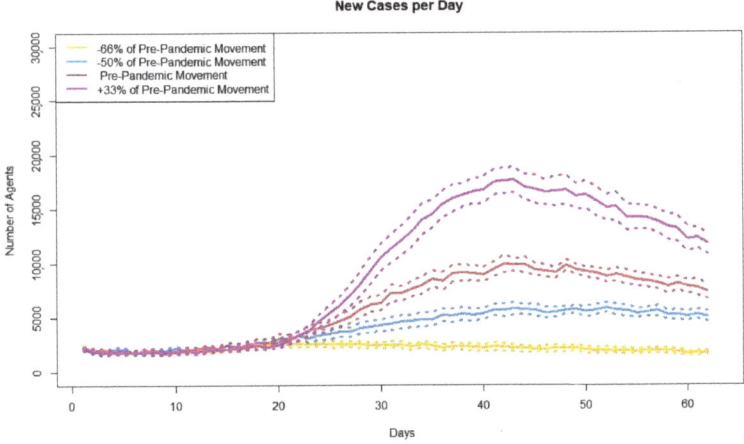

Figure 4. Plot showing the average simulated new cases per day across 30 runs for four different levels of movement. Dashed lines represent upper and lower bound of confidence intervals.

As the model output changes as expected, with the lowest number of new cases corresponding to the largest reduction in movements and then cases increasing as the agents level of movements increases, the model is considered validated through sensitivity analysis.

3.1.3. Comparison to Real Data

Figure 5 shows the average new cases per day across 30 simulation runs and the real Irish case counts during the same time period. Real cases are taken from the COVID-19 HPSC detailed statistics profile published by Ordnance Survey Ireland [34]. From the start of the model until April, the case counts are higher than the real cases and is likely due to a burn-in period of the model. During the summer months, from June to August, the case counts for the model are also higher than the real cases. This is likely due to the scaling of the model. From June to September, the number of new cases per day in Ireland is under 100, which is less than one agent with scaling. However, in order for the model to simulate the pandemic, there needs to be more than one agent infected and this likely leads to the difference in cases during the summer of 2020. However, we see a good match in the cases from October through December. Figure 5 also shows the confidence intervals around the average new cases per day. Although the average number of new cases per day matches closely with the real cases, the confidence intervals are relatively wide at the peaks. This is likely due to the fact that the case counts are around 1000, and as we saw in the cross validation, the scaling factor leads to large variations between runs when there is a smaller number of cases. However, based on the comparison between the average simulated cases and the real case counts and that the real cases are within the confidence intervals produced by the agent-based model we can consider that the model is validated through comparison to real data when there are 100 or more cases per day.

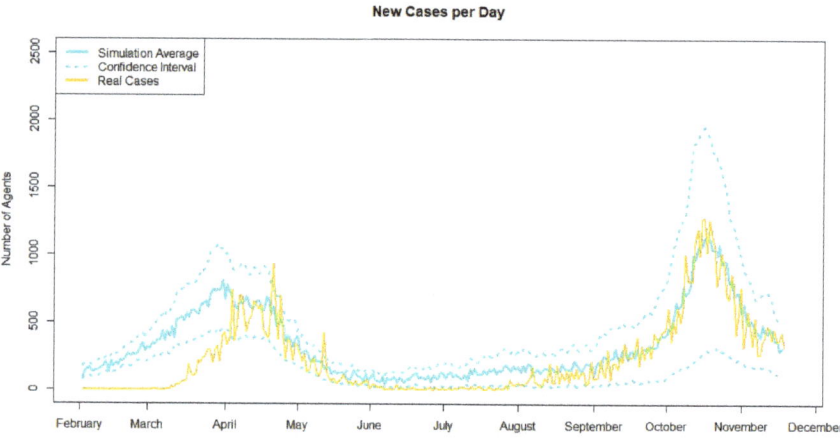

Figure 5. Plot showing the average simulated new cases per day across 30 runs in blue and the real Irish case counts in yellow. Upper and lower bounds of confidence intervals for the average simulated new cases are represented in blue dashed lines.

3.2. Testing

The previous sections discuss the scaled agent-based model for COVID-19 spread in Ireland and the validation of the model [33]. To show how the agent-based model is useful and can be used to better understand the pandemic we run an experiment that looks at opening schools after a period of closure, such as summer break, and the impact different levels of community mixing and return to work have on case numbers. During any infectious disease outbreak it is important to understand how changes to the current mixing and movement patterns will impact the number of cases. Re-opening schools post summer holidays is an important period of time with countries wanting to safely open the schools. This reopening will likely lead to an increase in cases but the size of the increase will be dependent on the movements of the other agents in the model. It is possible that as students go back to school, adults will see this as a return to normality and increase their movements as well.

To analyze the results of our model testing experiment, we first look at traditional output for infectious disease models, the number of new infectious cases per day, and then look at the output in more detail, analyzing the location where agents were infected and the age groups of the infected. Figure 6 shows the individual runs for the two scenarios and the average number of new infectious agents per day across the 30 runs in bold. In both plots the vertical lines indicate the day when schools reopen for the autumn term.

Looking at both plots, it can be seen that the increase in cases when schools reopen is much greater when the reopening coincides with an increase in agent movement in the community. The increased movement also appears to lead to a greater variation in individual runs as seen in Figure 6.

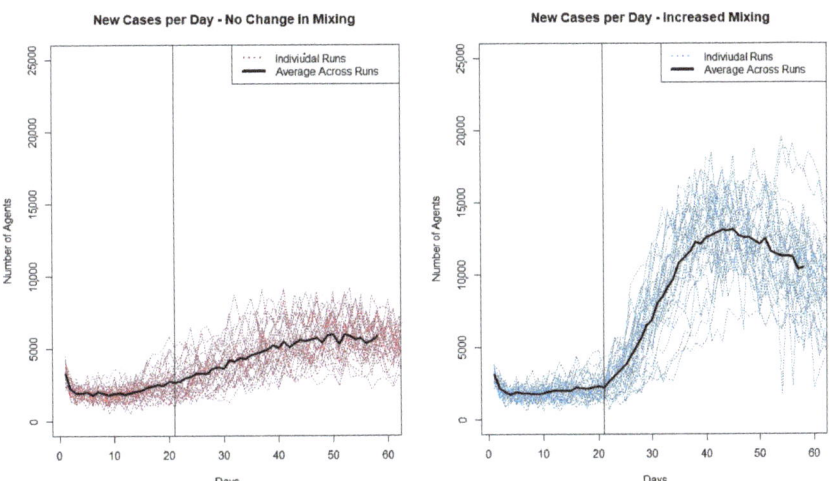

Figure 6. Plot showing the number of new infectious cases per day for the individual runs from the two scenarios.

This difference in increase in movement leads to a number of questions that the new cases per day metric cannot provide. While it is important to know that this increase in movement combined with the opening of schools leads to a greater number of cases, it might be important to understand where those cases are being infected. Are they all cases in the community? Or as community cases increase do cases that originate within the schools and home increase as well? Additionally, are certain age groups impacted more than others? These questions can help better understand the drivers of the spread of COVID-19 when schools reopen and can be better understood using the agent-based model. In the model agents keep track of if they were infected at home, school, work or in the community. Figure 7 shows the average number of infectious agents at a given time by their location of infection. When schools open but mixing does not increase, there is a slow, gradual increase in cases in schools, home and the community. There is little increase in the work setting, this is because in the model there are only a small percentage of agents who have returned to work in this scenario. An increase in agents returning to work may result in a larger increase in work cases. When school openings occur with an increase in community mixing, we still see little increase in cases at work, but the increased community mixing leads to a rapid increase in cases originating in the community and in homes. While there is a greater increase in cases originating in schools compared to when mixing does not increase, the greater levels of cases originating in schools only occur about 20 days after schools are open (the red lines for cases originating in schools only start to diverge at day 40). This suggests that there might be a delay in the impact of increased community mixing on cases in schools. There may be a threshold of cases that occur outside of schools before the higher cases spill over into the school setting.

The model output can also be used to look at the age groups of those infected. Figure 8 shows the average number of infectious agents by age group across the 30 runs for the two scenarios. The age groups are 0–9, 10–19, 20–29, 30–39, 40–49, 50–65, 66 plus. In the scenario where there is no change in community mixing when schools open while there is no considerable increase in the 20–65 year old age groups. However, when there is an increase in community mixing there is an immediate increase in cases in these age groups. In both scenarios, we see increases in the under 10 age group, the 10–19 age group and the over 65 age group. The increase in all three age groups is greater when community mixing increases. The increase in the over 65 group along with the student population is an interesting outcome from opening schools, especially as the cases in the other adult age groups do not increase in the no-change-in-mixing scenario. One possible reason for the increase in the over 65 population as schools open is that the grandparent caring that is built into the model. This could lead to the direct increase in transmission between children and the elderly that is seen in the model output. When the increase in cases due to schools opening in the over 65 age groups is paired with an increase in community mixing, we see the highest cases in any age group in the over 65 group.

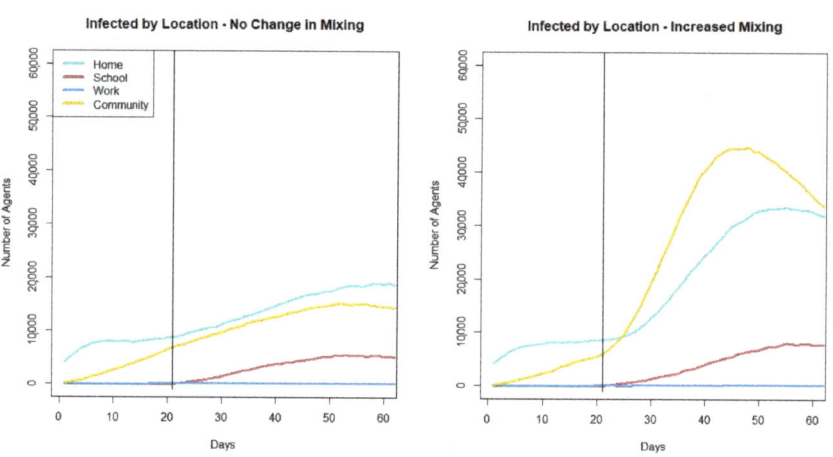

Figure 7. Plot showing average number of infectious agents at a given time based on their location of infection across 30 runs of the two mixing scenarios.

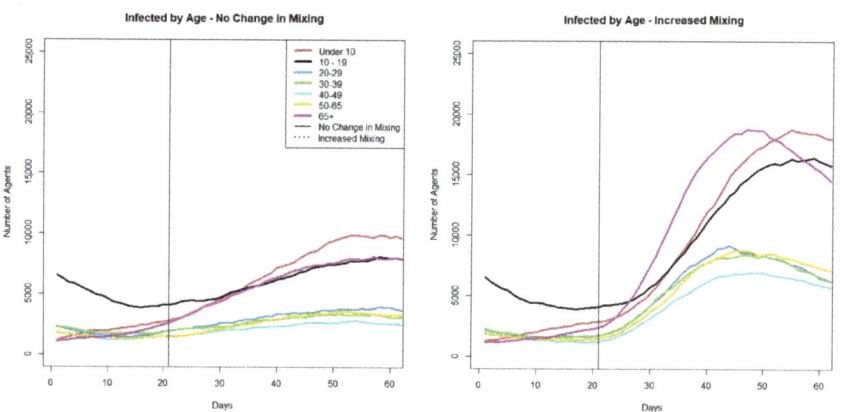

Figure 8. Plots showing average number of infectious agents at a given time based on their age across 30 runs of the two scenarios.

4. Discussion

Modeling the spread of COVID-19 has been a crucial piece in the pandemic response and agent-based models have played an important part of the modeling work done on COVID-19. The model presented in this paper is part of the literature surrounding models that were used during the COVID-19 pandemic. Models have been used to look at the effectiveness of contact tracing apps [15], or the impacts of interventions on ICU beds [14]. However, comparisons between model performance and model output are difficult to make, as there are no other agent-based models that simulate the spread of COVID-19 within Ireland, and it is not just the viral dynamics that allow for COVID-19 to spread as it has, but also the interactions of other factors, including the specific interventions a country put into place, the demographic makeup of a country, and the behaviors of the individuals. Additionally, as there is no set way to create an agent-based model for the spread of an infectious disease, parts of our model were designed to answer specific questions. For example, what was the impact of contact tracing or how does childcare by grandparents impact the number of cases in the over 65 population? Different models in the literature have included factors to address other questions. For example, Covasim looks at the health system capacity and thus has agents move from presymptomatic to mild, severe, and critical stages of infection [13]. We do not consider severity within our model but look at behaviors instead (not isolating, isolating, and waiting for a test). The Hoertel et al. model for France [14] also looks at health capacity and thus includes an agent's likelihood to have certain health conditions that might make COVID-19 more severe, such as obesity or diabetes. These factors are not included in our model, as we were not aiming to look at disease severity or health system capacity.

Agent-based models are computationally intensive and in some cases, work needs to be done to reduce the computing power needed to run the models. The scaling factor used in the model presented here reduces the number of agents needed to run the model which in turn decreases the memory needed to run the model. A scaling factor is used in other COVID-19 agent-based models, for example, the Covasim model [13] or the Thompson et al. model [16]; however, our scaling factor remains static while the factor used in the other models is dynamic. Although the scaling factor reduces the real-world fidelity of the model, we have shown through our model validation that the scaling of the model does not impact the average results. Thus the results produced by the model can help to better understand the COVID-19 pandemic and the impacts of different interventions.

The scaling factor does, however, lead to an increase in the variability in model output. The level of variability as well as how well the scaled model matches the output of an un-scaled model depends on the number of agents infected in the model. This suggests that there are thresholds above which the scaled model performs better. Future work on the scaling factor may involve investigating these thresholds in greater detail. For example, looking at different scaling factors, such as 1 agent to 50 people or 1 agent to 200 people, or alternative scaling methods, such as performing a clustering analysis on a set of individual characteristics, such as age, gender, family size, socioeconomic status, and geographic location, to find clusters of the population that can be represented by a single agent. This method would allow for variation in the 1 agent for X number of people scaling, such that 1 agent might represent 75 teenagers with one sibling in Dublin, but 1 agent might also represent 115 people who are 80 plus and living on their own in Leitrim. This clustered scaling would allow for a better representation of behavioral patterns among agent types and their importance to the course of the pandemic. For example, the 80 plus year old agents living in Leitrim might be greatly restricting their movements and thus not contributing as much to transmission, so their representation in the model would be down-weighted compared to the teenagers in Dublin who have higher levels of interactions and a greater contribution to transmission. A new method for scaling the results of the clustered model would need to be developed along with the model so as to not introduce artefactual results.

The results from our school opening experiment with the model shows how the agent-based model allows us to look at different scenarios and gain a deeper understanding of how changes in movements or interventions can impact an outbreak. With the agent-based model we can hold all other factors in the model constant and see how an increase in agent community mixing when schools reopen in the autumn impacts the number of cases. The agent-based model allows us to learn additional information about what might happen when schools open. When we do not have an increase in community mixing, we do not see a rapid increase of cases when schools open; as the model output when we do have increased community mixing does not show a large difference in cases originating within schools, this might suggest that opening schools might be relatively safe, and the resulting increase in cases around school opening might be more impacted by the actions outside of schools than within schools. This is likely because in Ireland during 2020 and 2021, schools were a controlled environment where students were required to wear masks and interact with pods of other students. Outside of school, students do not have to restrict their interactions with those within their school pod, leading to more contacts and increased chances of infection and are not required to wear masks. However, in both scenarios, we see an increase in cases in the over 65 population, which is one of the most vulnerable populations. This might suggest that in such a scenario, with schools reopening after summer holidays, it might be worthwhile to include some preventative measures to reduce cases in the older age groups. We can also compare the output of the test on school openings and background mixing to what really occurred in Ireland in September 2020. Real cases went up very gradually in the first 30 days after schools re-opened but then there was a large increase in cases by the end of October 2020. Based on our modeling results, this might suggest that there was an increase in mixing but the increase was between the two levels tested. Another possible explanation could be that initially when schools re-opened, the rest of the population continued to restrict their movements out of concern that cases would increase but when cases did not immediately increase in September, community mixing increased, leading to a rise in cases later.

The results of our validation and test experiment show that the model is both validated and useful. This gives a level of confidence in the model output, showing that the model results can be used in a pandemic or outbreak situation to help understand the spread of the disease. The agent-based model is not only able to provide information on the numbers infected, but also on the location of infection and the age groups infected. This additional information may be helpful in shaping policies or implementing restrictions.

There are a number of limitations of our model. No model is an exact replica of real life, and all models make assumptions. Some of the assumptions we have made should be considered when analyzing the results of the model. One example is that in the schools we model, we do not assign adult agents to be teachers. This could impact transmission between children and adults. In the real world, there is potential for transmission between students and staff in a school setting; however, some studies of COVID-19 transmission in schools in 2020 showed limited transmission in schools [35,36]. Additionally, the model only simulates the spread of COVID-19 in the Republic of Ireland and not in Northern Ireland. Because we do not simulate the spread of COVID-19 across the entirety of Ireland, there might be some key transportation patterns between border counties that are not included in the simulation that played a part in driving the pandemic in those border areas. Another limitation is in our generated contact networks. There is no existing data set for Ireland that provides contact patterns between age groups. We use the Netherlands POLYMOD data [27] to determine the number of contacts agents have. While we think these data are an OK approximation for Irish contact patterns, we are introducing some uncertainty into the model with this assumption. Model uncertainty is also introduced in the choice of parameters determining the dynamics of COVID-19. The parameters we use come from the literature and, where possible, from literature on the spread of COVID-19 in Ireland. However, even in the literature, there is a wide range of values for the different parameters, for example, in a review from 2020, published values for R_0 were found to range from 1.5 to 6.49 [37]. The selections we made for the model will impact the model output. The model was also created with the idea of looking at the short-term impacts of behavior changes or other interventions, so some assumptions, including assumptions around reinfections, were chosen with this in mind. This will likely impact the outcomes of the model if run for longer terms and for periods of the pandemic beyond 2020; thus, these assumptions would need to be adjusted.

It is important to note that this model was created during the COVID-19 pandemic as a tool designed to simulate the spread of COVID-19 in Ireland to better understand what might happen in the short term. In this paper, the model is validated off 2020 data, and we test the model on an example where initial conditions surrounding the model are based off of cases in 2020. For much of 2020 and 2021, Ireland was in strict lockdown, where non-essential workers were asked to work from home, and at times individuals were not allowed to go beyond 5 km from their homes. The lockdown interventions that can be implemented in the model reflect the strict nature of Ireland's lockdowns. At the time of publication, the situation is vastly different from that of 2020. While there are still many cases and deaths worldwide, vaccinations and previous infections have reduced the likelihood of contracting COVID-19 and the severity of the disease when contracted. Additionally, the strict lockdowns and travel restrictions have been lifted in most countries. While the model was validated on 2020 data, we included the ability to turn on a number of other other characteristics of the model, for example, multiple variants with different levels of infectiousness, or vaccinations that can take into account waning immunity. The model has and is evolving as the pandemic evolves. However, we feel that while having a model that is validated off 2020 data is a limitation, it is also important to have such a model and understand what we can learn from it to better prepare ourselves for the next potential pandemic.

5. Conclusions

Combined with other modeling techniques, such as a population level SEIR model, agent-based models can help to provide a greater picture of the future course of a pandemic and what the actual impact of interventions will be.

As it is possible that another pandemic will occur, it is necessary to take the lessons learned from the COVID-19 pandemic and create a better understanding of how modeling can help to respond to a pandemic situation. Additionally, looking at ways to make models that require high levels of resources, such as agent-based modeling, easier to run and use will improve their usability and uptake for future health crises.

Author Contributions: Conceptualization, E.H. and J.D.K.; methodology, E.H. and J.D.K.; software, E.H.; validation, E.H.; formal analysis, E.H.; writing—original draft preparation, E.H.; writing—review and editing, J.D.K. All authors have read and agreed to the published version of the manuscript.

Funding: This work was partly supported by the ADAPT Centre for Digital Content Technology which is funded under the SFI Research Centres Programme (Grant13/RC/2106_P2) and is co-funded under the European Regional Development Funds.

Institutional Review Board Statement: Not applicable.

Informed Consent Statement: Not applicable.

Data Availability Statement: Data available on request.

Acknowledgments: The model was constructed with the advice of members of the Irish Epidemiological Modelling Advisory Group (IEMAG). The authors wish to acknowledge the Irish Centre for High-End Computing (ICHEC) for the provision of computational facilities and support.

Conflicts of Interest: The authors declare no conflict of interest. The funders had no role in the design of the study; in the collection, analyses, or interpretation of data; in the writing of the manuscript; or in the decision to publish the results.

Abbreviations

The following abbreviations are used in this manuscript:

ABM	Agent-Based Model
IEMAG	Irish Epidemiological Modeling Advisory Group
SIR	Susceptible, Infected, Recovered
SEIR	Susceptible, Exposed, Infected, Recovered
CSO	Central Statistics Office
ODD	Overview, Design Concepts and Details

References

1. Department of Health. *Pandemic Flu—A National Framework for Responding to an Influenza Pandemic*; Technical Report; The Pandemic Influenza Preparedness Team Department of Health: London, UK, 2007.
2. Kao, R.R. The Role of Mathematical Modelling in the Control of the 2001 FMD Epidemic in the UK. *Trends Microbiol.* **2002**, *10*, 279–286. [CrossRef]
3. Simpson, C.R.; Beever, D.; Challen, K.; Angelis, D.D.; Fragaszy, E.; Goodacre, S.; Hayward, A.; Lim, W.S.; Rubin, G.J.; Semple, M.G.; et al. The UK's pandemic influenza research portfolio: A model for future research on emergin infections. *Lancet Infect. Dis.* **2019**, *19*, e295–e300. [CrossRef]
4. Ferguson, N.; Laydon, D.; Nedjati Gilani, G.; Imai, N.; Ainslie, K.; Baguelin, M.; Bhatia, S.; Boonyasiri, A.; Cucunuba Perez, Z.; Cuomo-Dannenburg, G.; et al. *Report 9: Impact of Non-Pharmaceutical Interventions (NPIs) to Reduce COVID19 Mortality and Healthcare Demand*; Technical Report; Imperial College: London, UK, 2020.
5. Gleeson, J.P.; Brendan Murphy, T.; O'Brien, J.D.; Friel, N.; Bargary, N.; O'Sullivan, D.J.P. Calibrating COVID-19 susceptible-exposed-infected-removed models with time-varying effective contact rates. *Philos. Trans. R. Soc. A Math. Phys. Eng. Sci.* **2022**, *380*, 20210120. [CrossRef]
6. Scott, N.; Palmer, A.; Delport, D.; Abeysuriya, R.; Stuart, R.M.; Kerr, C.C.; Mistry, D.; Klein, D.J.; Sacks-Davis, R.; Heath, K.; et al. Modelling the impact of relaxing COVID-19 control measures during a period of low viral transmission. *Med. J. Aust.* **2021**, *214*, 79–83. [CrossRef] [PubMed]
7. Hethcote, H.W. The Mathematics of Infectious Diseases. *Soc. Ind. Appl. Math. Rev.* **2000**, *42*, 599–653. [CrossRef]
8. Duan, W.; Fan, Z.; Gang, G.; Zhang, P.; Qiu, X. Mathematical and Computational Approaches to Epidemic Modeling: A Comprehensive Review. *Front. Comput. Sci.* **2015**, *9*, 806–826. [CrossRef] [PubMed]
9. Andrade, J.; Duggan, J. An evaluation of Hamiltonian Monte Carlo performance to calibrate age-structured compartmental SEIR models to incidence data. *Epidemics* **2020**, *33*, 100415. [CrossRef]
10. Pang, L.; Ruan, S.; Liu, S.; Zhao, Z.; Zhang, X. Transmission Dynamics and Optimal Control of Measles Epidemics. *Appl. Math. Comput.* **2014**, *256*, 131–147. [CrossRef]
11. Adam, D. Special report: The simulations driving the world's response to COVID-19. *Nature* **2020**, *580*, 316–318. [CrossRef] [PubMed]
12. Hunter, E.; Mac Namee, B.; Kelleher, J. An open-data-driven agent-based model to simulate infectious disease outbreaks. *PLoS ONE* **2018**, *13*, 1–35. [CrossRef]
13. Kerr, C.C.; Stuart, R.M.; Mistry, D.; Abeysuriya, R.G.; Rosenfeld, K.; Hart, G.R.; Núñez, R.C.; Cohen, J.A.; Selvaraj, P.; Hagedorn, B.; et al. Covasim: An agent-based model of COVID-19 dynamics and interventions. *PLoS Comput. Biol.* **2021**, *17*, 1–32. [CrossRef]
14. Hoertel, N.; Blachier, M.; Blanco, C.; Olfson, M.; Massetti, M.; Rico, M.S.; Limosin, F.; Leleu, H. A stochastic agent-based model of the SARS-CoV-2 epidemic in France. *Nat. Med.* **2020**, *26*, 1417–1421. [CrossRef]
15. Almagor, J.; Picascia, S. Exploring the effectiveness of a COVID-19 contact tracing app using an agent-based model. *Sci. Rep.* **2020**, *10*, 22235. [CrossRef]
16. Thompson, J.; McClure, R.; Blakely, T.; Wilson, N.; Baker, M.G.; Wijnands, J.S.; De Sa, T.H.; Nice, K.; Cruz, C.; Stevenson, M. Modelling SARS-CoV-2 disease progression in Australia and New Zealand: An account of an agent-based approach to support public health decision-making. *Aust. N. Z. J. Public Health* **2022**, *46*, 292–303. [CrossRef]
17. Bobashev, G.V.; Goedecke, D.M.; Yu, F.; Epstein, J.M. A Hybrid Epidemic Model: Combining The Advantages of Agent-Based and Equation Based-Approaches. In Proceedings of the 2007 Winter Simulation Conference, Washington, DC, USA, 9–12 December 2007; pp. 1532–1537. [CrossRef]
18. Hunter, E.; Mac Namee, B.; Kelleher, J. A Hybrid Agent-Based and Equation Based Model for the Spread of Infectious Diseases. *J. Artif. Soc. Soc. Simul.* **2020**, *23*, 14. [CrossRef]
19. Montañola-Sales, C.; Gilabert-Navarro, J.F.; Casanovas-Garcia, J.; Prats, C.; López, D.; Valls, J.; Cardona, P.J.; Vilaplana, C. Modeling tuberculosis in Barcelona. A solution to speed-up agent-based simulations. In Proceedings of the 2015 Winter Simulation Conference (WSC), Huntington Beach, CA, USA, 6–9 December 2015; pp. 1295–1306. [CrossRef]
20. Hunter, E.; Mac Namee, B.; Kelleher, J.D. A Model for the Spread of Infectious Diseases in a Region. *Int. J. Environ. Res. Public Health* **2020**, *17*, 3119. [CrossRef]
21. Wilensky, U. *Netlogo: Center for Connected Learning and Computer-Based Modeling*; Northwestern University: Evanston, IL, USA, 1999.
22. Hunter, E.; Kelleher, J.D. Adapting an Agent-Based Model of Infectious Disease Spread in an Irish County to COVID-19. *Systems* **2021**, *9*, 41. [CrossRef]
23. Hunter, E.; Mac Namee, B.; Kelleher, J.D. A Taxonomy for Agent-Based Models in Human Infectious Disease Epidemiology. *J. Artif. Soc. Soc. Simul.* **2017**, *20*, 2. [CrossRef]
24. CSO. Census 2011 Boundary Files. 2014. Available online: http://www.cso.ie/en/census/census2011boundaryfiles/ (accessed on 26 May 2016).
25. Central Statistics Office (CSO). Census 2016 Place of Work, School or College-Census of Anonymised Records (POWSCAR). 2017. Available online: https://www.cso.ie/en/census/census2016reports/powscar/ (accessed on 5 September 2018).
26. Hunter, E.; Kelleher, J.D. An ODD-Protocol for Agent-Based Model for the Spread of COVID-19 in Ireland. *Reports* **2022**, *1*. Available online: https://arrow.tudublin.ie/sknowmanrep/1/ (accessed on 14 April 2022).

27. Mossong, J.; Hens, N.; Jit, M.; Beutels, P.; Auranen, K.; Mikolajczyk, R.; Massari, M.; Salmaso, S.; Tomba, G.S.; Wallinga, J.; et al. Social Contacts and Mixing Patterns Relevant to the Spread of Infectious Diseases. *PLoS Med.* **2008**, *5*, e74. [CrossRef]
28. Hansen, C.H.; Michlmayr, D.; Gubbels, S.M.; Mølbak, K.; Ethelberg, S. Assessment of protection against reinfection with SARS-CoV-2 among 4 million PCR-tested individuals in Denmark in 2020: A population-level observational study. *Lancet* **2021**, *397*, 1204–1212. [CrossRef]
29. Thomas, J.C.; Weber, D.J. Concepts of Transmission and Dynamics. In *Epidemiologic Methods for the Study of Infectious Diseases*; Oxford University Press: New York, NY, USA, 2001; pp. 61–62.
30. Rodrigue, J.P.; Comtois, C.; Slack, B. *The Geography of Transport Systems*; Routledge, Taylor and Francis Group: London, UK, 2006.
31. Martin, J.; Carroll, C.; Khurshid, Z.; Moore, G.; Cosgrove, G.; Conway, R.; Buckley, C.; Browne, M.; Flynn, M.; Doyle, S. An overview of the establishment of a national contact tracing programme: A quality improvement approach in a time of pandemic. *HRB Open Res.* **2022**, *5*, 12. [CrossRef]
32. Carroll, C.; Conway, R.; O'Donnell, D.; Norton, C.; Hogan, E.; Browne, M.; Buckley, C.M.; Kavanagh, P.; Martin, J.; Doyle, S. Routine testing of close contacts of confirmed COVID-19 cases—National COVID-19 Contact Management Programme, Ireland, May to August 2020. *Public Health* **2021**, *190*, 147–151. [CrossRef] [PubMed]
33. Hunter, E.; Kelleher, J.D. A Framework for Validating and Testing Agent-based Models: A Case Study from Infectious Diseases Modelling. In Proceedings of the 34th annual European Simulation and Modelling Conference, Toulouse, France, 21–23 October 2020. [CrossRef]
34. OSI. COVID-19 HPSC Detailed Statistics Profile. 2022. Available online: https://data.gov.ie/dataset/covid-19-hpsc-detailed-statistics-profile?package_type=dataset (accessed on 10 March 2022).
35. Larosa, E.; Djuric, O.; Cassinadri, M.; Cilloni, S.; Bisaccia, E.; Vicentini, M.; Venturelli, F.; Rossi, P.G.; Pezzotti, P.; Bedeschi, E.; et al. Secondary transmission of COVID-19 in preschool and school settings in northern Italy after their reopening in September 2020: A population-based study. *Eurosurveillance* **2020**, *25*, 2001911. [CrossRef]
36. Heavey, L.; Casey, G.; Kelly, C.; Kelly, D.; McDarby, G. No evidence of secondary transmission of COVID-19 from children attending school in Ireland, 2020. *Eurosurveillance* **2020**, *25*, 2000903. [CrossRef]
37. Liu, Y.; Gayle, A.A.; Wilder-SMith, A.; Rocklov, J. The reproductive number of COVID-19 is higher compared to SARS coronavirus. *J. Travel Med.* **2020**. [CrossRef]

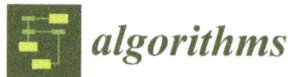

Article

Uncertainty in Visual Generative AI

Kara Combs [1], Adam Moyer [2] and Trevor J. Bihl [1,*]

[1] Sensors Directorate, Air Force Research Laboratory, Wright-Patterson Air Force Base, Dayton, OH 45322, USA; kara.combs.1@us.af.mil
[2] Analytics & Information Systems, Ohio University, Athens, OH 45701, USA; moyera@ohio.edu
* Correspondence: trevor.bihl.2@us.af.mil

Abstract: Recently, generative artificial intelligence (GAI) has impressed the world with its ability to create text, images, and videos. However, there are still areas in which GAI produces undesirable or unintended results due to being "uncertain". Before wider use of AI-generated content, it is important to identify concepts where GAI is uncertain to ensure the usage thereof is ethical and to direct efforts for improvement. This study proposes a general pipeline to automatically quantify uncertainty within GAI. To measure uncertainty, the textual prompt to a text-to-image model is compared to captions supplied by four image-to-text models (GIT, BLIP, BLIP-2, and InstructBLIP). Its evaluation is based on machine translation metrics (BLEU, ROUGE, METEOR, and SPICE) and word embedding's cosine similarity (Word2Vec, GloVe, FastText, DistilRoBERTa, MiniLM-6, and MiniLM-12). The generative AI models performed consistently across the metrics; however, the vector space models yielded the highest average similarity, close to 80%, which suggests more ideal and "certain" results. Suggested future work includes identifying metrics that best align with a human baseline to ensure quality and consideration for more GAI models. The work within can be used to automatically identify concepts in which GAI is "uncertain" to drive research aimed at increasing confidence in these areas.

Keywords: generative AI; image to text; computer vision; machine translation; uncertainty; text mining

Citation: Combs, K.; Moyer, A.; Bihl, T.J. Uncertainty in Visual Generative AI. *Algorithms* **2024**, *17*, 136. https://doi.org/10.3390/a17040136

Academic Editor: Alexander E.I. Brownlee

Received: 26 February 2024
Revised: 20 March 2024
Accepted: 25 March 2024
Published: 27 March 2024

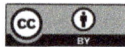

Copyright: © 2024 by the authors. Licensee MDPI, Basel, Switzerland. This article is an open access article distributed under the terms and conditions of the Creative Commons Attribution (CC BY) license (https://creativecommons.org/licenses/by/4.0/).

1. Introduction

Generative artificial intelligence (GAI) took the world by storm upon the public release of OpenAI's ChatGPT service in November 2022 [1]. Easily accessed for free through a chat-like web interface, it allowed for artificial intelligence (AI) to be seemingly available at anyone with an internet connection's fingertips. As opposed to scanning and searching several web pages for information, now, upon asking a question, its answer can be provided conveniently within a few seconds.

As its name suggests, GAI uses AI to create new results spanning applications in many different realms, such as text, images, videos, and audio [2]. As opposed to the original release of ChatGPT where only textual inputs and outputs were allowed, there has been a push to provide multi-modal support, especially on the outputs portion. The ability to automatically make AI-generated content (AIGC) has proven to be successful in many applications, including education [3,4], healthcare [5–7], engineering [8,9], and others. Shown in Table 1 are popular GAI language and image generator models. Language models are behind popular chatbots like ChatGPT, which uses GPT-3.5 (free) and GPT-4 (paid) [1,10], Bing Chat (GPT-4) [11], and Bard (PaLM 2) [12]. Image creation models allow users to input text to guide AI in the creation of an image. Not included in Table 1 are auditory applications (creation of audio or audio–visual content); however, this is an active area of research being explored. Given these models operate automatically, there is minimal human involvement after the training stage, which leads to concerns with these algorithms and models regarding their reliability, uncertainty, and accuracy [5,7].

Table 1. Generative AI models (modified from [13]).

Type	Model Family	Model Name	Release Date	Source(s)
Language models	OpenAI Generative Pre-Trained (GPT)	GPT-1	June 2018	[14,15]
		GPT-2	November 2019	[16]
		GPT-3	May 2020	[17]
		GPT-3.5	March 2022	[1]
		GPT-4	March 2023	[10,18]
	Google Language Model for Dialogue Applications (LaMDA)	LaMDA	May 2021	[19]
		LaMDA 2	May 2022	[20]
	Google Pathways Language Model (PaLM)	PaLM	March 2023	[21,22]
		PaLM 2	May 2023	[23,24]
	Meta Large Language Model Meta AI (LLaMA)	LLaMA	February 2023	[25,26]
	Inflection	Inflection-1	June 2023	[27]
Image generator models	OpenAI GLIDE	GLIDE	December 2021	[28]
	OpenAI DALL-E	DALL-E	February 2021	[29,30]
		DALL-E 2	April 2022	[31,32]
		DALL-E 3	October 2023	[33,34]
	Craiyon [1]	Craiyon [1]	July 2021	[35–37]
	Midjourney	Midjourney	February 2022	[38]
	Stability AI	Stable Diffusion	August 2022	[39,40]
	Google	Imagen	May 2022	[41]
		Parti	June 2022	[42]

[1] Craiyon was formerly known as DALL-E Mini until its name was changed in June 2022 at the request of OpenAI.

There has been reported dangerous and/or inappropriate behavior when interacting with GAI applications in general [43–45]. One individual reported that an early-access-version Bing Chat insisted that it was in love with the user and recommended that the individual leave his wife for it [46]. A chatbot trained for mental health agreed that the (artificial) patient should end their life within two message interchanges in one testing situation [47]. Several GAI chatbots also have preferences toward negative gender and racial stereotypes [45,48]. Though now corrected, ChatGPT provided inappropriate responses when prompted, exemplified by saying only men of particular ethnic backgrounds would make good scientists or by implying women in a laboratory environment were not there to conduct science [43]. These biases also carry over into the image-generation algorithms [49,50].

The literature attributes these biases to inherent issues with the image datasets they are trained upon, which include cultural underrepresentation/misrepresentation and content considered vulgar or violent (collectively titled "NSFW" or "Not safe for work") if not properly vetted [48,51]. This notably led to the removal of the MIT-produced 80 Million Tiny Images dataset (see [52]) in 2020 [53]. This issue continues to plague more recent datasets such as LAION-5B [54] (a subset of which was used to train Stable Diffusion), RedCaps [55], Google Conceptual Captions (GCC) [56], and more [51,57,58].

In August 2022, Prisma Labs released the app Lensa, a photo editor that used AI, specifically Stable Diffusion, on the backend, to alter photos [59]. Countless users complained that Lensa generated inappropriate versions of their fully clothed photos when uploaded [59,60]. Yet another photo editor, Playground AI (the Stable Diffusion backend for the free version), transformed an Asian MIT graduate into a blue-eyed and fair-skinned woman upon being asked to turn her photo into a "professional" photo [61]. When prompted to create a "photo portrait of a CEO", the average resulting faces as rendered by Stable Diffusion (V1.4 and V2) and DALL-E 2 all resembled fair-skinned males [49]. The volatile nature of GAI and its undesirable outcomes necessitates its regulation and guidance to ensure its ethical issue [48,62].

Future work with generative AI models needs to focus on eliminating unintentional biases or misrepresentations that have been the issue with previous versions. We propose the concept of "uncertainty" to measure where visual GAI is certain or uncertain regarding its inputs and outputs. Areas where GAI is uncertain are subject to more chaotic, stochastic results that can lead to unideal results related to the sensitive issues described earlier. To address these issues, we created three research questions:

1. How can GAI uncertainty be quantified?
2. How should GAI uncertainty be evaluated?
3. What text-to-image and image-to-text model combination performs best?

To answer these questions, we start with background on visual GAI, image quality assessment, and text evaluation methods. In Section 3, we describe the methodology used first in agnostic terms and then with details specific to this study. We propose a pipeline to compare the textual inputs and outputs of an image-to-text GAI algorithm, with the differences between the inputs and outputs representing GAI "uncertainty". The results are presented and discussed in Section 4, and then the paper wraps up with conclusions and future work in Section 5.

2. Background

Three fields were identified as foundational to this study. First, we discuss visual GAI including information from both text-to-image and image-to-text algorithms. Central to this paper is understanding how data can be fluid between their textual and visual states with minimal discrepancies. Therefore, we take advantage of multiple methods in both categories, text-to-image and image-to-text, within our data creation pipeline discussed in Section 3. Next, research in image quality assessment is discussed. Similar to the work of humans, just because an artistic rendition exists does not mean that it is a high-quality creation or even remotely what was commissioned in the first place. Addressing the text-to-image portion, an understanding of how image quality is quantified is presented to be compared later in the study. Finally, the background section concludes with text evaluation methods. To evaluate the pipeline's textual inputs and outputs, we explore the text mining field for how texts can be compared to one another as one answer.

2.1. Image Retrieval and Visual GAI

As GAI focuses on using AI to generate a new creation, visual GAI focuses on the translation between text and visualization [63]. The flow of translation can occur in either direction, either by taking text and transforming it into an image or by taking an image and deriving a description or caption [63–67]. Previous similar studies include [67,68]; however, we differentiate ourselves by utilizing different image-to-text and text-to-image generators, text prompts, and evaluation metrics.

2.1.1. Image-to-Text Generation

A significant amount of computer vision research is focused on classification; however, as an image has more complicated elements, a single label may not be appropriate to properly describe an image [69]. Therefore, some computer vision methods focus on creating a brief description of a given image [69–71]. Several datasets, such as the Microsoft Common Objects in Context (COCO) dataset (see [72]) and the Stanford image–paragraph dataset (see [73]), challenge researchers to create models that do this accurately and automatically [66,70,74]. Many other datasets also exist for the captioning of 2D images, 3D images, videos, and visual question answers [65]. Many techniques use the standard encoder and decoder architecture, growingly popular generative techniques (such as variational autoencoders (VAEs) and generative adversarial networks (GANs)), or reinforcement learning [70].

Recently, several large corporations have led the way in image-to-text research with several general-purpose image–text models capable of image captioning and visual question answering. In 2022, Microsoft released the Generative Image-to-text Transformer (GIT), which consists of one image encoder and one text decoder working together within a single task, as opposed to the historical setup where the encoder and decoder work on two separate tasks [75]. That same year, Salesforce developed an encoder–decoder model that works with a captioner that generates synthetic captions for images and a filter that removes irrelevant ones, called Bootstrapping Language-Image Pre-training for unified vision-language understanding and generation (BLIP) [76]. Google's DeepMind also joined with Flamingo, a family of visual language models that was trained using image–label pairs [77]. Later, in 2023, Microsoft presented the new Large Language and Vision Assistant (LLaVA) that combines the power of a vision encoder with a large language model [8], whereas in the same year, Salesforce built upon the earlier BLIP model with Bootstrapping Language-Image Pre-training with frozen unimodal models (BLIP-2), which combines frozen large language models and pre-trained image encoders via a "Querying Transformer" [78]. Additionally, in collaboration with academic partners, Salesforce also launched a fine-tuned version of BLIP-2 designed as an instruction tuning framework, InstructBLIP [79]. Image-to-text research is a growing field, like its related text-to-image methods.

2.1.2. Text-to-Image Generation

As pointed out in Table 2, there are several popular text-to-image diffusion models, which rapidly rose in popularity due to their accessibility and ease of use in 2021. Unlike popular generative adversarial networks (GANs) that consist of two neural networks (a discriminator and a generator) that are trained to create new images, a diffusion model adds or removes Gaussian noise to an image depending on the task [50,80].

Table 2. Comparison of text-to-image models (as of September 2023).

Model	Open-Source	Cost Structure	Tier/Image/Version	Cost
DALL-E 2	No	Pay-per-image	1024 × 1024 512 × 512 256 × 256	0.02 USD/image 0.018 USD/image 0.016 USD/image
DALL-E 3 (Quality: HD)	No No	Pay-per-image Pay-per-image	1024 × 1792 1792 × 1024 1024 × 1024	0.12 USD/image 0.12 USD/image 0.08 USD/image
DALL-E 3 (Quality: Standard)	No No	Pay-per-image Pay-per-image	1024 × 1792 1792 × 1024 1024 × 1024	0.08 USD/image 0.08 USD/image 0.04 USD/image
Craiyon	Yes	Free; Subscription	Free Supporter Professional	N/A 6 USD/mo or 60 USD/yr 24 USD/mo or 240 USD/yr
Stable Diffusion [1]	Yes	Free; Pay-per-image	Free Stable Diffusion XL 1.0 Stable Diffusion XL 0.9 Stable Diffusion XL 0.8 Stable Diffusion 2.1 [2] Stable Diffusion 1.5 [2]	N/A 0.016 USD/image 0.016 USD/image 0.005 USD/image 0.002 USD/image 0.002 USD/image
Midjourney	No	Subscription	Basic Standard Pro Mega	10 USD/mo or 96 USD/yr 30 USD/mo or 288 USD/yr 60 USD/mo or 576 USD/yr 120 USD/mo or 1152 USD/yr

[1] Cost depends on the number of denoising steps; the default number of 30 was used to estimate cost per image offered through Stability AI. [2] Regular Stable Diffusion models' cost depends on height and width; the default value of 512 × 512 was used to estimate cost per image.

OpenAI began the craze with its release of DALL-E in February 2021 [29]. DALL-E is a fine-tuned version of GPT-3 specifically for text-to-image generation through an autoregressive transformer architecture called the discrete variational autoencoder (dVAE) [29,30]. In response to this, an independent group of researchers introduced a smaller, open-source model originally called DALL-E Mini, but now known as Craiyon [36,37]. As opposed to DALL-E, Craiyon leverages a bidirectional encoder and pre-trained models to translate a textual prompt to an image [36]. Craiyon is a freemium service for which a free version exists for public use; however, a subscription plan can be purchased to remove the Craiyon logo and decrease generation time [35]. DALL-E 2 improves upon its earlier version by leveraging Contrastive Language-Image Pre-training (CLIP) embeddings before the diffusion step of the model [31,32].

In 2022, Google announced two models. First, they revealed Imagen, which is another diffusion model [30], but they later revealed a sequence-to-sequence model called Pathways AutoRegressive Text-to-Image Model (Parti) [42]. However, since Imagen and Parti have not been released for public use, little is known about their performance in comparison to the other models outside of the original conceptualization papers.

Yet another independent research laboratory produced the popular, Discord-hosted Midjourney, which is still operating under its open beta as of September 2023 [38]. Midjourney's software is proprietary, with limited public information about its internal mechanisms, but is only available through the purchase of a subscription plan.

Craiyon's greatest competitor yet for free open-source image generation was Stable Diffusion, which was released in August 2022 [39,40]. Stable Diffusion is a latent diffusion model, meaning the model works in a lower-dimensional latent space as opposed to the regular high-dimensional space in most other diffusion models, as shown in [40].

A comparison of the most popular models' fee structure breakdown is shown in Table 2. Since a human is not directly involved with the actual creation of an image (besides entering the prompt), the quality of AI-generated content has become another key point of interest.

2.2. Image Quality Assessment

Image quality assessment (IQA) is the evaluation of visual content [81]. Given that humans are typically the end users of such content, IQA is usually a subjective evaluation conducted by humans [81]. Traditional IQA focuses on the properties of the image itself as opposed to its visual context such as blurriness, noisiness, and distortion [81,82]. However, of interest to us is the evaluation of the content within AI-generated images—that is, how well is the information visually conveyed? To this aim, studies have identified subjective human-based methods for IQA [83]:

1. Single stimulus (Likert rating of a single image);
2. Double stimulus (Likert rating of two images presented one after another);
3. Forced choice (images are compared and the best one is selected);
4. Similarity judgment (given two images, the difference in quality between them is quantified).

IQA has the goal of facilitating the creation of representative AI-generated images that fit human alignment and perception [68]. Critical to evaluating this is the use of benchmark datasets, i.e., datasets that have previously been generated and have canonical truth identified. Several datasets exist for evaluation AIGC, such as TeTIm-Eval (Text-to-Image Evaluation), which was compared on DALL-E 2, Latent Diffusion, Stable Diffusion, GLIDE (Guided Language to Image Diffusion for Generation and Editing), and Craiyon [84]. Another dataset is the AGIQA-3K dataset (AI-generated Images Quality Assessment—3000), which aims to better capture both human perception and alignment following the Inception Score [85,86].

2.3. Text Evaluation Methods

Evaluation methods and metrics are needed to determine the validity of auto-generated captions [63,67]. Popular evaluation metrics are shown in Table 3, but more extensive reviews currently exist in the literature [63,87]. The MS COCO Dataset Challenge uses BLEU, ROUGE, METEOR, CIDEr, and SPICE to evaluate performance, so these have become the status quo for evaluating the similarity between texts [74]. Though not a text-to-text evaluation method, in the realm of automated image captioning, CLIPScore is worthy of mentioning due to being "reference-less" [88]. CLIPScore, based on the CLIP model originally proposed in [30], allows for the direct comparison of an image to its candidate caption via CLIP model embeddings [88].

Table 3. Popular text evaluation methods.

Metric	Description	Citation
Bilingual Evaluation Understudy (BLEU)	Focused on n-gram precision between reference and candidate	[89]
Recall-Oriented Understudy for Gisting Evaluation (ROUGE)	Based on the syntactic overlap, or word alignment, between references and candidates	[90]
Metric for Evaluation of Translation with Explicit Ordering (METEOR)	Measures based on unigram precision and recall	[91]
Translation Edit Rate (TER)	Calculated based on the number of operations needed to transform a candidate into a reference	[92]
TER-Plus (TERp)	Extension of TER that also factors in partial matches and word order	[93]
Consensus-based Image Description Evaluation (CIDEr)	Leverages term frequency-inverse document frequency (TF-IDF) as weights when comparing matching candidate and reference n-grams	[94]
Semantic Propositional Image Caption Evaluation (SPICE)	Determines similarity by focusing on comparing the semantically rich content of references and candidates	[95]
Bidirectional Encoder Representations from Transformers Score (BERTScore)	Utilizes BERT embeddings to compare the similarity	[96]

As text evaluation metrics have evolved, text mining has inspired the usage of cosine similarity metrics to measure how alike two texts may be. Over the past decade, word embedding models have become increasingly popular within the natural language processing field ever since the release of the vector space model Word2Vec in 2013 [97,98]. Though vector space models existed before 2013 (see [99]), the Word2Vec neural network approach to transforming varying lengths of text into a multi-dimension single vector was particularly exciting because of its ability to quantify semantic and syntactic information in a comparatively low-dimensional space. Vector space models allow for any word, sentence, or document to be represented and compared on a mathematical basis, usually to determine similarity or dissimilarity based on the cosine similarity metric [100].

As an alternative to the machine translation metrics above, cosine similarity is another evaluation metric of interest when comparing two texts. For two vectors, A and B, their cosine similarity is given by

$$CosineSimilarity(A, B) = \frac{A \cdot B}{\|A\| \|B\|}. \qquad (1)$$

Cosine similarity ranges from 0, meaning completely dissimilar, to 1, meaning exactly alike; although a negative cosine similarity is mathematically possible, it is considered to be 0. Word2Vec was followed by several other vector space models, with Global Vectors (GloVe) (see [101]) and FastText (see [102]) being the most prominent [103]. The embeddings of vector space models are static, meaning there is no variation for words with multiple meanings; however, this was addressed in more recent word embedding models that have contextualized vectors, such as Embeddings from Language Models (ELMo) [104], XLNet [105], and the Bidirectional Encoder Representations from Transformers (BERT) family of models [106]. BERT was released in 2018 (see [107]) and was soon followed by the Robustly optimized BERT pre-training Approach (RoBERTa) (see [108]), A Lite BERT (ALBERT) (see [109]), and a distilled version of BERT and RoBERTa (DistilBERT and DistilRoBERTa, respectively) (see [110]) [106]. Based on different pre-training data and international architecture, each word embedding model yields a different vector representation of a block of text, which thus yields different cosine similarity values when passed through each model.

3. Methodology

To measure uncertainty in visual GAI, we design an agnostic pipeline to compare textual image descriptions to the textual inputs (called "prompts") as shown in Figure 1. First, a database of prompts (green data block of Figure 1) is needed, which will be used as inputs into the text-to-image visual generative AI model. Next, this text-to-image (blue block of Figure 1) model generates an image based on the prompt. Then, the image that is produced is sent to an image-to-text (grey block of Figure 1) model to create an AI-generated caption of the image. Finally, the resulting caption is to be evaluated against the textual prompt used to originally generate the image (orange block of Figure 1). During the evaluation step, uncertainty is quantified as the similarity gap between the original textual prompt (from the database) and the resulting caption (provided by the image-to-text model). This is an agnostic, modular pipeline that can utilize different datasets, models, and evaluation methods to measure uncertainty in similar problems. The remainder of this section discusses the specific dataset, model, and evaluation used in this study.

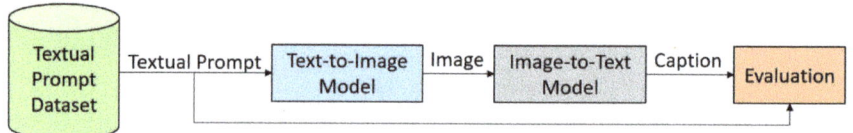

Figure 1. Uncertainty in visual GAI evaluation agnostic pipeline.

The pipeline in Figure 1 was customized for this study with the selected dataset, models, and evaluation methods shown in Figure 2. This process is explained more in-depth in Sections 3.1–3.4. The textual prompt dataset was provided by the modified version of the Sternberg and Nigro dataset used in [111], which produced 495 initial prompts.

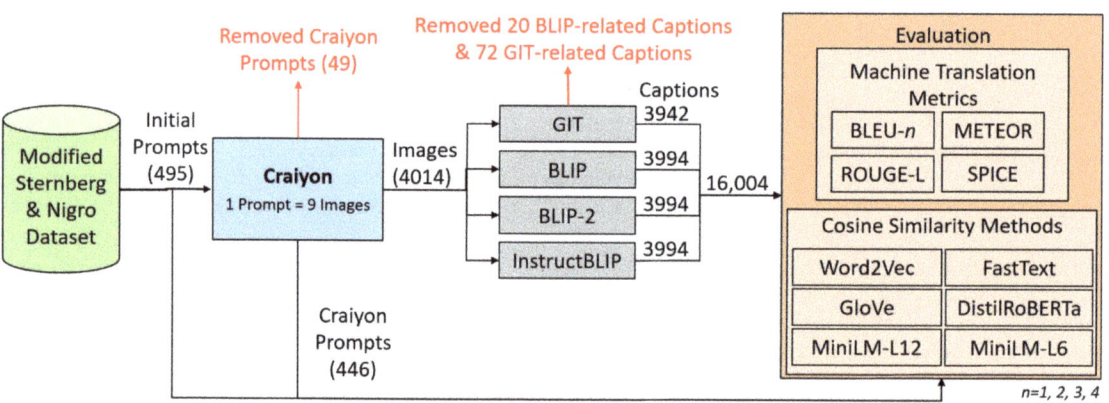

Figure 2. Customized pipeline for study.

The selected text-to-image model was Craiyon V3 [35–37]. Craiyon performs 2 unique steps. First, it creates its own version of the initial prompt, which we will call the "Craiyon prompt" (e.g., the initial prompt is "soap" and the Craiyon prompt adds details such that the new prompt is "a bar of soap on a white background"). This Craiyon prompt is used to create nine images by default. Therefore, every initial prompt yields 1 Craiyon prompt and 9 resulting images. Of the 495 initial problems, 49 were removed for quality reasons, leaving 446 initial prompts with corresponding Craiyon prompts. Craiyon creates 9 images per prompt, so the 446 remaining prompts were turned into 4014 images by Craiyon.

All 4014 images were passed through four image-to-text models—GIT [75], BLIP [76], BLIP-2 [78], and InstructBLIP [79]—for later comparison to one another. Due to various quality control reasons discussed in Section 3.3, not every image had a sufficient caption generated. Therefore, the insufficient captions were removed from the analysis. Thus, there were 16,004 total captions (3942 for GIT and 3994 for each BLIP-family model).

These captions were then evaluated on a variety of metrics, including machine translation methods and the cosine similarity of word embeddings. Seven machine translation methods were selected: Bilingual Evaluation Understudy (BLEU) (BLEU-1, BLEU-2, BLEU-3, and BLEU-4 were used, where the number represents the number of matching n-grams BLEU looks for) [89], Recall-Oriented Understudy for Gisting Evaluation—Longest common subsequence (ROUGE-L) [90], Metric for Evaluation of Translation with Explicit ORdering (METEOR) [91], and Semantic Propositional Image Caption Evaluation (SPICE) [95]. For the cosine similarity method, six models were selected: Word2Vec [97,98], Global Vectors (GloVe) [101], FastText [102], Distilled Robustly optimized Bidirectional Encoder Representations from Transformers approach (DistilRoBERTa) [110], Mini Language Model 12 Layer (MiniLM-L12) [112], and MiniLM 6 Layer (MiniLM-L6) [112].

3.1. Textual Prompts: Modified Sternberg and Nigro Dataset

The textual prompt dataset selected was a modified version of the Sternberg and Nigro textual analogy dataset used in [111]. The original Sternberg and Nigro dataset consisted of 197 word-based analogies in the "*A* is to *B* as *C* is to [what]?" form where the respondents had 4 options to choose from to complete the analogy [113]. Morrison modified this dataset so that respondents only had 2 options (the correct answer and the distractor) to pick from. The modified version of the dataset was selected due to the original dataset being lost. The modified Sternberg and Nigro dataset is particularly fascinating due to its inclusion of abstract and ambiguous concepts such as "true" and "false". The inability to visually represent these concepts has limited visual analogical reasoning research, which is intended to be expanded through the application of AIGC [114]. However, for this research, the individual words within the analogies were used as inputs to the text-to-image model. For example, analogy 157 is dirt is to soap as pain is to pill (correct answer) or hurt (distractor); this is stylized as Dirt:Soap::Pain:{Pill,Hurt}. Each word is used as a textual prompt to the text-to-image model. Due to time and resource limitations, only analogies 99–197 were considered for a total of 495 initial prompts.

3.2. Text-to-Image Model: Craiyon

The text-to-image model selected was Craiyon V3 (formerly known as DALL-E Mini), which uses a transformer and generator to create images from a textual prompt [35–37]. Craiyon was selected due to having a free tier (unlike Midjourney and DALL-E 2) and considering its previous success established in the literature [114–116]. Internally, Craiyon creates its prompt based on the initial prompt to generate nine images per prompt. The initial prompt, the Craiyon prompt, and the resulting nine images had five cases of coordination, as shown in Figure 3.

In Figure 3, well-coordinated prompts and corresponding images are highlighted in green. In Case A, we see the two prompts and the images all convey the same concept. In Case B, the two prompts align; however, the generated images are unrelated to either prompt. The initial prompt and the images are aligned in Case C, but in Case D, only the Craiyon prompt and images are aligned. Finally, in Case E, both prompts and the images appear to be unrelated to one another. Ideally, we would want all the data to fall in Case A; however, Cases C and D are better than the remaining two, Cases B and E, in this study. This is because we are comparing the prompts to the generated images, so if either of the prompts aligns with the images, the results will be inherently poor.

Case	A	B	C	D	E
Initial Prompt	Doctor	Arithmetic	Penny	Circle	See
Craiyon Prompt	A doctor in a white coat with a stethoscope	Mathematical symbols on white background	A smiling woman named Penny	Geometric abstract design with circles in vivid colors	A majestic fox with a fiery orange coat standing on a rocky ledge silhouetted against a setting sun
Craiyon Images	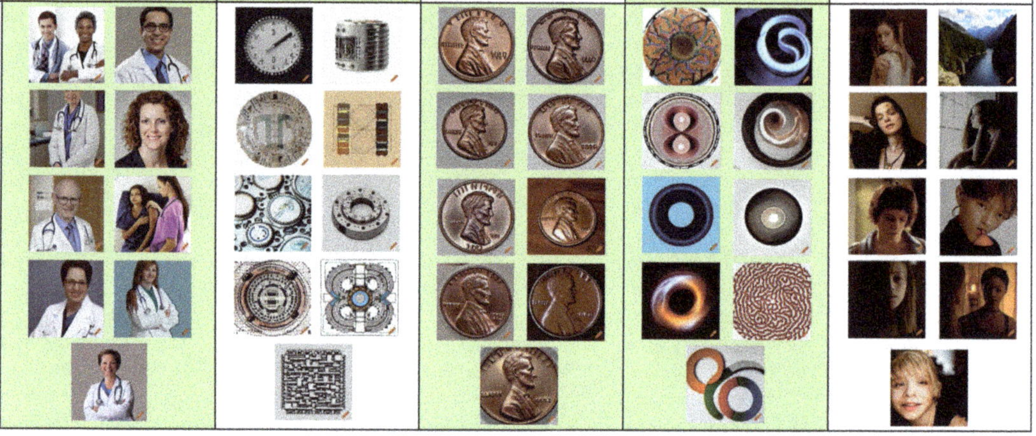				

Figure 3. Select initial and corresponding Craiyon prompts.

A total of 49 initial prompts were removed due to quality reasons, which reduced the number of Craiyon prompts created to 446. The quality reasons were often due to triggering a safety filter or due to Craiyon being unable to create its prompt from the given initial prompt. Examples of these prompts are shown in Table 4. Additionally, Craiyon generates 9 images per prompt; therefore, for the 446 prompts, there were 4014 images created.

Table 4. Initial prompts that produced removed Craiyon prompts.

Initial Prompt	Craiyon Prompt
Different	Sorry unable to determine the nature of the image
Worst	Invalid caption
New	Undefined
Defraud	Warning explicit content detected

3.3. Image-to-Text Models: GIT, BLIP, BLIP-2, and InstructBLIP

Four image-to-text models were selected for comparison: GIT [75], BLIP [76], BLIP-2 [78], and InstructBLIP [79]. All 4014 images were passed through each of the models. For some prompts, a caption could not be generated, or a blank caption was generated by the image-to-text model. Within the GIT model, this affected 72 captions, whereas for the BLIP family (BLIP, BLIP-2, and InstructBLIP), this occurred within 20 captions. Therefore, there were only 3942 GIT captions compared to the 3994 captions created by each BLIP-family model, for a total of 16,004 captions generated for comparison.

3.4. Textual Evaluation Metrics

To measure uncertainty, we survey a total of seven machine translation methods and we apply the cosine similarity metric to six word embedding models for a total of thirteen metrics for comparison to one another. We are interested in whether "uncertainty" is prominent when measured by these metrics. Textual evaluation is used to evaluate how similar two separate texts are; these can span from full documents to single lines. The "ground truth" text is called a "reference" and the text being compared to it is called a "candidate". Each image has two references, the initial and Craiyon prompts, which will be compared to the four candidates and the captions generated by the image-to-text models. In comparison to the cosine similarity metric, the machine translation metrics are better established and more direct.

Originally, machine translation metrics were used to evaluate automated translations; however, they also apply to automated image caption generation. Focusing on the latter, the machine translation methods used to separately compare each prompt (initial and Craiyon versions) as the references to the generated caption created by each of the image-to-text models were BLEU [89], ROUGE-L [90], METEOR [91], and SPICE [95]. These metrics, along with CIDEr, are the metrics used in the Microsoft Common Objects in Context (dubbed "MS COCO") Caption Evaluation challenge (see [117]); however, CIDEr was excluded as not applicable since it requires multiple candidate captions [94]. These methods allow for the consideration of multiple reference statements; therefore, each candidate caption was simultaneously compared to the initial and Craiyon prompts as shown in Figure 4. It is notable that there were four variants of the BLEU metric: BLEU-1, BLEU-2, BLEU-3, and BLEU-4. BLEU-1 looks for matching 1-gram, or words, between the texts. Then, BLEU-2 looks for matching 2-gram, where two words appear sequentially in order in both texts. For example, consider Phrase A, "pretty dog", and Phrase B, "pretty brown dog". Despite "pretty" and "dog" appearing sequentially in both phrases, the BLEU-2 score would be 0 because Phrase B breaks up the 2-gram, "pretty dog", with the word "brown". The case for BLEU-3 and BLEU-4 follows inductively. This process was repeated for each of the four machine translation metrics, whose scores ranged from 0, meaning dissimilar, to 1, meaning very similar. In total, each image had four caption candidates each evaluated by seven machine translation metrics for a total of 28 scores.

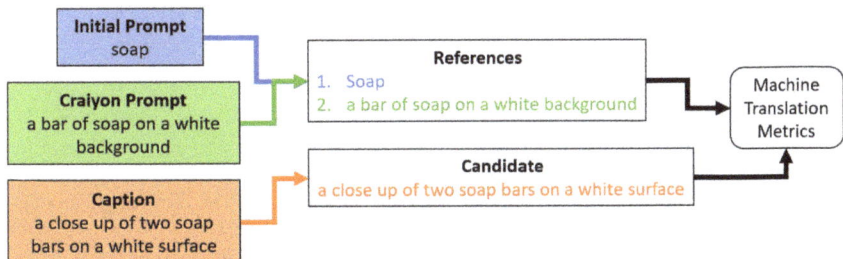

Figure 4. Machine translation input transformation.

The cosine similarity metrics are similar, as they range from 0 for dissimilar to 1 for highly similar; however, their implementation is different from the machine translation metrics. Cosine similarity is a popular metric for measuring similarity between vectors, such as word embeddings. However, to apply cosine similarity, it requires that the prompts and captions be transformed into their word embedding form(s), which is model-dependent. Six popular word embedding models were selected: Word2Vec [97,98], GloVe [101], FastText [102], DistilRoBERTa [110], MiniLM-L12 [112], and MiniLM-L6 [112].

Each prompt, the initial and Craiyon versions, and the four generated captions were transformed into their word embedding versions, visually represented in Figure 5. This transformation was performed by retrieving the word embedding for each word present in the prompt/caption from a pre-trained version of the models. In the event the prompt/caption had more than one word, each word in the prompt/caption's embedding was summed to create the overall prompt/caption embedding. Then, the caption embedding was compared separately to the initial prompt embedding and the Craiyon prompt embedding via their cosine similarity (see Equation (1)). In total, each image had its four captions and two prompts compared to one another (eight comparisons) in their six word embedding forms (i.e., eight comparisons by six forms) for a total of 48 cosine similarity scores.

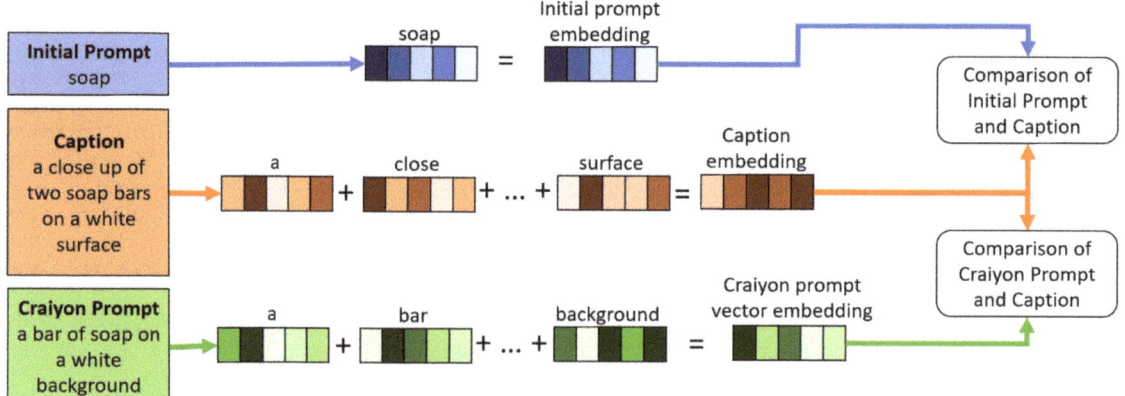

Figure 5. Cosine similarity input transformation.

4. Results and Discussion

The methodology described in Section 3 was applied to all prompt–caption pairs. An instance of the pipeline we used in this study is shown in Figure 6. An initial prompt is passed to Craiyon, which generates a Craiyon prompt and nine resulting images (for our purposes here, only one of those images is shown). Next, the generated image is passed onto our four image-to-text models, which each generate a caption. Finally, for the evaluation, this one image generates 76 similarity scores. There are 28 machine translation scores representing each of the seven machine translation metrics when evaluating each of the four image-to-text models. The remaining 48 scores are evenly split between those that were comparing the image caption to the initial and the Craiyon prompts. It is notable that Craiyon produces nine images for each prompt; therefore, this is repeated nine times for a total of 684 scores for each properly generated caption.

The results of the average evaluation score for each metric are shown in Tables 5–7. Table 5 shows the metrics for the machine translation methods since the initial and Craiyon prompts were used as references for the candidate (generated caption) to be compared at once. The BLEU, ROUGE, METEOR, and SPICE scores range from 0 (least ideal) to 1 (most ideal). Since this ability was not available for the cosine similarity results, the generated captions' cosine similarities to the initial prompt are shown in Table 6 and their cosine similarity to the Craiyon prompt is shown in Table 7. Due to how cosine similarities are calculated, a negative value is possible, but the effective scale ranges from 0 (completely dissimilar) to 1 (exactly alike). Despite the metrics being measured on the same scale, machine translation scores look at the replication of words, phrases, etc., in the prompts and captions, whereas cosine similarity considers how similar the prompt and caption are to one another.

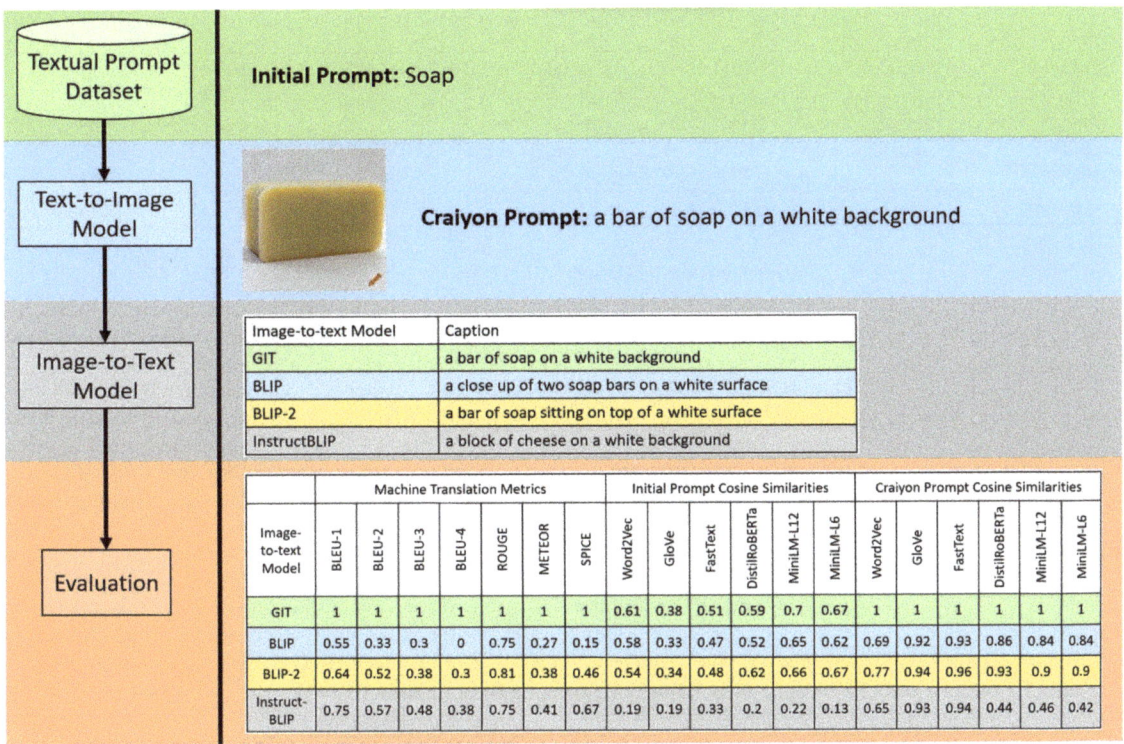

Figure 6. Metric calculation example walkthrough.

Table 5. Machine translation metrics and scores.

Model	BLEU-1	BLEU-2	BLEU-3	BLEU-4	ROUGE	METEOR	SPICE
GIT	19.4%	4.4%	1.2%	0.4%	23.6%	9.9%	7.1%
BLIP	15.1%	3.4%	0.8%	0.2%	20.3%	9.3%	6.6%
BLIP-2	20%	4.4%	1.4%	0.4%	24.3%	10.1%	7.2%
InstructBLIP	19.4%	4.5%	1.4%	0.5%	23.5%	10%	7.3%
Average	18.5%	4.2%	1.2%	0.4%	22.9%	9.8%	7.2%

Table 6. Average cosine similarity between initial prompt and generated captions.

Model	Word2Vec	GloVe	FastText	DistilRoBERTa	MiniLM-L12	MiniLM-L6
GIT	32.2%	40%	47.7%	22.3%	24.7%	25.3%
BLIP	31.7%	39.5%	50.2	18.3%	20.3%	20.4%
BLIP-2	32.4%	40.1%	48.1%	21.3%	23.3%	24%
InstructBLIP	32.5%	40.3%	49.8%	21.8%	24%	24.5%
Average	32.2%	40%	49%	20.9%	23.1%	23.6%

Table 7. Average cosine similarity between Craiyon prompt and generated captions.

Model	Word2Vec	GloVe	FastText	DistilRoBERTa	MiniLM-L12	MiniLM-L6
GIT	41.7%	72.1%	78.1%	28.2%	27.1%	28.1%
BLIP	42.5%	73.8%	79.2%	25.5%	24.3%	25.3%
BLIP-2	42.3%	73.2%	79.4%	27.6%	26.5%	27.5%
InstructBLIP	43.8%	72.1%	78.4%	28.7%	27.4%	28.6%
Average	42.6%	72.8%	78.8%	27.5%	26.3%	27.4%

4.1. Machine Translation Results

In Table 5, we see the BLEU-1 score is highest compared to the remaining BLEU scores, which is as expected since the prompts/captions were relatively short (typically less than ten words before the removal of stop words). Given the very small values for BLEU-2 through BLEU-4 (cosine similarity less than 0.05), they may not be appropriate to consider for future similar analyses. ROUGE consistently scored the four image-to-text models the highest, being in the 20–25% range. METEOR scored the captions around the 10% value and SPICE was lower, around the 60–70% range. BLIP consistently scored slightly lower than the remaining three on all the machine translation metrics; however, on average all the metrics scored the prompt–caption comparison relatively low.

4.2. Cosine Similarity Results

When using the initial prompt to compare the cosine similarity to the captions in Table 6, we had a wide variety of scores based on the word embeddings from various vector space models (Word2Vec, GloVe, and FastText) and pre-trained language models (DistilRoBERTa, MiniLM-L12, and MiniLM-L6). There is a clear gap of at least 0.05 between the vector space models and the pre-trained language models. Word2Vec scored the captions the lowest of the vector space models, but higher than any of the pre-trained language models, with values around 32%. GloVe scored captions higher, around the 40% similarity mark, but FastText gave the highest similarity scores, near 50% similarity. Though these scores are higher than the machine translation values, 50% would correspond with a neutral prompt/caption, meaning they are neither dissimilar nor similar. All the pre-trained language models gave relatively low similarity scores within the 18–26% range. This performance is expected to a degree since a one-word initial prompt is typically being compared to a multi-word sentence. Using the example from Figure 6, the initial prompt is "soap" and the GIT-created caption is "a bar of soap on a white background". Even though "soap" is in the caption, there are several other words that influence the sentence vector, which would have to cancel one another out perfectly to be left with a vector equivalent to the word embedding for "soap".

Table 7 includes the highest scores from this study across the board. Opposed to comparing the initial prompt, the Craiyon prompt is used for comparison to the generated caption. Since the Craiyon prompts were structured more similarly to the generated captions, it is not surprising that the values in Table 7 are higher than those in Table 6. However, similar behaviors exist between the models presented in both tables; vector space models provide higher similarities to the pre-trained language models. Word2Vec still assigned the lowest similarity scores amongst the vector space models, but there is about a 10% increase from the average similarity using the initial prompt. We see more significant jumps into the 70s for GloVe and FastText, which is approximately a 30% increase from the initial prompt scores in Table 6. All the pre-trained language models remained in the 20–30% range with single-digit increases from when the initial prompt was used.

4.3. Major Results

Although Tables 5–7 all have scores within the same range, they cannot necessarily be compared directly to one another given they each have different inputs that affect their resulting output. However, several high-level conclusions can be drawn:

1. Machine translation methods yielded consistently low scores in comparison to the cosine similarity scores;
2. For the cosine similarity metrics, the Craiyon prompts yielded higher scores than the initial prompts when comparing them with the generated captions;
3. Vector space models (Word2Vec, GLoVe, and FastText) were most generous with their similarity scores compared to pre-trained language models;
4. Image-to-text models minimally affected the similarity scores.

These major results show how various text evaluation methods can be used to evaluate "uncertainty" within generative AI models. As the various image-to-text models did not seem to impact the uncertainty quantification, the evaluation metrics are what researchers should study. The "best" evaluation metric is dependent on validation by human judgment and how much "uncertainty" a human believes to be associated with a prompt–caption pair.

These results suggest there is a significant amount of uncertainty within the AIGC based on our metrics. One potential explanation for this is the existence of many data elements classified as Case B (the prompts do not align with the images) or E (neither the prompts nor the images align with one another) from Figure 3. The detrimental results of this can be seen in Figure 6, where the Craiyon prompt was "a bar of soap on a white background" and the InstructBLIP caption was "a block of cheese on a white background". Though these two sentences have different subjects, they share six out of eight words, yet still received low cosine similarity scores from the pre-trained language models and no score exceeding 0.75 for the machine translation metrics. Minimizing, if not eliminating, any data point that falls into Case B or E (see Figure 3) would assist in ensuring these scores are meaningful.

5. Conclusions and Future Work

AI-generated content (AIGC), especially its visual variety, has had an unprecedented rate of production with the rise of high-quality and easy-to-use interfaces exemplified by DALL-E 2, Midjourney, and Craiyon. Despite many astounding results, there are still areas where these generative AI (GAI) models show "uncertainty" when transforming a textual prompt into its corresponding visual counterpart. We first propose a generic pipeline that has four main modules: text-to-image, image-to-text, image quality assessment, and text evaluation methods. The textual prompt dataset is used to prompt the text-to-image generator to create a corresponding image. This image is passed to an image-to-text model to produce a corresponding caption, which is compared to the initial textual prompt used for that particular image.

This generic pipeline was specified in this study such that the textual prompt dataset was the Sternberg and Nigro analogy dataset originally used in [111], but for accessibility, we used its modified version proposed in [113]. The image-to-text model selected was Craiyon V3 due to its cost and versatility [35–37]. Four image-to-text models were selected, which each produced one caption per image: GIT [75], BLIP [76], BLIP-2 [78], and InstructBLIP [79]. Several evaluation metrics were selected for comparison, split between typical machine translation metrics (BLEU [89], ROUGE-L [90], METEOR [91], and SPICE [95]) and cosine similarity based on various word embedding models (Word2Vec [97,98], GLoVe [101], FastText [102], DistilRoBERTa [110], MiniLM-L12 [112], and MiniLM-L6 [112]). Each evaluation metric was calculated for each prompt–caption pair.

To answer the primary question of how to quantify uncertainty, we used the scores from the evaluation metrics ranging from 0 (dissimiSlar) to 1 (exactly alike). The four image-to-text models behaved comparably to one another across all the metrics used. The machine translation scores on average were lower than the cosine similarity methods, with BLEU-1 scoring the hisghest. There was more variation within the cosine similaritsy metrics. FastText provided the highest similarity scores across all the other metrics; however, GLoVe was close behind. Vector space models (Word2Vec, GLoVe, and FastText) appeared to give higher similarity scores compared to the word embedding models (DistilRoBERTa,

MiniLM-12, and MiniLM-6). In conclusion, it appears that the image-to-text model has a limited impact on the analysis, whereas the evaluation metrics differ greatly. The quantification of where AI is certain or uncertain is an important step in the creation of usage guidance and policy.

Regarding future work, one idea would be to eliminate elements of the dataset that fall within Cases B or E to minimize the number of "garbage in, garbage out" results. The ultimate goal is to better engineer the prompts such that the images are always representative of the intended concept. Further exploration into prompt engineering is needed to help eliminate some of these issues and minimize the amount of uncertainty with AIGC. Of the metrics used to evaluate the results, for shorter prompts/captions, as in our case, there is little value added to the BLEU-3 and BLEU-4 scores. These scores may provide more insights when used to evaluate longer prompts/captions. Considering other image-to-text models that provide greater details or longer captions would also be interesting in a later study. Within image quality assessment, a human baseline is often established to which the automated metrics are to be compared in determining which one reflects human judgment the best. A human factors study to establish this quality baseline is currently being conducted by the researchers. Upon the establishment of a baseline, other popular text evaluation metrics may be of interest to explore on the dataset as well.

Author Contributions: Conceptualization: K.C., A.M. and T.J.B. Data curation: K.C., A.M. and T.J.B. Methodology: K.C., A.M. and T.J.B. Writing—original draft: K.C., A.M. and T.J.B. Writing—review and editing: K.C., A.M. and T.J.B. All authors have read and agreed to the published version of the manuscript.

Funding: This research received no external funding.

Data Availability Statement: The modified Sternberg and Nigro dataset from [111] will be made available by the authors on request. The images presented in this article are not readily available because of Department of Defense data and information sharing restrictions.

Acknowledgments: The authors would like to thank Arya Gadre and Isaiah Christopherson for generating the image dataset used in this study during the 2023 AFRL Wright Scholars Research Assistance Program. The views expressed in this paper are those of the authors and do not necessarily represent any views of the U.S. Government, U.S. Department of Defense, or U.S. Air Force. This work was cleared for Distribution A: unlimited release under AFRL-2023-5966.

Conflicts of Interest: The authors declare no conflicts of interest.

References

1. OpenAI Introducing ChatGPT. 2022. Available online: https://openai.com/blog/chatgpt (accessed on 24 March 2024).
2. Google. Generative AI Examples. 2023. Available online: https://cloud.google.com/use-cases/generative-ai (accessed on 24 March 2024).
3. Baidoo-Anu, D.; Ansah, L.O. Education in the era of generative artificial intelligence (AI): Understanding the potential benefits of ChatGPT in promoting teaching and learning. *J. AI* **2023**, *7*, 52–62. [CrossRef]
4. Lodge, J.M.; Thompson, K.; Corrin, L. Mapping out a research agenda for generative artificial intelligence in tertiary education. *Australas. J. Educ. Technol.* **2023**, *39*, 1–8. [CrossRef]
5. Mesko, B.; Topol, E.J. The imperative for regulatory oversight of large language models (or generative AI) in healthcare. *NPJ Digit. Med.* **2023**, *6*, 120. [CrossRef] [PubMed]
6. Godwin, R.C.; Melvin, R.L. The role of quality metrics in the evolution of AI in healthcare and implications for generative AI. *Physiol. Rev.* **2023**, *103*, 2893–2895. [CrossRef] [PubMed]
7. Oniani, D.; Hilsman, J.; Peng, Y.; Poropatich, R.K.; Pamplin, J.C.; Legault, G.L.; Wang, Y. From military to healthcare: Adopting and expanding ethical principles for generative artificial intelligence. *arXiv* **2023**, arXiv:2308.02448. [CrossRef] [PubMed]
8. Liu, Y.; Yang, Z.; Yu, Z.; Liu, Z.; Liu, D.; Lin, H.; Li, M.; Ma, S.; Avdeev, M.; Shi, S. Generative artificial intelligence and its applications in materials science: Current situation and future perspectives. *J. Mater.* **2023**, *9*, 798–816. [CrossRef]
9. Regenwetter, L.; Nobari, A.H.; Ahmed, F. Deep generative models in engineering design: A review. *J. Mech. Design.* **2022**, *144*, 071704. [CrossRef]
10. OpenAI Introducing ChatGPT Plus. 2023. Available online: https://openai.com/blog/chatgpt-plus (accessed on 24 March 2024).
11. Microsoft. Bing Chat. 2023. Available online: https://www.microsoft.com/en-us/edge/features/bing-chat (accessed on 24 March 2024).

12. Pichai, S. An Important Next Step on Our AI Journey. 2023. Available online: https://blog.google/technology/ai/bard-google-ai-search-updates/ (accessed on 24 March 2024).
13. Combs, K.; Bihl, T.J.; Ganapathy, S. Utilization of Generative AI for the Characterization and Identification of Visual Unknowns. *Nat. Lang. Process. J.* 2024, in press. [CrossRef]
14. Vaswani, A.; Shazeer, N.; Parmer, N.; Uszkoreit, J.; Jones, L.; Gomez, A.N.; Kaiser, L.; Polosukhin, I. Attention is all you need. In Proceedings of the 31st Conference on Neural Information Processing Systems (NeurIPS 2017), Long Beach, CA, USA, 4–9 December 2017.
15. Radford, A.; Narasimhan, K.; Salimans, T.; Sutskever, I. Improving Language Understanding by Generative Pre-Training. OpenAI White Paper. 2018. Available online: https://s3-us-west-2.amazonaws.com/openai-assets/research-covers/language-unsupervised/language_understanding_paper.pdf (accessed on 24 March 2024).
16. Radford, A.; Wu, J.; Child, R.; Luan, D.; Amodei, D.; Sutskever, I. Language models are unsupervised multitask learners. *OpenAI Blog* 2019, 1, 9.
17. Brown, T.B.; Mann, B.; Ryder, N.; Subbiah, M.; Kaplan, J.; Dhariwal, P.; Neelakantan, A.; Shyam, P.; Sastry, G.; Askell, A.; et al. Language models are few-shot learners. In Proceedings of the 34th Conference on Neural Information Processing Systems (NeurIPS 2020), Virtual, 6–12 December 2020.
18. OpenAI. GPT-4 Technical Report. *arXiv* 2023, arXiv:2303.08774v4.
19. Collins, E.; Ghahramani, Z. LaMDA: Our Breakthrough Conversation Technology. 2021. Available online: https://blog.google/technology/ai/lamda/ (accessed on 24 March 2024).
20. Pichai, S. Google I/O 2022: Advancing Knowledge and Computing. 2022. Available online: https://blog.google/technology/developers/io-2022-keynote/ (accessed on 24 March 2024).
21. Narang, S.; Chowdhery, A. Pathways Language Model (PaLM): Scaling to 540 Billion Parameters for Breakthrough Performance. 2022. Available online: https://ai.googleblog.com/2022/04/pathways-language-model-palm-scaling-to.html (accessed on 24 March 2024).
22. Chowdhery, A.; Narang, S.; Devlin, J.; Bosma, M.; Mishra, G.; Roberts, A.; Barham, P.; Chung, H.W.; Sutton, C.; Gehrmann, S.; et al. PaLM: Scaling language modeling with pathways. *J. Mach. Learn. Res.* 2023, 24, 1–113. Available online: https://jmlr.org/papers/volume24/22-1144/22-1144.pdf (accessed on 24 March 2024).
23. Google. PaLM 2 Technical Report. *arXiv* 2023, arXiv:2305.10403.
24. Ghahramani, Z. Introducing PaLM 2. 2023. Available online: https://blog.google/technology/ai/google-palm-2-ai-large-language-model/ (accessed on 24 March 2024).
25. Meta, A.I. Introducing LLaMA: A Foundational, 65-Billion-Parameter Large Language Model. 2023. Available online: https://ai.facebook.com/blog/large-language-model-llama-meta-ai/ (accessed on 24 March 2024).
26. Touvron, H.; Lavril, T.; Izacard, G.; Martinet, X.; Lachaux, M.-A.; Lacroix, B.; Roziere, B.; Goyal, N.; Hambro, E.; Azhar, F.; et al. LLaMA: Open and efficient foundation language model. *arXiv* 2023, arXiv:2302.13971.
27. Inflection, A.I. Inflection-1. 2023. Available online: https://inflection.ai/assets/Inflection-1.pdf (accessed on 24 March 2024).
28. Nichol, A.; Dhariwal, P.; Ramesh, A.; Shyam, P.; Mishkin, P.; McGrew, B.; Sutskever, I.; Chen, M. GLIDE: Toward photorealistic image generation and editing with text-guided diffusion models. In Proceedings of the 39th International Conference on Machine Learning, Baltimore, MD, USA, 17–23 July 2022. Available online: https://proceedings.mlr.press/v162/nichol22a/nichol22a.pdf (accessed on 24 March 2024).
29. OpenAI. DALL-E: Creating Images from Text. 2021. Available online: https://openai.com/research/dall-e (accessed on 24 March 2024).
30. Radford, A.; Kim, J.W.; Hallacy, C.; Ramesh, A.; Goh, G.; Agarwal, S.; Sastry, G.; Askell, A.; Mishkin, P.; Clark, J.; et al. Learning transferable visual models from natural language supervision. In Proceedings of the 38th International Conference on Machine Learning, Virtual, 18–24 July 2021. Available online: https://proceedings.mlr.press/v139/radford21a/radford21a.pdf (accessed on 24 March 2024).
31. OpenAI. DALL-E 2. 2022. Available online: https://openai.com/dall-e-2 (accessed on 24 March 2024).
32. Ramesh, A.; Dhariwal, P.; Nichol, A.; Chu, C.; Chen, M. Hierarchical text-conditional image generation with CLIP latents. *arXiv* 2022, arXiv:2204.06125.
33. OpenAI. DALL-E 3. 2023. Available online: https://openai.com/dall-e-3 (accessed on 24 March 2024).
34. Betker, J.; Goh, G.; Jing, L.; Brooks, T.; Wang, J.; Li, L.; Ouyang, L.; Zhuang, J.; Lee, J.; Guo, Y.; et al. Improving Image Generation with Better Captions. 2023. Available online: https://cdn.openai.com/papers/dall-e-3.pdf (accessed on 24 March 2024).
35. Dayma, B.; Patril, S.; Cuenca, P.; Saifullah, K.; Ahraham, T.; Le Khac, P.; Melas, L.; Ghosh, R. DALL-E Mini. 2021. Available online: https://github.com/borisdayma/dalle-mini (accessed on 24 March 2024).
36. Dayma, B.; Patril, S.; Cuenca, P.; Saifullah, K.; Abraham, T.; Le Khac, P.; Melas, L.; Ghosh, R. DALL-E Mini Explained. Available online: https://wandb.ai/dalle-mini/dalle-mini/reports/DALL-E-Mini-Explained--Vmlldzo4NjIxODA (accessed on 24 March 2024).
37. Dayma, B.; Cuenca, P. DALL-E Mini—Generative Images from Any Text Prompt. Available online: https://wandb.ai/dalle-mini/dalle-mini/reports/DALL-E-mini-Generate-images-from-any-text-prompt--VmlldzoyMDE4NDAy (accessed on 24 March 2024).
38. Midjourney. 2022. Available online: https://www.midjourney.com/ (accessed on 24 March 2024).

39. StabilityAI Stable Difussion Launch Announcement. 2022. Available online: https://stability.ai/blog/stable-diffusion-announcement (accessed on 24 March 2024).
40. Rombach, R.; Blattmann, A.; Lorenz, D.; Essert, P.; Ommer, B. High-resolution image synthesis with latent diffusion models. In Proceedings of the IEEE/CVF Conference on Computer Vision and Pattern Recognition, New Orleans, LA, USA, 19–23 June 2022. Available online: https://openaccess.thecvf.com/content/CVPR2022/html/Rombach_High-Resolution_Image_Synthesis_With_Latent_Diffusion_Models_CVPR_2022_paper.html (accessed on 24 March 2024).
41. Saharia, C.; William, C.; Saxena, S.; Li, L.; Whang, J.; Denton, E.; Ghasemipour, S.K.S.; Ayan, B.K.; Mahdavi, S.S.; Lopes, R.G.; et al. Photorealistic text-to-image diffusion models with deep language understanding. In Proceedings of the 36th Conference on Neural Information Processing Systems (NeurIPS 2022), New Orleans, LA, USA, 28 November–9 December 2022. Available online: https://proceedings.neurips.cc/paper_files/paper/2022/hash/ec795aeadae0b7d230fa35cbaf04c041-Abstract-Conference.html (accessed on 24 March 2024).
42. Yu, J.; Xu, Y.; Koh, J.Y.; Luong, T.; Baid, G.; Wang, Z.; Vasudevan, V.; Ku, A.; Yang, Y.; Ayan, B.K.; et al. Scaling autoregressive models for content-rich text-to-image generation. *Trans. Mach. Learn. Res.* **2022**. Available online: https://openreview.net/pdf?id=AFDcYJKhND (accessed on 24 March 2024).
43. Alba, D. OpenAI Chatbot Spits out Biased Musings, Despite Guardrails. Bloomberg. 2022. Available online: https://www.bloomberg.com/news/newsletters/2022-12-08/chatgpt-open-ai-s-chatbot-is-spitting-out-biased-sexist-results (accessed on 24 March 2024).
44. Wolf, Z.B. AI Can Be Racist, Sexist and Creepy. What Should We Do about It? CNN Politics: What Matters. 2023. Available online: https://www.cnn.com/2023/03/18/politics/ai-chatgpt-racist-what-matters/index.html (accessed on 24 March 2024).
45. Weidinger, L.; Mellor, J.; Rauh, M.; Griffin, C.; Uesato, J.; Huang, P.; Cheng, M.; Glaese, M.; Balle, B.; Kasirzadeh, A.; et al. Ethical and social risks of harm from language models. *arXiv* **2021**, arXiv:2112.04359.
46. CNN Journalist Says He Had a Creepy Encounter with New Tech that Left Him Unable to Sleep. 2023. Available online: https://www.cnn.com/videos/business/2023/02/17/bing-chatgpt-chatbot-artificial-intelligence-ctn-vpx-new.cnn (accessed on 24 March 2024).
47. Daws, R. Medical Chatbot Using OpenAI's GPT-3 Told a Fake Patient to Kill Themselves. 2020. Available online: https://www.artificialintelligence-news.com/2020/10/28/medical-chatbot-openai-gpt3-patient-kill-themselves/ (accessed on 24 March 2024).
48. Chen, C.; Fu, J.; Lyu, L. A pathway towards responsible AI generated content. In Proceedings of the Thirty-Second International Joint Conference on Artificial Intelligence, Macao, China, 19–25 August 2023. Available online: https://www.ijcai.org/proceedings/2023/0803.pdf (accessed on 24 March 2024).
49. Luccioni, A.S.; Akiki, C.; Mitchell, M.; Jernite, Y. Stable bias: Analyzing societal representations in diffusion models. In Proceedings of the 37th Conference on Neural Information Processing Systems (NeurIPS 2023), New Orleans, LA, USA, 10–16 December 2023. Available online: https://proceedings.neurips.cc/paper_files/paper/2023/file/b01153e7112b347d8ed54f317840d8af-Paper-Datasets_and_Benchmarks.pdf (accessed on 24 March 2024).
50. Bird, C.; Ungless, E.L.; Kasirzadeh, A. Typology of risks of generative text-to-image models. In Proceedings of the 2023 AAAI/ACM Conference on AI, Ethics, and Society, Montreal, QC, Canada, 8–10 August 2023. [CrossRef]
51. Garcia, N.; Hirota, Y.; Wu, Y.; Nakashima, Y. Uncurated image-text datasets: Shedding light on demographic bias. In Proceedings of the IEEE/CVF Conference on Computer Vision and Pattern Recognition, Vancouver, BC, Canada, 17–24 June 2023. Available online: https://openaccess.thecvf.com/content/CVPR2023/papers/Garcia_Uncurated_Image-Text_Datasets_Shedding_Light_on_Demographic_Bias_CVPR_2023_paper.pdf (accessed on 24 March 2024).
52. Torralba, A.; Fergus, R.; Freeman, W.T. 80 Million tiny images: A large dataset for non-parametric object and scene recognition. *IEEE Trans. Pattern Anal. Mach. Intell.* **2008**, *30*, 1958–1970. [CrossRef] [PubMed]
53. Prabhu, V.U.; Birhane, A. Large datasets: A pyrrhic win for computer vision? *arXiv* **2020**, arXiv:2006.16923.
54. Shuhmann, C.; Beaumont, R.; Vencu, R.; Gordon, C.; Wightman, R.; Cherti, M.; Coombes, T.; Katta, A.; Mullis, C.; Wortsman, M.; et al. LAION-5B: An open large-scale dataset for training next generation image-text models. In Proceedings of the 36th Conference on Neural Information Processing Systems (NeurIPS 2022), New Orleans, LA, USA, 28 November–9 December 2022. Available online: https://proceedings.neurips.cc/paper_files/paper/2022/file/a1859debfb3b59d094f3504d5ebb6c25-Paper-Datasets_and_Benchmarks.pdf (accessed on 24 March 2024).
55. Desai, K.; Kaul, G.; Aysola, Z.; Johnson, J. RedCaps: Web-curated image-text data created by the people, for the people. In Proceedings of the 35th Conference on Neural Information Processing Systems (NeurIPS 2021), Virtual, 6–12 December 2021. Available online: https://datasets-benchmarks-proceedings.neurips.cc/paper/2021/file/e00da03b685a0dd18fb6a08af0923de0-Paper-round1.pdf (accessed on 24 March 2024).
56. Sharma, P.; Ding, N.; Goodman, S.; Soricut, R. Conceptual captions: A cleaned, hypernymed, image alt-text dataset for automatic image captioning. In Proceedings of the 56th Annual Meeting of the Association for Computational Linguistics (Volume 1: Long Papers), Melbourne, Australia, 15–20 July 2018. [CrossRef]
57. Birhane, A.; Prabhu, V.U.; Kahembwe, E. Multimodal datasets: Misogyny, pornography, and malignant stereotypes. *arXiv* **2021**, arXiv:2110.01963.
58. Fabbrizzi, S.; Papadopoulos, S.; Ntoutsi, E.; Kompatsiaris, I. A survey on bias in visual datasets. *Comput. Vis. Image Underst.* **2022**, *223*, 103552. [CrossRef]

59. Sottile, Z. What to Know about Lensa, the AI Portrait App All over Social Media. CNN Style. 2023. Available online: https://www.cnn.com/style/article/lensa-ai-app-art-explainer-trnd/index.html (accessed on 24 March 2024).
60. Heikkila, M. The Viral AI Avatar App Lensa Undressed Me—Without My Consent. 2022. Available online: https://www.technologyreview.com/2022/12/12/1064751/the-viral-ai-avatar-app-lensa-undressed-me-without-my-consent/ (accessed on 24 March 2024).
61. Buell, S. An MIT Student Asked AI to Make Her Headshot More 'Professional'. It Gave Her Lighter Skin and Blue Eyes. The Boston Globe. 2023. Available online: https://www.bostonglobe.com/2023/07/19/business/an-mit-student-asked-ai-make-her-headshot-more-professional-it-gave-her-lighter-skin-blue-eyes/ (accessed on 24 March 2024).
62. Hacker, P.; Engel, A.; Mauer, M. Regulating ChatGPT and other large generative AI models. In Proceedings of the 2023 ACM Conference on Fairness, Accountability, and Transparency, Chicago, IL, USA, 12–15 June 2023.
63. Ullah, U.; Lee, J.; An, C.; Lee, H.; Park, S.; Baek, R.; Choi, H. A review of multi-modal learning from the text-guided visual processing viewpoint. *Sensors* **2022**, *22*, 6816. [CrossRef] [PubMed]
64. Baraheem, S.S.; Le, T.; Nguyen, T.V. Image synthesis: A review of methods, datasets, evaluation metrics, and future outlook. *Artif. Intell. Rev.* **2023**, *56*, 10813–10865. [CrossRef]
65. Elasri, M.; Elharrouss, O.; Al-Maadeed, S.; Tairi, H. Image generation: A review. *Neural Process. Lett.* **2022**, *54*, 4609–4646. [CrossRef]
66. Cao, M.; Li, S.; Li, J.; Nie, L.; Zhang, M. Image-text retrieval: A survey on recent research and development. In Proceedings of the Thirty-First International Joint Conference on Artificial Intelligence, Vienna, Austria, 23–29 July 2022. Available online: https://www.ijcai.org/proceedings/2022/0759.pdf (accessed on 24 March 2024).
67. Bithel, S.; Bedathur, S. Evaluating Cross-modal generative models using retrieval task. In Proceedings of the 46th International ACM SIGIR Conference on Research and Development in Information Retrieval, Taipei, Taiwan, 23–27 July 2023. [CrossRef]
68. Borji, A. How good are deep models in understanding the generated images? *arXiv* **2022**, arXiv:2208.10760.
69. He, X.; Deng, L. Deep learning for image-to-text generation: A technical overview. *IEEE Signal Process. Mag.* **2017**, *34*, 109–116. [CrossRef]
70. Żelaszczyk, M.; Mańdziuk, J. Cross-modal text and visual generation: A systematic review. Part 1—Image to text. *Inf. Fusion.* **2023**, *93*, 302–329. [CrossRef]
71. Combs, K.; Bihl, T.J.; Ganapathy, S. Integration of computer vision and semantics for characterizing unknowns. In Proceedings of the 56th Hawaii International Conference on System Sciences, Maui, HI, USA, 3–6 January 2023. [CrossRef]
72. Lin, T.; Maire, M.; Belongie, S.; Bourdev, L.; Girshick, R.; Hays, J.; Perona, P.; Ramanan, D.; Zitnick, C.L.; Dollar, P. Microsoft COCO: Common objects in context. In Proceedings of the 13th European Conference Proceedings, Zurich, Switzerland, 6–12 September 2014. [CrossRef]
73. Krause, J.; Johnson, J.; Krishna, R.; Li, F. A hierarchical approach for generating descriptive image paragraphs. In Proceedings of the IEEE Conference on Computer Vision and Pattern Recognition, Honolulu, HI, USA, 21–26 July 2017. Available online: https://openaccess.thecvf.com/content_cvpr_2017/html/Krause_A_Hierarchical_Approach_CVPR_2017_paper.html (accessed on 24 March 2024).
74. Bernardi, R.; Cakici, R.; Elliott, D.; Erdem, A.; Erdem, E.; Ikizler-Cinbis, N.; Keller, F.; Muscat, A.; Plank, B. Automatic description generation from images: A survey of models, datasets, and evaluation measures. *J. Artif. Intell. Res.* **2016**, *55*, 409–442. [CrossRef]
75. Wang, J.; Yang, Z.; Hu, X.; Li, L.; Lin, K.; Gan, Z.; Liu, Z.; Liu, C.; Wang, L. GIT: A generative image-to-text transformer for vision and language. *arXiv* **2022**, arXiv:2205.14100.
76. Li, J.; Li, D.; Xiong, C.; Hoi, S. Bootstrapping language-image pre-training for unified vision-language understanding and generation. In Proceedings of the 39th International Conference on Machine Learning, Baltimore, MD, USA, 17–23 July 2022. Available online: https://proceedings.mlr.press/v162/li22n.html (accessed on 24 March 2024).
77. Alayrax, J.; Donahue, J.; Luc, P.; Miech, A.; Barr, I.; Hasson, Y.; Lenc, K.; Mensch, A.; Millican, K.; Reyolds, M.; et al. Flamingo: A visual language model for few-shot learning. In Proceedings of the 36th Conference on Neural Information Processing Systems (NeurIPS 2022), New Orleans, LA, USA, 28 November–9 December 2022. Available online: https://proceedings.neurips.cc/paper_files/paper/2022/hash/960a172bc7fbf0177ccccbb411a7d800-Abstract-Conference.html (accessed on 24 March 2024).
78. Li, J.; Li, D.; Savarese, S.; Hoi, S. BLIP-2: Bootstrapping language-image pre-training with frozen image encoders and large language models. *arXiv* **2023**, arXiv:2301.12597.
79. Dai, W.; Li, J.; Li, D.; Tiong, A.M.H.; Zhao, J.; Wang, W.; Li, B.; Fung, P.; Hoi, S. InstructBLIP: Toward general-purpose vision-language model with instruction tuning. *arXiv* **2023**, arXiv:2304.08485.
80. Xu, M.; Yoon, S.; Fuentes, A.; Park, D.S. A comprehensive survey of image augmentation technics for deep learning. *Pattern Recognit.* **2023**, *137*, 109347. [CrossRef]
81. Zhai, G.; Min, X. Perceptual image quality assessment: A survey. *Sci. China Inf. Sci.* **2020**, *63*, 211301. [CrossRef]
82. Chandler, D.M. Seven challenges in image quality assessment: Past, present, and future research. *Int. Sch. Res. Not.* **2013**, *2013*, 905685. [CrossRef]
83. Mantiuk, R.K.; Tomaszewska, A.; Mantiuk, R. Comparison of four subjective methods for image quality assessment. *Comput. Graph. Forum.* **2012**, *31*, 2478–2491. [CrossRef]
84. Galatolo, F.A.; Gimino, M.G.C.A.; Cogotti, E. TeTIm-Eval: A novel curated evaluation data set for comparing text-to-image models. *arXiv* **2022**, arXiv:2212.07839.

85. Salimans, T.; Goodfellow, I.; Wojciech, Z.C.V.; Radford, A.; Chen, X. Improved techniques for training GANs. In Proceedings of the 30th Conference on Neural Information Processing Systems (NeurIPS 2016), Barcelona, Spain, 5–10 December 2016. Available online: https://proceedings.neurips.cc/paper_files/paper/2016/hash/8a3363abe792db2d8761d6403605aeb7-Abstract.html (accessed on 24 March 2024).
86. Li, C.; Zhang, Z.; Wu, H.; Sun, W.; Min, X.; Liu, X.; Zhai, G.; Lin, W. AGIQA-3K: An open database for AI-generated image quality assessment. *arXiv* **2023**, arXiv:2306.04717. [CrossRef]
87. Gehrmann, S.; Clark, E.; Thibault, S. Repairing the cracked foundation: A survey of obstacles in evaluation practices for generated text. *J. Artif. Intell. Res.* **2023**, *77*, 103–166. [CrossRef]
88. Hessel, J.; Holtzman, A.; Forbes, M.; Le Bras, R.; Choi, Y. CLIPscore: A reference-free evaluation metric for image captioning. In Proceedings of the 2021 Conference on Empirical Methods in Natural Language Processing, Punta Cana, Dominican Republic, 7–11 November 2021. [CrossRef]
89. Papineni, K.; Roukoas, S.; Ward, T.; Zhu, W. Bleu: A method for automatic evaluation of machine translation. In Proceedings of the 40th Annual Meeting of the Association for Computational Linguistics, Denver, CO, USA, 7–12 July 2002. [CrossRef]
90. Lin, C. Rouge: A package for automatic evaluation of summaries. In Proceedings of the ACL Workshop on Text Summarization Branches Out Workshop, Barcelona, Spain, 25–26 July 2004. Available online: https://aclanthology.org/W04-1013 (accessed on 24 March 2024).
91. Banerjee, S.; Lavie, A. METEOR: An automatic metric for MT evaluation with improved correlation with human judgments. In Proceedings of the ACL Workshop on Intrinsic and Extrinsic Evaluation Measures for Machine Translation and/or Summarization, Ann Arbor, MI, USA, 29 June 2005. Available online: https://aclanthology.org/W05-0909 (accessed on 24 March 2024).
92. Snover, M.; Door, B.; Schwartz, R.; Micciulla, L.; Makhoul, J. A study of translation edit rate with targeted human annotation. In Proceedings of the 7th Conference of the Association for Machine Translation in the Americas: Technical Papers, Cambridge, MA, USA, 8–12 August 2006. Available online: https://aclanthology.org/2006.amta-papers.25 (accessed on 24 March 2024).
93. Snover, M.; Madnani, N.; Dorr, B.; Schwartz, R. TERp system description. In Proceedings of the ACL Workshop on Statistical Machine Translation and MetricsMATR, Uppsala, Sweden, 15–16 July 2008.
94. Vedantam, R.; Zitnick, C.L.; Parikh, D. CIDEr: Consensus-based image description evaluation. In Proceedings of the IEEE Conference on Computer Vision and Pattern Recognition, Boston, MA, USA, 7–12 June 2015. Available online: https://openaccess.thecvf.com/content_cvpr_2015/html/Vedantam_CIDEr_Consensus-Based_Image_2015_CVPR_paper.html (accessed on 24 March 2024).
95. Anderson, P.; Fernando, B.; Johnson, M.; Gould, S. SPICE: Semantic propositional image caption evaluation. In Proceedings of the 14th European Conference on Computer Vision, Amsterdam, The Netherlands, 11–14 October 2016. [CrossRef]
96. Zhang, T.; Kishore, V.; Wu, F.; Weinberger, K.Q.; Artzi, Y. BERTScore: Evaluating text generation with BERT. In Proceedings of the International Conference on Learning Representations, Virtual, 26 April–1 May 2020. Available online: https://arxiv.org/abs/1904.09675 (accessed on 24 March 2024).
97. Mikolov, T.; Sutskever, I.; Chen, K.; Corrado, G.S.; Dean, J. Distributed representations of words and phrases and their compositionality. In Proceedings of the 26th International Conference on Neural Information Processing Systems, Lake Tahoe, CA, USA, 5–8 December 2013. Available online: https://proceedings.neurips.cc/paper/2013/file/9aa42b31882ec039965f3c4923ce901b-Paper.pdf (accessed on 24 March 2024).
98. Mikolov, T.; Yih, W.; Zweig, G. Linguistic regularities in continuous space word representations. In Proceedings of the 2013 Conference of the North American Chapter of the Association for Computational Linguistics: Human Language Technologies, Atlanta, GA, USA, 9–14 June 2013. Available online: https://aclanthology.org/N13-1090.pdf (accessed on 24 March 2024).
99. Gunther, F.; Rinaldi, L.; Marelli, M. Vector-space models of semantic representation from a cognitive perspective: A discussion of common misconceptions. *Perspect. Psychol. Sci.* **2019**, *14*, 1006–1033. [CrossRef]
100. Shahmirazadi, O.; Lugowski, A.; Younge, K. Text similarity in vector space models: A comparative study. In Proceedings of the 18th IEEE International Conference on Machine Learning and Applications, Pasadena, CA, USA, 13–15 December 2021. [CrossRef]
101. Pennington, J.; Socher, R.; Manning, C.D. Glove: Global vectors for word representation. In Proceedings of the 2014 Conference on Empirical Methods in Natural Language Processing (EMNLP), Doha, Qatar, 25–29 October 2014. [CrossRef]
102. Bojanowski, P.; Grave, E.; Joulin, A.; Mikolov, T. Enriching word vectors with subword information. *Trans. Assoc. Comput. Linguist.* **2017**, *5*, 135–146. [CrossRef]
103. Wang, C.; Nulty, P.; Lillis, D. A comparative study on word embeddings in deep learning for text classification. In Proceedings of the 4th International Conference on Natural Language Processing and Information Retrieval, Seoul, Republic of Korea, 18–20 December 2020. [CrossRef]
104. Peters, M.E.; Neumann, M.; Iyyer, M.; Gardner, M.; Clark, C.; Lee, K.; Zettlemoyer, L. Deep contextualized word representations. In Proceedings of the North American Chapter of the Association for Computational Linguistics: Human Language Technology, New Orleans, LA, USA, 1–6 June 2018. Available online: https://arxiv.org/abs/1802.05365 (accessed on 24 March 2024).
105. Yang, Z.; Dai, Z.; Yang, Y.; Carbonell, J.; Salakhutdinov, R.; Le, Q.V. XLnet: Generalized autoregressive pretraining for language understanding. In Proceedings of the 33rd Conference on Neural Information Processing Systems (NeurIPS 2019), Vancouver, BC, Canada, 8–14 December 2019. Available online: https://proceedings.neurips.cc/paper/2019/hash/dc6a7e655d7e5840e66733e9ee67cc69-Abstract.html (accessed on 24 March 2024).

106. Combs, K.; Lu, H.; Bihl, T.J. Transfer learning and analogical inference: A critical comparison of algorithms, methods, and applications. *Algorithms* **2023**, *16*, 146. [CrossRef]
107. Devlin, J.; Chang, M.; Lee, K.; Toutanova, K. BERT: Pre-training of deep bidirectional transformers for language understanding. In Proceedings of the 2019 Annual Conference of the North American Chapter of the Association for Computational Linguistics: Human Language Technologies, Minneapolis, MN, USA, 2–7 June 2019. [CrossRef]
108. Liu, Y.; Ott, M.; Goyal, N.; Du, J.; Joshi, M.; Chen, D.; Levy, O.; Lewis, M.; Settlemoyer, L.; Stoyanov, V. RoBERTa: A robustly optimized bert pretraining approach. *arXiv* **2019**, arXiv:1907.11692.
109. Lan, Z.; Chen, M.; Goodman, S.; Gimpel, K.; Sharma, P.; Soricut, R. ALBERT: A lite BERT for self-supervised learning of language representations. In Proceedings of the International Conference on Learning Representations, Virtual, 26 April–1 May 2020. Available online: https://arxiv.org/abs/1909.11942 (accessed on 24 March 2024).
110. Sanh, V.; Debut, L.; Chaumond, J.; Wolf, T. DistilBERT, a distilled version of BERT: Smaller, faster, cheaper and lighter. *arXiv* **2019**, arXiv:1910.01108.
111. Morrison, R.G.; Krawczyk, D.C.; Holyoak, K.J.; Hummel, J.E.; Chow, T.W.; Miller, B.L.; Knowlton, B.J. A neurocomputational model of analogical reasoning and its breakdown in frontotemporal lobar degeneration. *J. Cogn. Neurosci.* **2004**, *16*, 260–271. [CrossRef] [PubMed]
112. Wang, W.; Wei, F.; Dong, L.; Bao, H.; Yang, N.; Zhou, M. MiniLM: Deep self-attention distillation for task-agnostic compression of pre-trained transformers. In Proceedings of the 34th Conference on Neural Information Processing Systems (NeurIPS 2020), Virtual, 6–12 December 2020. Available online: https://proceedings.neurips.cc/paper/2020/hash/3f5ee243547dee91fbd053c1c4 a845aa-Abstract.html (accessed on 24 March 2024).
113. Sternberg, R.J.; Nigro, G. Developmental patterns in the solution of verbal analogies. *Child Dev.* **1980**, *51*, 27–38. [CrossRef]
114. Combs, K.; Bihl, T.J. A preliminary look at generative AI for the creation of abstract verbal-to-visual analogies. In Proceedings of the 57th Hawaii International Conference on System Sciences, Honolulu, HI, USA, 3–6 January 2024. Available online: https://hdl.handle.net/10125/106520 (accessed on 24 March 2024).
115. Reviriego, P.; Merino-Gomez, E. Text to image generation: Leaving no language behind. *arXiv* **2022**, arXiv:2208.09333.
116. O'Meara, J.; Murphy, C. Aberrant AI creations: Co-creating surrealist body horror using the DALL-E Mini text-to-image generator. *Converg. Int. J. Res. New Media Technol.* **2023**, *29*, 1070–1096. [CrossRef]
117. Chen, X.; Fang, H.; Lin, T.; Vedantam, R.; Gupta, S.; Dollar, P.; Zitnick, C.L. Microsoft COCO captions: Data collection and evaluation server. *arXiv* **2015**, arXiv:1504.00325.

Disclaimer/Publisher's Note: The statements, opinions and data contained in all publications are solely those of the individual author(s) and contributor(s) and not of MDPI and/or the editor(s). MDPI and/or the editor(s) disclaim responsibility for any injury to people or property resulting from any ideas, methods, instructions or products referred to in the content.

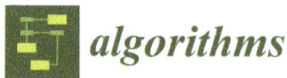 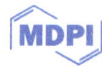

Article

Framework Based on Simulation of Real-World Message Streams to Evaluate Classification Solutions

Wenny Hojas-Mazo [1], Francisco Maciá-Pérez [2], José Vicente Berná Martínez [2], Mailyn Moreno-Espino [3], Iren Lorenzo Fonseca [2] and Juan Pavón [4,*]

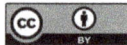

Citation: Hojas-Mazo, W.; Maciá-Pérez, F.; Berná Martínez, J.V.; Moreno-Espino, M.; Lorenzo Fonseca, I.; Pavón, J. Framework Based on Simulation of Real-World Message Streams to Evaluate Classification Solutions. *Algorithms* **2024**, *17*, 47. https://doi.org/10.3390/a17010047

Academic Editor: Nuno Fachada

Received: 30 December 2023
Revised: 18 January 2024
Accepted: 19 January 2024
Published: 21 January 2024

Copyright: © 2024 by the authors. Licensee MDPI, Basel, Switzerland. This article is an open access article distributed under the terms and conditions of the Creative Commons Attribution (CC BY) license (https://creativecommons.org/licenses/by/4.0/).

[1] Departamento de Inteligencia Artificial e Infraestructura de Sistemas Informáticos, Facultad de Ingeniería Informática, Universidad Tecnológica de La Habana, José Antonio Echeverría, Calle 114 #11901, entre 119 y 127, CUJAE, Marianao, La Habana 19390, Cuba; whojas@ceis.cujae.edu.cu

[2] Department of Computer Science and Technology, University of Alicante, 03690 Alicante, Spain; pmacia@ua.es (F.M.-P.); jvberna@ua.es (J.V.B.M.); iren.fonseca@ua.es (I.L.F.)

[3] Centro de Investigación en Computación, Instituto Politécnico Nacional, Ciudad de México 07738, Mexico; mmorenoe2022@cic.ipn.mx

[4] Instituto de Tecnología del Conocimiento, Universidad Complutense de Madrid, 28040 Madrid, Spain

* Correspondence: jpavon@fdi.ucm.es

Abstract: Analysing message streams in a dynamic environment is challenging. Various methods and metrics are used to evaluate message classification solutions, but often fail to realistically simulate the actual environment. As a result, the evaluation can produce overly optimistic results, rendering current solution evaluations inadequate for real-world environments. This paper proposes a framework based on the simulation of real-world message streams to evaluate classification solutions. The framework consists of four modules: message stream simulation, processing, classification and evaluation. The simulation module uses techniques and queueing theory to replicate a real-world message stream. The processing module refines the input messages for optimal classification. The classification module categorises the generated message stream using existing solutions. The evaluation module evaluates the performance of the classification solutions by measuring accuracy, precision and recall. The framework can model different behaviours from different sources, such as different spammers with different attack strategies, press media or social network sources. Each profile generates a message stream that is combined into the main stream for greater realism. A spam detection case study is developed that demonstrates the implementation of the proposed framework and identifies latency and message body obfuscation as critical classification quality parameters.

Keywords: classification; evaluation; non-stationary message streams; simulation

1. Introduction

Information exchange through multiple communication channels (mail, SMS, internal applications, RSS, etc.) from different senders and to one or more recipients plays a key role in institutions [1] and companies [2] and generates a large, dynamic message stream. An example context of relevance to institutions and companies is to better understand how rational and emotional postings on social media influence customer behaviour [3,4].

The underlying characteristics of these dynamic message streams pose some serious challenges to effective classification, such as concept drift, concept evolution, latency and adversarial attacks [5,6]. First, the concepts embedded in a stream change over time. This is known as concept drift and requires a classifier to adapt to the current concepts. For example, a reader's topic of interest may change over time after reading a large number of messages with different topics. Second, a message stream usually consists of a large number of objects (instances), and these objects are characterised by a high-dimensional feature space (e.g., the message topics referred to in a message stream are described by a large vocabulary). Third, latency, verification latency or delay, is the time between the availability of an unlabelled instance and its actual labelling [7]. This period can be measured in terms of time or number of instances. Since most benchmark datasets do not have time stamps, the number of instances is usually used in the literature as a measure of latency. The occurrence of such latencies has a direct impact on the model update strategy during drift events, which can lead to a decrease in classifier accuracy [8]. The latency can be divided into null latency, extreme latency and intermediate latency [8]. At null latency, the real labels of the instances are always available immediately after classification. At extreme latency the real labels are never available to the classifier, requiring an unsupervised approach or an incremental update of the model over time. At intermediate latency, an intermediate delay time L, where $0 < L < \infty$, is considered until the real labels are available. This time can be constant (the same for all stream instances) or variable. If the delay is variable, the time of availability of the real labels may differ from the arrival order of the examples, and therefore, the classifier may receive the label of the instance $\vec{x}_{t+5}$ before receiving the label of $\vec{x}_{t+2}$. Fourth, the adversarial attacks in the context of the message stream are carried out by the adversarial character known as the spammer. Spammers try to evade the classifier while maintaining the readability of the message content, for example, by including certain misspellings or authentic words in the message [9]. As a result, spam messages may contain malicious information strategically inserted by spammers to corrupt the data used to train classifiers. In [6], a detailed analysis is made of the tricks used by spammers to evade spam filters, such as text poisoning, obfuscated words or hidden text salting.

In order to evaluate the performance of classifiers on dynamic message streams, different corpus [6,10], different measures [6,10] and evaluation methods [6,11] have been published. In general, most models show high accuracy when evaluated on known and relevant public datasets [6,11]. This situation contributes to the generation of overly optimistic results and makes the actual deployment of message classification solutions uncertain, since the problems of adversarial data manipulation by spammers and concept drift are often ignored [6,11]. However, some proposals have presented forms of evaluation that take these aspects into account [6,11–15].

Proposals for evaluating adversarial data manipulation by spammers in the message stream context have not been found. However, proposals have been identified in other contexts that attempt to measure classifier stability in the face of adversarial attacks [12,13]. In [12], the stability of the classifier under adversarial contamination of the training data is quantified by introducing a metric to classify its robustness. In [13], frameworks for security analysis and evaluation of classification algorithms are proposed by simulating attack scenarios.

Regarding the evaluation of concept drift in the message stream context, two were found, specifically in spam detection [6,11]. In [11], the SDAI methodology is proposed, based on the measurement of classifier accuracy in four different but complementary scenarios: static, dynamic operations, adaptive capabilities and internationalisation. The static scenario evaluates the overall performance of the classifier in a controlled environment, while the dynamic operation scenario measures its behaviour under automatic updating schemes. The adaptive capabilities scenario simulates the operation of the classifier in a server context, categorising messages from multiple senders and covering different subject areas, and the internationalisation scenario evaluates the ability of the classifier to classify incoming messages in different languages, whether in standalone or server mode. In [6], a strategy very similar to the adaptive scenario of [11] is proposed, where the classifier is trained on a corpus (SpamAssassin corpus) and tested on another corpus (Ling-Spam corpus), which covers different topics than the training corpus. The main differences of the variant in [6] are the algorithms used to process and classify the messages and the corpora used for training and testing. In [6], four spam filters trained on five email datasets collected from different sources at different times are evaluated to see if the spam filters maintain their generalisation performance. Both proposals essentially try to deal with concept drift and spammer influence, ref. [11] in the dynamic scenario and both in the adaptive scenario. However, in the dynamic scenario, the following perspective is oriented towards the action of the classifier rather than the generation of the stream. The stream is generated using cross-validation by segmenting the base corpus into 10 partitions and selecting 9 for training and 1 for testing. This procedure does not allow adequately modelling environments with intermediate and extreme latency; the behaviour of the different spammers and other message sources that may exist is limited to what is reflected in the messages of the corpus used and does not allow adapting the behaviour by adjusting parameters such as spammer strategies, message sending ratio, message batch size and other parameters that make the stream more realistic; and the configuration to evaluate different types of message processing services, classifiers or a combination of both can become complex.

In addition, several frameworks have been proposed to assist users in carrying out specific aspects of the stream classification process [16]. These frameworks allow the integration of different stream classification tasks, improve interoperability and include all necessary components for algorithm development [17]. A stream classification framework may include data generators or real-world datasets for benchmarking, data processing, classifier algorithms, and testing of classification results [16]. Existing frameworks that have been used to classify text messages include Jubatus [14] and Massive Online Analysis (MOA) [15]. Jubatus, a framework that emerged from a Japanese research project [14], emphasises distributed processing and features a model-sharing architecture to support practical training and collaboration of classification models. This aims to reduce the network costs and latency associated with distributed environments. The framework incorporates test datasets from various sources and includes features for feature space simplification and textual data preprocessing. It also integrates basic stream classification algorithms, provides minimal evaluation and monitoring functionality, and is compatible with the Spark analytics engine or the Python sci-kit-learn library [18]. MOA [15] is derived from WEKA, the Waikato Environment for Knowledge Analysis framework, written in Java and accessible via a graphical user interface (GUI) or command line. Originally developed to assess stream classification performance and manage algorithm speed, memory usage and accuracy MOA includes numerous datasets, preprocessing approaches, stream-classification-related algorithms and evaluation methods. Advanced applications include extensions for tweet collection, sentiment analysis and data reduction techniques in evolving streams. Both frameworks do not allow adequate modelling of environments where multiple message stream generators are simultaneously configured to emulate the behaviour of spammers and other message sources that may exist and contribute to the main message stream (limited to what is reflected in the messages of the corpus used).

This research hypothesises that the modelling of the sources of message emission to the main stream as profiles with configurable behaviours, and the modelling of the stream according to simulation techniques and queueing theory, will provide a message stream to evaluate message processing and/or classification solutions closer to the real one, thus allowing to detect in advance possible problems of processors and/or classifiers and to avoid degradation of their performance during their operation.

This paper presents a framework that simulates real-world message streams to evaluate classification solutions. The framework consists of four modules: message stream simulation, processing, classification and evaluation. The first module uses simulation techniques and queueing theory to replicate real-world message streams. The next module enhances the input messages for effective classification. The third module applies existing classification solutions to categorise the generated stream. Finally, the fourth module evaluates the performance of the classification solutions by measuring various metrics.

The rest of the paper is structured as follows: Section 2 describes the details of the proposed framework. Section 3 develops a case study in the spam detection environment to evaluate the proposed framework. Finally, Section 5 summarises the main conclusions.

2. Proposed Framework

This paper proposes a framework based on the simulation of real message streams for the evaluation of classification solutions. The proposed framework aims to provide researchers (especially data scientists) in the area of text stream classification with an environment that facilitates the evaluation of text message processing and/or classification solutions. The proposal is designed to facilitate the integration of existing processing and/or classification solutions, mainly in the form of web services, for evaluation with the generated message streams or as a basis for comparison with other solutions. Figure 1 shows a view of the framework architecture, which aims to make this framework as versatile as possible, with the ability to adapt and readjust the technological resources to the changing situation at any time, and which follows a similar scheme to the architecture proposed in [19]. An architectural style based on n-layer architectures has been used, structuring the elements into levels.

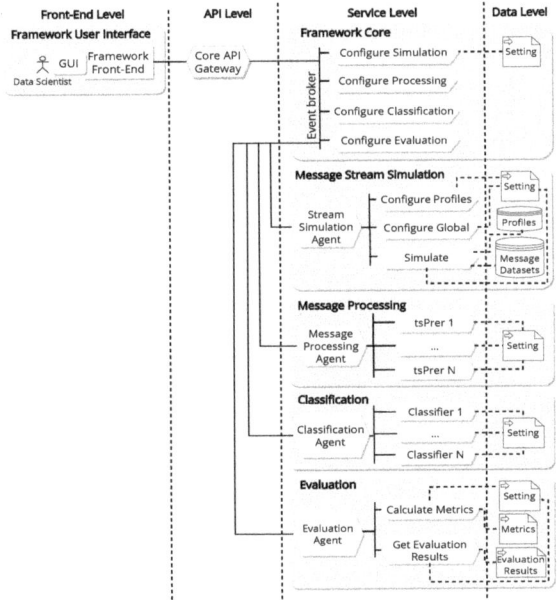

Figure 1. Framework architecture view.

The front-end level defines the elements needed to interact with end users, grouped under the concept of the framework user interface and organised according to the model, view, controller (MVC) architectural pattern. The framework front-end is intended for the data scientists, and is based on a graphical user interface (GUI). The API level contains the service that acts as an application programming interface (API) for the other of the services. This allows for the centralised exposure of all the endpoints defined in the backend. This level is the core of the solution and consists of five main modules: Framework Core, Message Stream Simulation, Message Processing, Classification, and Evaluation. Each of the modules in the service level accesses the data level through the persistence services in the service layer (Figure 1 shows the relationship between the services and their main data sources, with dashed lines to indicate that this relationship is indirect). The following is a description of each of the core-level modules that make up the proposed framework.

2.1. Framework Core

The Framework Core consists of a set of services that provide the basic functionality of the Framework Service: Configure Simulation, Configure Processing, Configure Classification and Configure Evaluation. All these services are connected to the Gateway and to each other via an Event Broker that manages the messages.

2.2. Message Stream Simulation

Message Stream Simulation, using the simulation technique [20] and the queueing theory [21], attempts to mimic the generation of a message stream, similar to a real-world environment. The goal of this module is to generate a message stream S that is as close as possible to a real scenario. To achieve this goal, profiles are modelled. A profile p is considered in this paper as an abstract entity that can have n instances, each of which generates a message stream S_{p_n}. Profiles can be used to model thematic sources and/or user profiles. A thematic source generates a message stream about one or more topics such as Computers, Science, Society and others. A user profile generates a message stream with similar characteristics to user/entity types of the web such as Spammer, Social Network, Personal, Marketing, Information and others. A profile instance is defined as $p_n = (name, svb, mc, S_{p_n})$, where $name$ is the identifier of each instance profile, svb is a set of variable behaviours that can be different for each profile instance, mc is a message corpus and S_{p_n} is the generated message stream.

The set of variable behaviours (svb) are parameters that can change the way a profile instance generates a message stream. When simulating non-stationary message streams to closely emulate message sending sources, the variables message send rate, message batch size, message size and message obfuscation play an essential role. The message send rate represents the frequency with which messages are sent by the source, and in a non-stationary environment, the message send rate can fluctuate over time. By adjusting this variable in the simulation, one can capture the varying intensity of message traffic. Similarly, the message batch size, which refers to the number of messages sent together as a batch, affects the burstiness and temporal patterns of the message streams. In non-stationary scenarios, batch size can change, and adjusting this variable in the simulation allows for the replication of such dynamics. Message size refers to the size in digital units of the content of each message. In non-stationary message streams, the size distribution of messages may change, and incorporating this variability into the simulation will affect the processing of message content, as the content and size of the context to be analysed by the word processor will vary. In addition, message obfuscation is one of the tricks used by spammers to evade spam filters and is relevant to the evaluation of solutions to be developed in the context of spam detection. Future versions of the framework could include the modelling of other tricks used by spammers. Based on that, the svb Message Send Rate (msr), Message Batch Size (mbs), Message Size (ms) and Message Obfuscation (mo) are defined. msr is equal to mean arrival rate λ, which is the time between sending messages. λ can be a constant or a random value that can change in a constant time t_λ. In mbs, the size s of the message batch mb can be a constant, or it can change randomly in a constant time t_{mb}. To change s, an integer uniform random number is generated with an interval $[0, z]$, where z is the maximum value of the size for mb. In mbs, before forming each mb, the input source can be filtered by a minimum message size ms that changes in constant time t_{ms}. This reduces the input source to form the mb to the message with a size equal to or greater than ms. To change ms, a uniform integer random number is generated with an interval $[1, k]$, where k is the maximum value of KB for ms. The mo consists of replacing the letters i and l in the body of the message with the characters ¡ and 1, respectively. Before sending each mb, q message from the batch of messages can be selected and obfuscated. To select the q messages, an integer uniform random number with an interval $[0, v]$ is generated, first to select the set of messages to be obfuscated, and second to select the q messages to be obfuscated (the last time with an interval $[1, v]$ without repetitions).

The mc form a message corpus about the profile class, which can receive messages from the public corpus or from personal sources (e.g., emails from a mailbox). A message corpus is defined as $mc = \{m_1, m_2, \ldots, m_n\}$, where m_i is the i-th message in the corpus.

S_{p_n} is defined as:

$$S_{p_n} = \begin{pmatrix} m_{1,1}, & m_{1,2}, & \cdots & m_{1,r_1}; \\ m_{2,1}, & m_{2,2}, & \cdots & m_{2,r_2}; \\ \cdots; & & & \\ m_{n,1}, & m_{n,2}, & \cdots & m_{n,r_n}; \\ \cdots; & & & \end{pmatrix}$$

Here, $m_{i,j}$ represents the j-th text at the i-th time. The union of the message streams generated by each profile instance forms the message stream, so it is defined as $S = \cup_{p=1}^{l} S_p \mid p \in P$, where $S_p = \cup_{n=1}^{q} S_{p_n}$.

The general modelling of profile behaviour is based on simulation concepts [20] and the M/M/1 queueing model (Poisson input, exponential service times and single server) [21]. To summarise the physical operation of the system, incoming messages enter the queue, are eventually served, and then leave. It is therefore necessary for the simulation model to describe and synchronise the arrival of messages and the serving of messages. The general behaviour of the profile instance is shown in Figure 2.

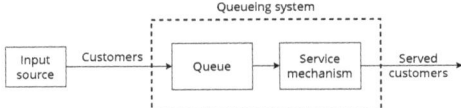

Figure 2. General behaviour of profile instance.

Starting at time 0, the simulation clock records the (simulated) time t that has elapsed during the simulation run so far. The information about the queueing system that defines its current status, i.e., the state of the system, is $N(t) = $ number of messages in the system at time t. The events that change the state of the system are the arrival of messages or a service completion for the messages currently in service (if any). The values of mean arrival rate λ and mean service rate μ are $t_{ms}/h * r$ and t_{ms}, respectively. Each profile instance has independent t_{ms}, r and h values. The state transition formula is:

$$\text{Reset } N(t) = \begin{cases} N(t) + n & \text{if the arrival of } n \text{ texts occurs at time } t \\ N(t) - n & \text{if service completion of } n \text{ messages occurs at time } t \end{cases}$$

The event generation method consists in forming a message batch $mb = \{m_1, m_2, \ldots, m_r\}$, where m_i represents the i-th message in the batch, selecting from n messages of the input source by generating an integer uniform random number for each message and sending it to the queue. The random numbers have an interval of $[1, n]$. This method of event generation allows us to assume that the input source is infinite, since n messages can be selected from each element of mb, generating n^r batches, which tend to be infinite. In the queue system, the queue discipline is first-come-first-served. The service mechanism consists in sending a message batch $mb = \{m_1, m_2, \ldots, m_r\}$ in a μ.

The training examples profile will have a single instance that generates a message stream by selecting message examples and their real classes from the messages sent by the created profile instances. The examples in this stream can be used by the evaluated solutions in the learning process. The latency lat is the time between the prediction of an unlabelled instance by a classifier and the availability of its real label by the environment, and is classified as either null, intermediate or extreme latency.

2.3. Message Processing

Message Processing transforms the message input into a high-quality one that is suitable for the learning process to follow, using techniques such as integration, normalisation, cleaning, transformation and reduction. Data processing [22] stands out as a crucial stage in the knowledge discovery process. Although often overlooked in comparison to other phases such as data mining, data processing typically requires a greater investment of time and effort, accounting for more than 50% of the overall undertaking [23]. Raw data typically contain numerous imperfections, including inconsistencies, missing values, noise and redundancies. Consequently, the effectiveness of successive learning algorithms is inevitably compromised in the presence of poor data quality [24]. It follows that the application of appropriate processing measures has a significant impact on the quality and reliability of the resulting automated insights and decisions.

The message stream processing module consists of a set of text stream preprocessors, denoted as $TsPre = \{tsPre_1, tsPre_2, \ldots, tsPre_n\} | n \geq 1$, which typically employ natural language processing techniques and feature analysis (lexical terms). Commonly used natural language processing techniques include text content extraction, tokenisation and part-of-speech tagging. Following the application of natural language processing techniques, feature analysis is used to reduce the dimensionality of the set of features present in the texts through selection and/or reduction, with the aim of representing the content in a structure that is amenable to classification solutions. This module can be used for the following purposes:

- Evaluate the message stream processing solutions to be developed. To perform this evaluation, several processing solutions are selected that will process the same message stream to obtain the feature sets that will then be used by one or more classification algorithms. Since what would vary in the classification process is the way the message stream is preprocessed, the better the quality of the results, the better the processing solution used.
- Focus the evaluation on the classification process. One of the solutions available in the module is used for all classification solutions used, which means that the quality of the result depends on the classification algorithm used. Therefore, this approach allows the comparison of classification algorithms without the need to preprocess the message stream.
- Identifying the correlation between variants of text processing solutions and classification algorithms. This makes it possible to identify the best-performing combinations of classification algorithms and text stream processing solutions.

The use of this module is optional, as classification solutions may internally include a message stream processing component. This variant is also taken into account in the proposed evaluation framework by disabling the use of this module. The main value of this module is not the text processing algorithms it uses, but the possibility of integrating existing or developing text processing algorithms into the framework through the use of web services and their joint evaluation. This variant makes it possible to distribute the execution load of the sorting processing algorithms to different computing nodes, which process the messages of the stream sent to them and return the sorting result to the framework.

2.4. Classification

Based on learning algorithms, Classification classifies the messages of the generated stream. The classification module can aggregate different classification solutions that exist in the literature or are proprietary. The module consumes these solutions as web services that are available and comply with an input and output format. The solutions of the module to be evaluated classify the generated message streams into different categories. The same message stream can be classified by more than one classification solution, which allows comparing the performance of n solutions with the same message stream generated in the simulation. In this framework, classification solutions that include a text processing component can be evaluated. To train these classifiers, 90% of a set of messages, such as the messages in the SpamAssassin corpus, is used. The main value of this module is not the classification algorithms it uses, but the possibility of integrating existing or developing classification algorithms into the framework through the use of web services and their joint evaluation. This approach allows the execution load of sorting and classification algorithms to be distributed across different computing nodes. These nodes process the messages within the stream sent to them and then send the sorting results back to the framework.

2.5. Evaluation

Evaluation evaluates the performance of the learners used to classify the stream by measuring accuracy, precision, recall, positive true, positive false, negative true and negative false. The evaluation module receives the output of the classifiers used and the real classes of each message in the stream generated in the simulation. From this information, measures of accuracy, precision, recall, true positives, false positives, true negatives and false negatives are applied to obtain the performance of the different classification solutions. This allows comparisons to be made with other classifiers using the same input parameters.

The evaluation module allows you to design and run experiments to evaluate message stream analysis solutions and analyse the results. Designing experiments involves organising the following initial elements: setting the simulation time, configuring the message stream generator, configuring text processing (if enabled), configuring classification and configuring the evaluation process.

By setting the simulation time it is possible to regulate the duration of the experiment to be carried out. The configuration of the message stream generator consists of defining and/or creating the profile instances that will constitute the source that generates the message streams to be processed in the simulation. Instances may exist previously or be created in the same design of the experiment, although the instance of training examples is unique, as explained in the description of the Message Stream Simulation module. Existing instances can be selected without further adjustment of the *sub* parameters, although they can be changed at the experimenter's discretion. To create a profile instance, it is first named, classified according to profile types, and it is decided which messages will form the corpus. Parameter values are then set to adjust the various *sub* of the profile instance to suit the experimenter.

In the processing configuration, you can choose whether to use the processing module or not. The classification solutions to be evaluated may include the processing stage and therefore the use of this module would not be necessary. On the other hand, the choice to use the processing module may be due to the use of a basic processing that allows to focus only on the evaluation of the classification process, or to evaluate a processing solution by comparing it with other solutions and seeing the classification behaviour when receiving the outputs of the different preprocessors that can be compared by one or more available classification solutions.

3. Case Study: Spam Email Detection

This section presents a case study, Spam Email Detection, where an implementation (https://github.com/Cujae-IF/FrameworkToEvaluateMessageClassification.git accessed on 16 January 2024) of the proposed framework is used to evaluate solutions in spam detection scenarios. The Spam Email Detection case study aims to measure the influence of email streams on the quality (accuracy, precision and recall) of spam email detection. For this purpose, the proposed framework will be implemented to generate mail streams from the SpamAssassin corpus [25] using the Message Stream Simulation module, to classify them using a built-in test classifier (LearningAntiSpamServer) in the Classification module, and finally to evaluate the quality of the classification using the Evaluation module.

While email recipients may have historically viewed spam as nothing more than an annoying intrusion, unwanted advertising or a waste of time, they now commonly associate it with complex and potential threats to their online security, integrity and trustworthiness [26]. Approximately 50% to 85% of the world's daily email traffic is now generated by spam [6], although spam is not exclusive to email and can also be found in other contexts such as social networks [27]. The negative impact of spam has resulted in billions of dollars of economic loss every year. Several proposed spam detection techniques have been developed to determine the authenticity of the emails [6,10,28]. To evaluate the performance of the filters, various corpus, measures and evaluation methods have been published [6,10]. Although the evaluation of spam filters seems to be quite consolidated from an academic point of view, the current methods do not simulate the real environment correctly. Among the factors that are often not taken into account when evaluating spam filters are the combination in the stream of email clusters with different characteristics (e.g., social networking, marketing and informational), the arrival frequency of the emails to be filtered, the size of the emails, the number of emails per arrival, and the obfuscation of the email body by spammers.

3.1. Materials and Methods

In order to perform an analysis of the features included in the evaluation framework, the Spam Email Detection case study was performed in the Spam Email Detection scenario. The case study focuses on running simulations to analyse the performance behaviour with respect to the factors involved in the generation of the email stream. The LearningAntiSpamServer classifier is initially trained on 500 spam and 500 ham mails from the SpamAssassin corpus [25] in all simulation runs.

In the case study the factors considered for the simulation are Message Send Rate (MSR), Message Batch Size (MBS), Message Size (MS), Message Obfuscation (MO) and Latency (LAT). The levels for each of these factors are MSR: 1-constant or 2-random; MBS: 1-constant or 2-random; MS: 1-Without limit or 2-With lower limit; MO: 1-Without obfuscation or 2-With obfuscation; and LAT: 1-Null, 2-Intermediate or 3-Extreme. Spammer (SP), Social Network (SNP), Personal (PP), Marketing (MP) and Informational (IP) profiles are modelled for the spam detection environment; however, the proposed solution allows the modelling of other profiles for this and other message analysis contexts. These profiles form clusters in which you can group different types of emails that occur in real-world scenarios. The characterisation of the email corpus used by each profile modelled for the spam detection environment is shown in Table 1.

Table 1. Characterisation of email records by profile.

Profile	Source	Instances	Spam	Ham
Spammer	Personal email accounts	150	150	0
Social Network	Personal email accounts	300	300	0
Personal	Personal email accounts	450	425	25
Marketing	Personal email accounts	500	500	0
Informational	Personal email accounts	500	240	260

In order to determine the constant values of the message send rate and message batch size factors to be used in the experiment, a small study was conducted with 30 university students. These students were asked how many emails they had received per hour during the day from sources associated with the defined profiles. In addition, the category other sources (Others) were included for those emails that were not included in the profiles. From the data, we obtained the average number of emails received per hour for each of the sources, which is shown in Table 2.

Table 2. Average number of emails received per hour.

	SNP	IP	MP	PP	SP	Others
Mean	30	14	36	2	6	1

As can be seen, social networks and news media have the highest average email traffic. Taking into account the data collected, the following values of the levels were tested in the simulation for the experiment with the highest number of emails in the shortest time:

- Message send rate constant: 5 min.

- Message batch size constant: The average number of emails received per hour from each source. In the case of source Others it was not taken into account as it was not covered by the profiles.

In addition, the lower limit value of the MS factor was chosen to be 10 KB.

Obfuscation, which is applied to the body of the mail, models one of the behaviours of a spammer and is only applied to mails with a real spam class. The time variation in the sending of training instances aims to evaluate the quality of the response as the arrival time of the [instance, class] pair increases. In the experiment, the time variation has two possible values: higher frequency (sending training instances with a random frequency between [0:1] min) and lower frequency (sending training instances with a random frequency between [5:20] min). This variable is a fundamental aspect for semi-supervised learning solutions. The duration of each of the simulations will be 1 h. Given the factors and their levels, Table 3 represents the experimental units in arrays, where the value is the treatment given to the factor. For example, the value 2 in MO means that the treatment for the variable "Message Obfuscation" will be "With Obfuscation". In addition, changes from one experimental unit to another are highlighted.

Table 3. Description of the experimental units.

Factors	Unit Number												
	01	02	03	04	05	06	07	08	09	10	11	12	13
MSR	1	2	1	1	1	1	2	1	1	1	1	1	1
MBS	1	1	2	1	1	1	1	2	1	1	1	1	1
MS	1	1	1	2	1	1	1	1	2	1	1	2	1
MO	1	1	1	1	2	1	1	1	1	2	1	1	2
LAT	1	1	1	1	1	2	2	2	2	2	3	3	3

The combination of the extreme level of the Latency factor with the random levels of the Message Send Rate and Message Batch Size factors was not included in these experimental units. These combinations were not included on the assumption that by not learning during classification, the frequency of mail arrivals or the amount of mail received by the classifiers would not affect the quality of classification and would be similar to using the constant level.

3.2. Analysis of the Results

The aim of this section is to analyse the results obtained by classifying the generated email streams into spam and ham. Based on the analysis of the traces generated by the 13 simulations, the email streams are characterised in Table 4.

Figures 3 and 4 show the results obtained for accuracy, precision and recall for each experimental unit.

In Figure 4, it can be seen that as latency decreases, so do the values of all the measures. This suggests an influence of latency on the quality of results, which may be due to a low ability to adapt to possible concept drift with few training instances of the used processor and/or message classifier. A variation of this may be the use of semi-supervised or unsupervised learning approaches to learn from unlabelled instances. On the other hand, in Experimental Units 5, 10 and 13, there is a significant decrease that coincides with the introduction of obfuscation in the emails, suggesting its significant influence on the classification quality. One of the reasons for this reduction in the quality of results may be that terms that the user recognises as having similar or the same meaning, even if they have different spellings, are not recognised by the processor used and are treated as different terms. In addition, the other three factors have a similar level of influence, regardless of the level of sending training instances. For a better understanding of the results, the experimental units are divided into the three levels of the Latency factor as shown in Figure 4 and detailed below:

- Experimental Units 1–5: Null.
- Experimental Units 6–10: Intermediate.
- Experimental Units 11–13: Extreme.

Table 4. Characterisation of simulated email streams.

Stream	Profiles					Training Instances	Total Emails
	SNP	IP	MP	PP	SP		
S01	360	168	432	24	72	1284	2340
S02	270	168	324	18	72	2126	2978
S03	57	168	96	42	72	2713	3148
S04	360	168	432	24	72	905	1961
S05	360	168	432	24	72	1388	2444
S06	360	168	432	24	72	410	1466
S07	390	168	468	26	72	321	1445
S08	48	168	74	56	72	115	533
S09	360	168	432	24	72	86	1142
S10	360	168	432	24	72	529	1585
S11	360	168	432	24	72	-	1056
S12	360	168	432	24	72	-	1056
S13	360	168	432	24	72	-	1056
Total emails	4005	2184	4850	358	936	9877	

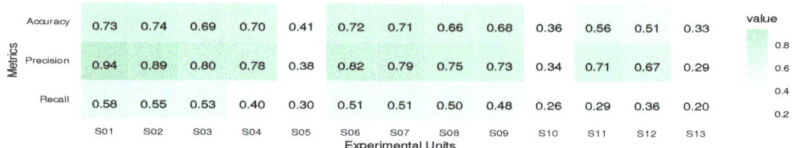

Figure 3. Heat map of general results of the experiment.

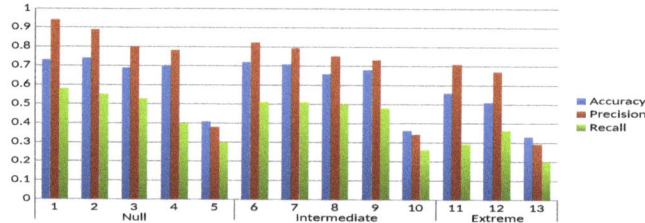

Figure 4. Graphical representation of the overall results of the experiment.

To better see the influence of the factors for each level of the Latency factor, separate analyses are performed. Figure 5 illustrates the behaviour of the quality measures for the experimental units corresponding to the null level.

The first experimental unit is taken as the baseline, as none of the first four factors are changed. In almost all cases there is a tendency for the quality of the result to decrease with respect to the baseline, except for accuracy, where Factor 1 (Experimental Unit 2) shows a slight increase. On the other hand, for most measures, the order of influence of the factors is Factor 4, 3, 2 and 1, with Factor 4 (obfuscation of the body of the mail) having the most significant influence. This order is not true for the accuracy of Factors 2 and 3 (Experimental Units 3 and 4, respectively).

Figure 6 illustrates the behaviour of the quality measures for the experimental units corresponding to the intermediate level.

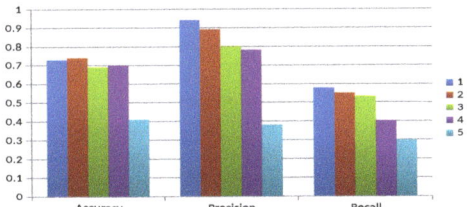

Figure 5. Graphical representation of the null level latency results.

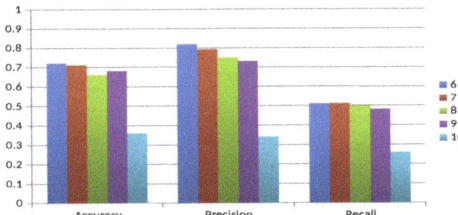

Figure 6. Graphical representation of the intermediate level latency results.

The sixth experimental unit is taken as the baseline, as none of the first four factors are changed. In almost all cases there is a tendency for the quality of the result to decrease with respect to the baseline, except for recall, where Factor 1 (Experimental Unit 7) is the same. On the other hand, for most of the measures, the order of influence of the factors is Factor 4, 3, 2 and 1, with Factor 4 (obfuscation of the body of the mail) having the most significant influence. Factors 2 and 3 (Experimental Units 8 and 9, respectively) do not follow this order for accuracy.

Figure 7 illustrates the behaviour of the quality measures for the experimental units corresponding to the extreme level.

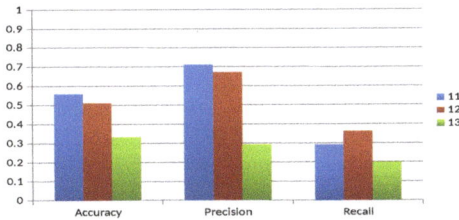

Figure 7. Graphical representation of the extreme level latency results.

The eleventh experimental unit is taken as the baseline, as none of the first four factors are changed. In almost all cases there is a tendency for the quality of the result to decrease with respect to the baseline, except for recall, where Factor 3 (Experimental Unit 12) shows an increase with respect to the baseline. On the other hand, for all measures, the order of influence of the factors is Factor 4 and 3, with Factor 4 (obfuscation of the body of the mail) having the most significant influence. Overall, the experimental results show that in most cases the second levels of the identified factors tend to decrease the classification quality values. Factor 1, however, exceeds the baseline in one case and is equal to the baseline in another, and Factor 3 exceeds the baseline in one case. On the other hand, the order of influence of the first four factors is almost always Factor 4, 3, 2 and 1. From the results obtained, it could be said that the factors with the most notable influence are Factors 4 and 5 (message obfuscation and latency, respectively).

4. Discussion

Current approaches focus on evaluating classification solutions with message streams generated from a cross-validation strategy or with different message corpora. This reduces the ability to adequately model dynamic environments with varying latency and limits the representation of different behaviours of message sources such as spammers. In contrast, the present proposal generates the message streams following a profiling approach of the message sending sources together with the use of simulation techniques and queueing theory. This gives the possibility to model the different behaviours that different sources may have, be it different spammers with different adversarial attack strategies, press media or social network sources. Each of these profile instances generates its own stream of messages, which are then combined into the main stream, which is closer to the real stream. For example, in the study case presented, it was found that the evaluated classification solution degrades in its quality results as the latency increases and when message obfuscation strategies are used by spammers. This suggests that the classification solution should be improved to better adapt to message streams where training message latency increases and spammers use message obfuscation strategies. A possible solution to the latency problem could be the use of a semi-supervised or unsupervised classification approach and, for obfuscated messages, the improvement of the text processor used by means of a term similarity approach. However, these sources may have social and proactive behaviours that influence the generation of the stream and are not covered by the proposed solution. An example of this is the spammers themselves, who may proactively vary their attack strategy so that their target cannot evade them, sometimes forming communities of spammers. Furthermore, the proposed solution only considers obfuscation of the message body as an adversarial attack strategy for this type of source, and there are others.

On the other hand, in the developed study case, the latency in sending training instances and the obfuscation of the body of the messages were identified as the parameters with the greatest impact on the quality of the classification. This case study demonstrated the performance of the proposed framework. However, the dataset used for the evaluation was small, as were the processing and classification solutions used, suggesting a larger-scale evaluation at the level of the volume of messages used and a wider range of classifiers and text processors. Furthermore, the framework was only evaluated in the context of spam detection, although it can be used in other contexts, such as news analysis, where sources are modelled as thematic profiles that may constitute digital news media.

5. Conclusions

In this work, we present a framework based on message stream simulation to evaluate solutions of classification. The use of the queueing theory in the modelling of the user profiles contributed a bigger formalism to the proposed solution. The incorporation of randomness in some of the events of the simulation allowed approximating the generation of the message stream to a real scenario. The evaluation module provides the ability to apply the evaluation measures to analyse the behaviour of the classifiers under the same input conditions. The case study demonstrates an evaluation design that allows identifying the factors present in real contexts that most influence the quality of classification solutions, and thus knowing how to adapt the solution. For the evaluated solution, the factors that most influenced the quality were message obfuscation and latency. Future work is planned to perform a robustness or sensitivity analysis to better understand how changes in simulation parameters affect the reliability of the proposed framework; to develop new test cases and/or scenarios in contexts such as news analysis, unanswered message identification, social media message classification, and others that demonstrate greater versatility and applicability of the proposed framework to a wider range of message classification challenges; to use the proposed framework to evaluate and compare solutions from the literature for semi-supervised text classification in intermediate and extreme latency scenarios; and to make social modelling of message delivery sources to identify social and proactive behaviours, which can then be implemented using an intelligent multi-agent approach.

Author Contributions: Conceptualization, W.H.-M. and M.M.-E.; methodology, F.M.-P. and J.V.B.M.; validation, M.M.-E., F.M.-P. and J.V.B.M.; formal analysis, W.H.-M., F.M.-P. and M.M.-E; writing—original draft preparation, W.H.-M.; writing—review and editing, I.L.F. and J.P. All authors have read and agreed to the published version of the manuscript.

Funding: This research received no external funding.

Data Availability Statement: The data presented in this study are available in http://mlkd.csd.auth.gr/datasets.html.

Conflicts of Interest: The authors declare no conflicts of interest.

References

1. Bularca, M.; Nechita, F.; Sargu, L.; Motoi, G.; Otovescu, A.; Coman, C. Looking for the Sustainability Messages of European Universities' Social Media Communication during the COVID-19 Pandemic. *Sustainability* **2022**, *14*, 1554. [CrossRef]
2. Bui, Q.; Lyytinen, K. Aligning adoption messages with audiences? priorities: A mixed-methods study of the diffusion of enterprise architecture among the US state governments. *Inf. Organ.* **2022**, *32*, 100423. [CrossRef]
3. Hemker, S.; Herrando, C.; Constantinides, E. The Transformation of Data Marketing: How an Ethical Lens on Consumer Data Collection Shapes the Future of Marketing. *Sustainability* **2021**, *13*, 11208. [CrossRef]
4. Anastasiei, B.; Dospinescu, N.; Dospinescu, O. The impact of social media peer communication on customer behaviour—Evidence from Romania. *Argum. Oecon.* **2022**, *1*, 247–264. [CrossRef]
5. Zheng, X.; Li, P.; Wu, X. Data Stream Classification Based on Extreme Learning Machine: Review. *Big Data Res.* **2022**, *30*, 100356. [CrossRef]
6. Jáñez Martino, F.; Alaiz-Rodríguez, R.; González-Castro, V.; Fidalgo, E.; Alegre, E. A review of spam email detection: Analysis of spammer strategies and the dataset shift problem. *Artif. Intell. Rev.* **2023**, *56*, 1145–1173. [CrossRef]
7. Marrs, G.; Hickey, R.; Black, M. The impact of latency on online classification learning with concept drift. In Proceedings of the Knowledge Science, Engineering and Management 2010 (KSEM 2010), Belfast, Northern Ireland, UK, 1–3 September 2010; Bi, Y., Williams, M., Eds.; Springer: Berlin/Heidelberg, Germany, 2010; Volume 6291, pp. 459–469. [CrossRef]
8. Souza, V.; Pinho, T.; Batista, G. Evaluating Stream Classifiers with Delayed Labels Information. In Proceedings of the 7th Brazilian Conference on Intelligent Systems (BRACIS), Sao Paulo, Brazil, 22–25 October 2018; pp. 408–413. [CrossRef]
9. Biggio, B.; Roli, F. Wild Patterns: Ten Years after the Rise of Adversarial Machine Learning. *Pattern Recogn.* **2018**, *84*, 317–331. [CrossRef]
10. Dada, E.; Bassi, J.; Chiroma, H.; Abdulhamid, S.; Adetunmbi, A.; Ajibuwa, O. Machine learning for email spam filtering: Review, approaches and open research problems. *Heliyon* **2019**, *5*, e01802. [CrossRef] [PubMed]
11. Pérez-Díaz, N.; Ruano-Ordás, D.; Fdez-Riverola, F.; Méndez, J. SDAI: An integral evaluation methodology for content-based spam filtering mode. *Expert Syst. Appl.* **2012**, *39*, 12487–12500. [CrossRef]
12. Nelson, B.; Biggio, B.; Laskov, P. Understanding the Risk Factors of Learning in Adversarial Environments. In Proceedings of the 4th ACM Workshop on Security and Artificial Intelligence; AISec '11, Chicago, IL, USA, 21 October 2011; ACM: New York, NY, USA, 2011; pp. 87–92. [CrossRef]
13. Biggio, B.; Corona, I.; Maiorca, D.; Nelson, B.; Šrndić, N.; Laskov, P.; Giacinto, G.; Roli, F. Evasion Attacks against Machine Learning at Test Time. In Proceedings of the Machine Learning and Knowledge Discovery in Databases, Prague, Czech Republic, 23–27 September 2013; Blockeel, H., Kersting, K., Nijssen, S., Železný, F., Eds.; Springer: Berlin/Heidelberg, Germany, 2013; pp. 387–402.
14. Jubatus: Distributed Online Machine Learning Framework. Available online: http://jubat.us/en/ (accessed on 16 January 2024).
15. Bifet, A.; Holmes, G.; Kirkby, R.; Pfahringer, B. MOA: Massive Online Analysis. *J. Mach. Learn. Res.* **2010**, *11*, 1601–1604.
16. Clever, L.; Pohl, J.; Bossek, J.; Kerschke, P.; Trautmann, H. Process-Oriented Stream Classification Pipeline: A Literature Review. *Appl. Sci.* **2022**, *12*, 9094. [CrossRef]
17. Gartner IT Glossary. Frameworks. 2021. Available online: https://www.gartner.com/en/information-technology/glossary/framework (accessed on 5 September 2022).
18. Apache Software Foundation. *Apache Spark—Unified Analytics Engine for Big Data*; Apache Software Foundation: Forest Hill, MD, USA, 2021.
19. Pérez, F.M.; Fonseca, I.L.; Martínez, J.V.B.; Maciá-Fiteni, A. Distributed Architecture for an Elderly Accompaniment Service Based on IoT Devices, AI, and Cloud Services. *IEEE MultiMedia* **2023**, *30*, 17–27. [CrossRef]
20. Hiller, F.; Lieberman, G. *Introduction to Operations Research*; Raghothaman Srinivasan; McGraw-Hill Science: New York, NY, USA, 2010; Chapter Simulation, pp. 934–990.
21. Hiller, F.; Lieberman, G. *Introduction to Operations Research*; Raghothaman Srinivasan; McGraw-Hill Science: New York, NY, USA, 2010; Chapter Queueing Theory, pp. 759–827.

22. García, S.; Luengo, J.; Herrera, F. *Data Preprocessing in Data Mining*, 1st ed.; Springer: Cham, Switzerland, 2015. [CrossRef]
23. Pyle, D. *Data Preparation for Data Mining*, 1st ed.; Morgan Kaufmann Publishers Inc.: San Francisco, CA, USA, 1999.
24. Ramírez-Gallego, S.; Krawczyk, B.; García, S.; Woźniak, M.; Herrera, F. A survey on data preprocessing for data stream mining: Current status and future directions. *Neurocomputing* **2017**, *239*, 39–57. [CrossRef]
25. Katakis, I.; Tsoumakas, G.; Banos, E.; Bassiliades, N.; Vlahavas, I. An adaptive personalized news dissemination system. *J. Intell. Inf. Syst.* **2009**, *32*, 191–212. [CrossRef]
26. Gangavarapu, T.; Jaidhar, C.; Chanduka, B. Applicability of machine learning in spam and phishing email filtering: Review and approaches. *Artif. Intell. Rev.* **2020**, *53*, 5019–5081. [CrossRef]
27. Ali, S.; Islam, N.; Rauf, A.; Din, I.; Guizani, M.; Rodrigues, J. Privacy and Security Issues in Online Social Networks. *Future Internet* **2018**, *10*, 114. [CrossRef]
28. Yang, H.; Liu, Q.; Zhou, S.; Luo, Y. A Spam Filtering Method Based on Multi-Modal Fusion. *Appl. Sci.* **2019**, *9*, 1152. [CrossRef]

Disclaimer/Publisher's Note: The statements, opinions and data contained in all publications are solely those of the individual author(s) and contributor(s) and not of MDPI and/or the editor(s). MDPI and/or the editor(s) disclaim responsibility for any injury to people or property resulting from any ideas, methods, instructions or products referred to in the content.

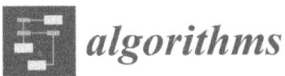

Article

CNN Based on Transfer Learning Models Using Data Augmentation and Transformation for Detection of Concrete Crack

Md. Monirul Islam [1], Md. Belal Hossain [2], Md. Nasim Akhtar [3], Mohammad Ali Moni [4] and Khondokar Fida Hasan [5,*]

1. Department of Computer Science and Engineering, University of Information Technology and Sciences, Baridhara J Block, Dhaka 1212, Bangladesh; monirul.islam@uits.edu.bd
2. Department of Computer Science and Engineering, Pabna University of Science and Technology, Pabna 6600, Bangladesh; belal.cseai@gmail.com
3. Department of Computer Science and Engineering, Dhaka University of Engineering and Technology, Gazipur 1707, Bangladesh; drnasim@duet.ac.bd
4. Artificial Intelligence and Data Science, School of Health and Rehabilitation Science, Faculty of Health and Behavioural Sciences, The University of Queensland, Brisbane, QLD 4072, Australia; m.moni@uq.edu.au
5. School of Computer Science, Queensland University of Technology, Brisbane, QLD 4001, Australia
* Correspondence: fida.hasan@qut.edu.au

Citation: Islam, M.M.; Hossain, M.B.; Akhtar, M.N.; Moni, M.A.; Hasan, K.F. CNN Based on Transfer Learning Models Using Data Augmentation and Transformation for Detection of Concrete Crack. *Algorithms* 2022, 15, 287. https://doi.org/10.3390/a15080287

Academic Editor: Frank Werner

Received: 26 June 2022
Accepted: 12 August 2022
Published: 15 August 2022

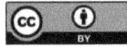

Copyright: © 2022 by the authors. Licensee MDPI, Basel, Switzerland. This article is an open access article distributed under the terms and conditions of the Creative Commons Attribution (CC BY) license (https:// creativecommons.org/licenses/by/ 4.0/).

Abstract: Cracks in concrete cause initial structural damage to civil infrastructures such as buildings, bridges, and highways, which in turn causes further damage and is thus regarded as a serious safety concern. Early detection of it can assist in preventing further damage and can enable safety in advance by avoiding any possible accident caused while using those infrastructures. Machine learning-based detection is gaining favor over time-consuming classical detection approaches that can only fulfill the objective of early detection. To identify concrete surface cracks from images, this research developed a transfer learning approach (TL) based on Convolutional Neural Networks (CNN). This work employs the transfer learning strategy by leveraging four existing deep learning (DL) models named VGG16, ResNet18, DenseNet161, and AlexNet with pre-trained (trained on ImageNet) weights. To validate the performance of each model, four performance indicators are used: accuracy, recall, precision, and F1-score. Using the publicly available CCIC dataset, the suggested technique on AlexNet outperforms existing models with a testing accuracy of 99.90%, precision of 99.92%, recall of 99.80%, and F1-score of 99.86% for crack class. Our approach is further validated by using an external dataset, BWCI, available on Kaggle. Using BWCI, models VGG16, ResNet18, DenseNet161, and AlexNet achieved the accuracy of 99.90%, 99.60%, 99.80%, and 99.90% respectively. This proposed transfer learning-based method, which is based on the CNN method, is demonstrated to be more effective at detecting cracks in concrete structures and is also applicable to other detection tasks.

Keywords: transfer learning; alexnet; crack detection

1. Introduction

Concrete cracks are a common indication of concrete defects in civil engineering structures. It affects structural health and induces an additional risk of unexpected breakdowns and accidents [1,2]. Hence, detecting cracks regularly and taking appropriate actions for the safety of the concrete structure is of great significance. The traditional method of detecting cracks on concrete structures relies on professional observation. Such conventional methods are not only costly but also laborious, time-consuming, and on many occasions, dangerous too [3]. However, the recent advancement of machine learning-based image processing technologies has gained attention as an efficient and automated method to detect cracks on concrete structures that also overcome the cons of manual methods [4].

The growing computer vision community working on different image-detection methods. It has proposed many techniques over the decades, including thresholding [5], edge detection [6], and wavelet transforms [7], to name a few, where some of these methods address concrete crack detection problems. However, this field needs an efficient and reliable solution as the concrete images are challenged with various surface textures, irregularity of cracks, and background complexity that differs crack detection from other image analysis applications.

Recently, deep learning-based models, predominantly neural networks with multiple layers, are playing a significantly successful role in feature learning [8]. On top of that, the availability of high-performing computing facilities and ongoing improvement of excellent training methods on available datasets drive the rapid development of deep learning. In this saga, the convolutional neural network (CNN) is a feed-forward neural network that performs excellently in large-scale image processing [9,10]. Although some of these models proved excellent in feature extractions on different applications, their accuracy requires improvement for concrete crack detection. To achieve efficient performance, reduce training time, and overcome the lack of a humongous dataset, in this paper, we have proposed a method of transfer learning-based CNN with the pre-trained model that shows significant improvement [11]. Our work has made the following contribution:

- We conduct experiments on the CCIC dataset with four different CNN models (VGG16, ResNet18, DenseNet161, and AlexNet), applying the transfer learning technique for detecting concrete surface cracks from images and examination with other models to demonstrate the success of the suggested model.
- We designed our model such that every CNN model has only one fully connected (FC) layer, having two output features for binary classification. We modified the VGG16 and AlexNet models by replacing the last three FC layers with only one FC layer.
- Our strategy is the most compatible with AlexNet, and it outperforms the competition. AlexNet achieves 99.90% accuracy on the validation set on the CCIC dataset.
- The proposed method demonstrates superior crack detection for concrete structures, which can efficiently be utilized for other detection purposes.

The paper is now organized as follows. We provided a brief review of the literature in Section 2. Section 3 includes methodology, which describes experimental Setup, Model Training, and Evaluation. Section 4 presents the result analysis and discussions. The paper is concluded in Section 5.

2. Literature Review

Sometimes, some research work has been done based on transfer learning for various types of crack detection. In [12], the authors presented a practical deep-learning-based crack detection model for three types of crack images, including concrete pavement, asphalt pavement, and bridge deck cracks. Also, they proposed an encoder-decoder structural model with a fully convolutional neural network, named PCSN, also known as SegNet, and achieved 99% accuracy. In [13], the MobileNet-based transfer learning model is proposed for wall crack detection as well as authors got 99.59% accuracy. In [14], a transfer learning approach was applied to the VGG16 model to recognize structural damage and achieved 90% accuracy. In [15], a deep transfer learning method based on YOLOv3 and RetinaNet models, pre-trained on the COCO dataset, was proposed for detecting rail surface cracks. In 2021, a novel method, FF-BLS, was proposed that could accurately classify crack and non-crack images with an accuracy of 96.72% [16]. In 2019, a transfer learning approach on the VGG16 pre-trained model achieved 94% accuracy, and slightly fine-tuning a well-trained FC layer with VGG16 achieved 98% accuracy [17]. In 2018, a transfer learning method on the VGG16 pre-trained model gained 92.27% accuracy after training with less than 3500 images [18]. They conclude the transfer learning approach is suitable to train on limited datasets. In [19], an image segmentation model based on ResNet101 was proposed for concrete crack detection with 94.52% precision and 95.25% recall accuracy in 2021. In 2021, a deep learning model was proposed, and although they achieved good accuracy on training, validation accuracy was 97.7% for the CCIC [20] dataset [21]. A deep, fully convolutional neural network named CrackSegNet with dilated convolution, spatial pyramid pooling, and skip connection modules was proposed to detect concrete cracks in tunnels [22]. In 2021, three kinds of deep neural networks, AlexNet, ResNet18, and VGGNet13, were compared and found ResNet18 (accuracy 98.8%) performs well compared with the remaining two models [23]. In 2021, the transfer learning method was applied on GoogLeNet Inception V3 and CNN-Crack; GoogLeNet Inception V3 performs well compared to the other one with an accuracy of 97.3% on drone cameras [24]. In [25], vision-based metal crack detection was proposed. In 2021, a pavement crack detection method based on the YOLOv5 model was proposed with 88.1% accuracy [26]. Recently in 2021, a railway slab crack detection method was proposed based on the VGG16 model and achieved 81.84%, 67.68%, and 84.55% in precision, IoU, and F1-score, respectively [27]. In [28], a deep learning model was developed for ceramic crack segmentation. In [29], a concrete air voids detection and segmentation method was proposed based on the path aggregation network (PANet). In [30], a thermal crack detection method, U-Net, was proposed to be used in fire-exposed concrete structures and achieved 78.12% Intersection over Union (IoU). In [31], a dilated convolution with Resnet-18 as the basic network model was proposed for detecting concrete cracks. In [32], a concrete crack detection method using a U-net fully convolutional network was proposed in this paper.

In this experiment, we built a concrete cracks detection model using the transfer learning (TL) approach on various well-known CNN models. We applied four available CNN models named VGG16, ResNet18, DenseNet161, and AlexNet with pre-trained (trained on ImageNet) weights for utilizing the transfer learning approach. TL-based CNN approach achieves over 99% accuracy for all the models. Our approach fits well with AlexNet most, and its performance outweighs others. AlexNet achieves 99.90% accuracy on the validation set after only 13 epochs of training. The training duration provides better timing over VGG16, ResNet18, and DenseNet161 models.

3. Materials and Methods

In this work, we presented a transfer learning method for detecting concrete surface cracks with high accuracy. Figure 1 illustrates the detailed block diagram of the methodology.

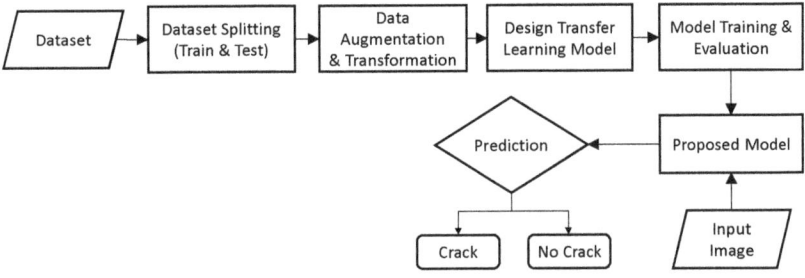

Figure 1. A block diagram of the proposed methodology.

We divided our collected dataset into two sets: train and test. The train set is used for method training, while the test set is used for model validation and model testing. The splitting procedure was carried out at random. On the training dataset, data augmentation, and transformations take place. Following that, we designed transfer learning models. On designed TL models, model training and evaluation take place. Then we compare the TL methods before displaying the best TL method proposed. Finally, we feed the input images into the best TL model that has been proposed, and it produces the expected result, which is either crack or non-crack.

3.1. Dataset Description

The utilized dataset in this research paper is Concrete Crack Images for Classification (CCIC) [20]. It contains concrete images having cracks and non-cracks, collected from various METU Campus Buildings. The dataset is classified into positive and negative classes, referring to cracks and non-cracks images, respectively. There are 40,000 images with 227 × 227 pixels with RGB channels, and each type has 20,000 images. The dataset is generated from 458 high-resolution (4032 × 3024 pixels) images taken from floors and walls of various concrete buildings. Images are taken with the camera facing directly to the concrete surfaces keeping about a one-meter distance. The images are captured on the same day with similar illumination conditions. The concrete surface has variation because of plastering, paint, exposure, etc. But no data augmentation is applied [33]. Some cracks and non-cracks images of the used dataset are shown in Figure 2.

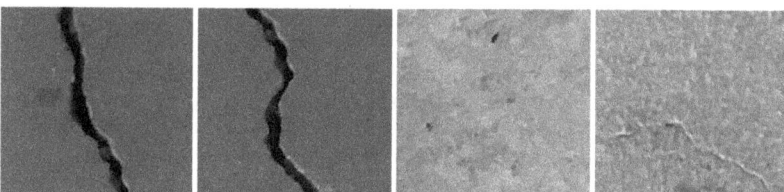

Figure 2. Sample crack and non-crack images of the CCIC dataset.

3.2. Dataset Splitting

Our dataset consists of 20,000 cracks and 20,000 non-cracks images, in a total of 40,000 images. We split the datasets into 2 groups, with ratios of 80% and 20% for the Train set as well as the Test or Validation set, respectively. After randomly splitting the dataset into train along with test sets, we obtained 31,999 images (16,000 cracks and 15,999 non-cracks images) in the train set and 8001 (4000 cracks and 4001 non-cracks) images in the test set. After using the test dataset for validation of the model, the training dataset is used for training the model and calculating various evaluation matrices. Dataset splitting is shown in Table 1 briefly.

Table 1. Dataset Test-train splitting.

	Crack	Non-Crack	Total
Train	16,000	15,999	31,999
Test	4000	4001	8001
Total	20,000	20,000	40,000

3.3. Data Augmentation and Transformation

Deep learning models perform very well on large datasets. Data augmentation is a crucial technique in deep learning for a limited dataset that enhances the size and quality of a training dataset to build a better deep learning model. There are various data augmentation techniques like flipping, cropping, rotation, color space transformation, noise injection, etc. [34]. We used data augmentation and transfer learning to overcome the lack of training data as well as get rid of overfitting. In our training dataset, we use some of the data augmentation techniques, which are described below.

3.3.1. Random-Resized-Crop Method

The random-Resized-Crop method is an augmentation method that crops a random portion of the image and resizes it according to the desired size. Such a crop is made by a random area depending on a scale and an arbitrary aspect ratio. The scale specifies a lower and upper bound for the arbitrary location of the crop, and the ratio specifies required bounds from the random aspect ratio of the yield before resizing. In our training dataset, scale = (0.8, 1.0), ratio = (0.75, 1.33) and size = (227, 227) are used. Figure 3 shows an example of this technique.

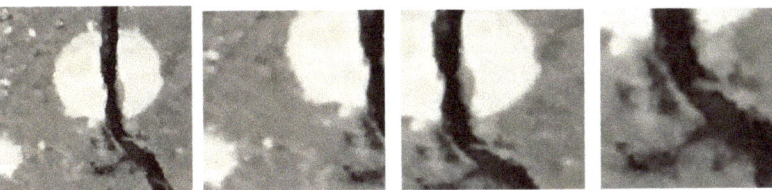

Figure 3. Example of Random Resized Crop transformation. (Left is the original image).

3.3.2. Random-Rotation Method

This augmentation method rotates the image by randomly selected angles from a specific range of degrees. In our training dataset, angles are selected between −15 degrees and +15 degrees. The area outside the rotated image is filled with pixel value 0. Figure 4 shows an example of the Random Rotation technique.

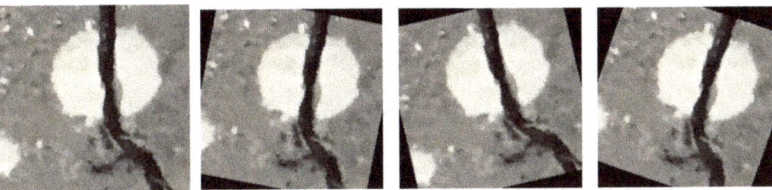

Figure 4. Example of Random Rotation transformation. (Left is the original image).

3.3.3. Color-Jitter Method

This augmentation method randomly changes the brightness, contrast, saturation, and hue of an image. An example of this method is shown in Figure 5.

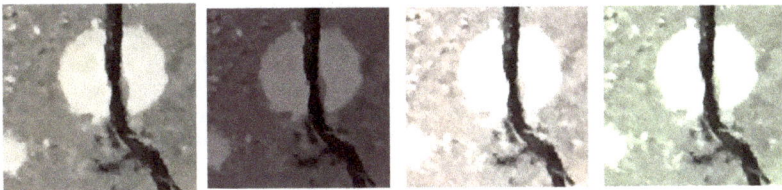

Figure 5. Example of Color Jitter transformation. (Left is the original image).

3.3.4. Random-Horizontal-Flip Method

This augmentation method horizontally flips the given image randomly with a specified probability. Our training dataset has been flipped with 50% probability. An example of a Random Horizontal Flip is exhibited in Figure 6.

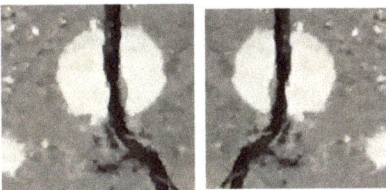

Figure 6. Example of Random Horizontal Flip transformation. (Left is the original image).

We used the above data augmentation techniques for training datasets and did not use data augmentation techniques for testing test data. Besides, some preprocessing stages are applied to both train and test datasets. CCIC dataset's image dimension is 227 × 227. But the desired input image dimension of our proposed model is 224 × 224. For this reason, preprocessing is applied to achieve desired image dimensions. Center cropping is applied on the 227 × 227 dimension image for getting a 224 × 224 dimension image. Also, we apply normalization to all images. Our pre-trained models expect input 3-channel RGB images normalized using mean of [0.485, 0.456, 0.406] and standard deviation of [0.229, 0.224, 0.225].

3.4. Design Transfer Learning Model

Image recognition has advanced remarkably, mostly because deep learning (DL) and deep convolutional neural networks (CNNs) with large-scale annotated datasets are now widely available. With enough training data, CNNs can learn data-driven, highly representative, hierarchical image characteristics. Currently, there are three main methods for effectively employing CNNs for image classification: building the CNN from scratch, using pre-trained CNN features that are available for purchase, and using unsupervised CNN pre-training with supervised fine-tuning. Transfer learning, or fine-tuning CNN models pre-trained from natural image datasets to image problems, is another efficient technique. A step in the process by which computers may examine a picture and assign it the proper label is image categorization [35–37].

Overall, CNN and deep learning (DL) are key components of image categorization nowadays. DL methods can tackle issues with increasingly complicated, highly variable functions. It also involves a sizable picture dataset, even one without labels. Machines can recognize and extract characteristics from images with the aid of DL. The image categorization [35,38] on CNN, therefore, generates a lot of attention. To perform tasks correctly, DL approaches need a lot of data [8]. Having access to a wealth of knowledge is not necessarily true. Pre-trained models are applied in this situation. In this study, transfer learning (TL) is the reuse of a deep learning pre-trained approach where knowledge is driven from one model to another [39].

Several well-known pre-trained models exhibit excellent performance across a range of computer vision issues. Some of them are VGG [40], ResNet [41], DenseNet [42], AlexNet [43], Inception v3 [44], GoogLeNet [45], MobileNet [46] etc. These models are trained on extensive datasets with various classes of images. Using TL methods, it is now possible to achieve very good performance on several computer vision issues with a lack of data and computing power. This paper experimented on four well-known models named VGG, ResNet, DenseNet, and AlexNet. In the following sections, we discuss these transfer learning models.

3.4.1. VGG16

VGG16 is a CNN model trained on the ImageNet dataset of over 1.2 million images from 1000 classes [40]. The architecture of the VGG16 model is depicted in Figure 7.

There are several convolutional (conv) layers, where filters with 3 × 3 kernels are used. The convolution stride and padding are fixed to 1 pixel. Max-pooling is applied, followed by some conv layers with 2 × 2 kernels, a stride of 2, and padding of 0. The input to conv layer is of fixed size 224 × 224 RGB image.

Three FC layers are added in the last part of the architecture, and the last layer is configured for 1000 classes. The Rectified Linear Unit (ReLU), a non-linear activation function is used by all hidden layers.

We apply the pre-trained VGG16 model to the proposed Transfer Learning (TL) model. We call it TL VGG16. We remove the last three FC layers and replace them with an FC2 layer such that output features match for binary classification.

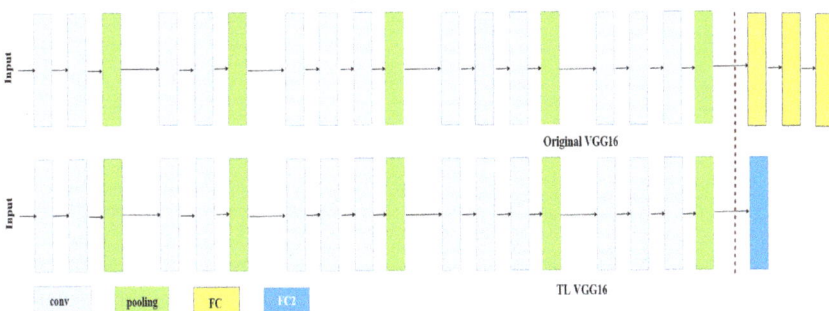

Figure 7. VGG16 and TL VGG16 architectures.

3.4.2. ResNet18

ResNet is a CNN technique presented in the paper titled Deep Residual Learning for Image Recognition' [41]. The model trained on ImageNet dataset of over 1.2 million images belonging to 1000 classes. The architecture of the ResNet18 model is depicted in Figure 8.

There are several convolutional (conv) layers. Filters with 7×7 kernels, strides of 2, and padding of 3 are used in the first conv layer. In the remaining conv layers, filters with 3×3 kernels, strides of 1, and padding of 1 are used except for some down-sampling conv with 1×1 kernels and stride of 2. The pattern remains the same, bypassing the input every 2 convolutions. Max-pooling is applied following the 1st conv layer with 3×3 kernels, a stride of 2 as well as padding of 1. The input to conv layer is of fixed size 224×224 RGB image.

Three FC layers are added in the last part of the architecture, and the last layer is configured for 1000 classes. Most hidden layers employ Batch Normalization, and a convolutional layer after ReLU.

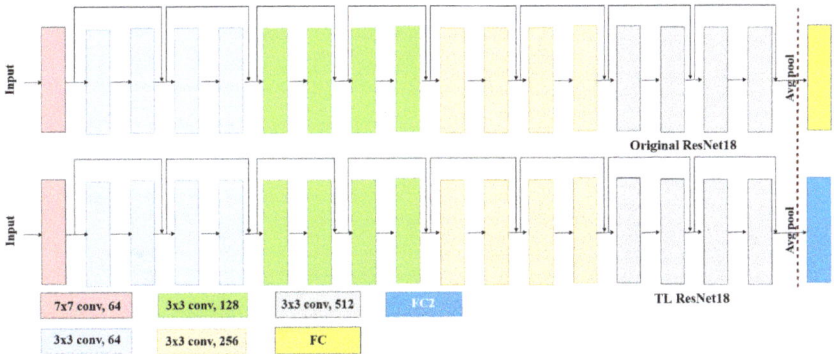

Figure 8. ResNet18 and TL ResNet18 architecture.

We use the pre-trained ResNet18 method for the proposed TL ResNet18 model. We replace the last FC layer with a Fully-Connected FC2 layer such that output features match for binary classification.

3.4.3. DenseNet161

DenseNet161 is a CNN model proposed by Zhuang et al. [42]. They have trained their model on an ImageNet dataset of over 1.2 million images from 1000 classes. A typical architecture of the DenseNet161 model is shown in Figure 9. It can be seen that there are a series of convolution (conv) layers within it, where every layer has access to its preceding feature maps. In the first conv layer, filters with 7×7 kernels, strides of 2, and padding of 3 are used. Then Normalization, ReLU, and max-pooling with 3×3 kernels, a stride of 2, and padding of 1 are used. After the first conv layer, there are four dense blocks and each block has corresponding 6, 12, 36, and 24 dense layers. Each dense layer consists of two conv layers; the preceding conv layer has a filter with 1×1 kernels and stride of 1 and, the latter conv layer has a filter with 3×3 kernels, a stride of 1, and padding of 1. Before conv layer, Batch Normalization, and ReLU are used. In the middle of two dense-blocks transition layers with Batch Normalization, ReLU, conv layer with 1×1 kernels and a stride of 1 and then an AvgPool with 2×2 kernels, a stride of 2, and padding of 0 are used. After the 4th dense-block Batch, normalization is applied.

An FC layer is added in the last part of the architecture and configured for 1000 classes.

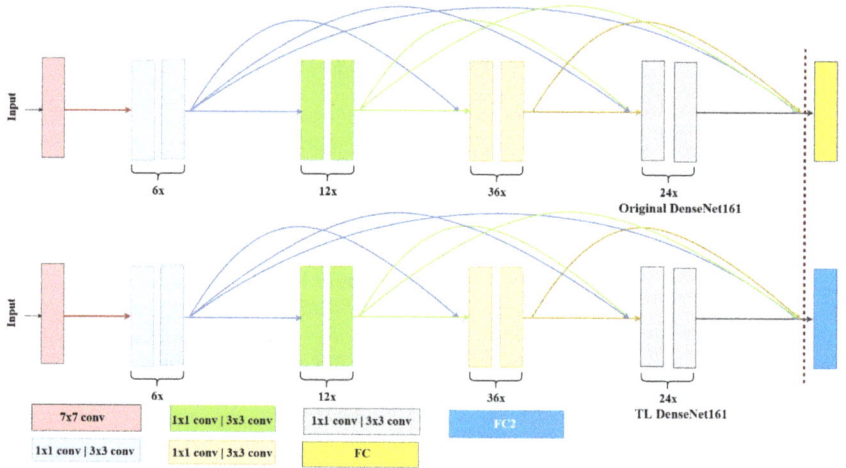

Figure 9. DenseNet161 and TL DenseNet161 architectures.

We used the pre-trained DenseNet161 model for the proposed TL DenseNet161 model. We have replaced the last FC layer with an FC2 layer such that output features match binary classification. The input to conv layer is of fixed size 224×224 RGB image.

3.4.4. AlexNet

AlexNet is a CNN model proposed by Alex Krizhevsky [43]. The model trained on ImageNet dataset of over 1.2 million images belonging to 1000 classes. The architecture of the AlexNet model is depicted in Figure 10. There are several convolutional (conv) layers. In the conv layer, filters with 11×11 kernels, strides of 4, and padding of 2 are used. In the 2nd conv layer, filters with 5×5 kernels, strides of 1, and padding of 2 are used. In the remaining three conv layers, filters with 3×3 kernels, strides of 1, and padding of 1 are used. Max-pooling is applied, followed by conv layers with 3×3 kernels, a stride of 2, and padding of 0.

Three FC layers are added in the last part of the architecture. All hidden layers use the ReLU, a non-linear activation function. Dropout with the possibility of 0.5 is utilized before the first two FC layers. The last layer is configured for 1000 classes.

We use the pre-trained AlexNet model for the proposed TL AlexNet model. We remove the last three FC layers and replace them with an FC2 layer such that output features match for binary classification. The input to conv layer is of fixed size 224×224 RGB image.

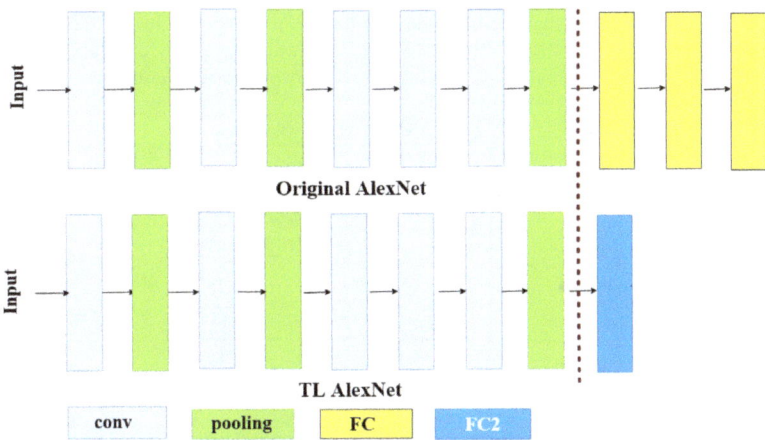

Figure 10. AlexNet and TL AlexNet architecture.

3.5. Experimental Setup, Model Training, and Evaluation

All the experiments take place in a Google Colaboratory notebook with a GPU runtime. Training is taken repeatedly throughout a number of epochs. We train our models for 30 epochs. After using the test dataset for validation of the model, the training dataset is applied for training the model. We use the PyTorch library primarily developed by the AI Research lab of Facebook. We implement the PyTorch data loader to take data of 128 batch size. We utilize the same hyperparameters optimization setup for all architectures. Table 2 shows the used hyperparameters in the experimental setup.

Table 2. Hyperparameters of different TL methods.

Parameters	Parameters Value
Batch size	128
Optimizer	Adam
Learning rate	0.001
Betas	(0.9, 0.999)
Eps	1×10^{-8}
Weight decay	0
Criterion	Cross Entropy Loss

We determine the cross-entropy loss on the train as well as test sets for each epoch. We employ the Adam optimizer [47] using the mentioned parameters value.

In Figure 11, train losses, validation losses along with train accuracies as well as validation accuracies of each TL method are depicted. In the experimental observation, we see that there is no over-fitting occurring in any of the TL models. In the first row of Figure 11, the TL VGG16 models show that both train and validation loss is reduced very quickly, and they do not improve for a higher number of epochs. The TL ResNet18 model's train and validation loss are decreased gradually and the validation loss is always lower than the training loss with very little difference. The TL DenseNet161 model's train and validation loss follow an almost similar pattern to the TL ResNet18 model. On the other hand, we see in the training and validation loss of TL AlexNet that the bare difference between the two lines, unlike ResNet18 and DenseNet161. Hence, we can conclude this model converge quickly with very good generalization capability. Whereas, train along with validation accuracy of several TL methods are presented in the second row Figure 11. We see a similar pattern like the train and validation loss of different TL models. The ResNet18 and DenseNet161 follow the same pattern: validation accuracy is always greater than the training accuracy. Also, train accuracy is always less than the validation accuracy in the VGG16 model. But the TL AlexNet model shows the different patterns, the train, and validation accuracy overlap, and achieves high accuracy among other models. The AlexNet shows good generalization among others.

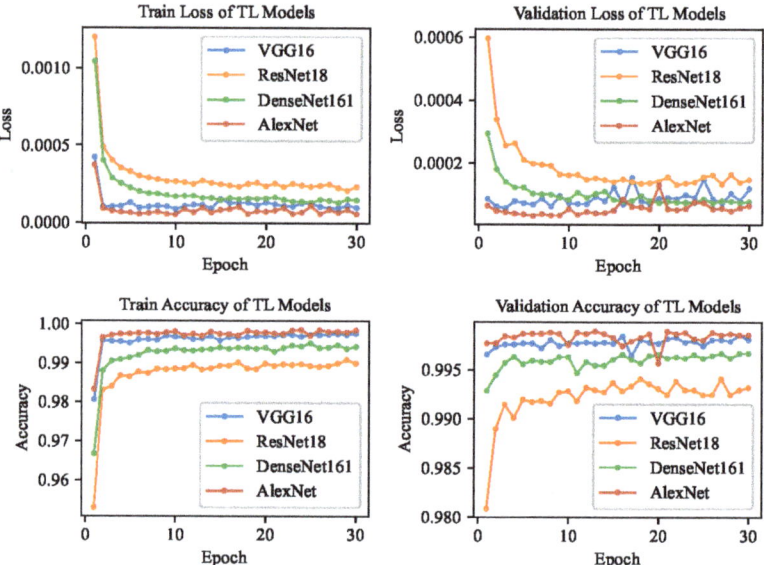

Figure 11. Loss and accuracy of all TL models both in Train and validation.

We clearly see that AlexNet achieves the best score for the lowest training and validation losses among all other models. Also, we clearly see that AlexNet achieves the best score for the highest training and validation accuracies among all other models.

4. Result Exploration and Argument

Through the confusion matrix, we can find out the P, R, F1, and Accuracy. These are the criteria for evaluating the classification model. Confusion matrix has four keywords of this including True Positive, False Positive, False Negative, and True Negative [48].

We can define **Precision**, **Recall**, **F1-score**, and **Accuracy** mathematically by using the Equations (1)–(4) respectively.

$$Precision, P = \frac{TP}{TP + FP} \quad (1)$$

$$Recall, R = \frac{TP}{TP + FN} \quad (2)$$

$$F1 - score, F1 = 2 \times \frac{P \times R}{P + R} \quad (3)$$

$$Accuracy = \frac{Number\ of\ correct\ predictions}{Total\ number\ of\ predictions\ made} \quad (4)$$

After 30 epochs of training of all TL models, an evaluation is made on a test dataset consisting of 8001 images where 4000 images are cracks and 4001 images are non-cracks. Figure 12 illustrates the confusion matrix of all models.

The TL VGG16 predicts 3996 (TP) cracks and 3990 (TN) non-cracks images correctly, as well as 4 (FN) cracks images predicted as non-crack, and 11 (FP) non-cracks images predicted as cracks Figure 12a. The number of FN is minimum among other models.

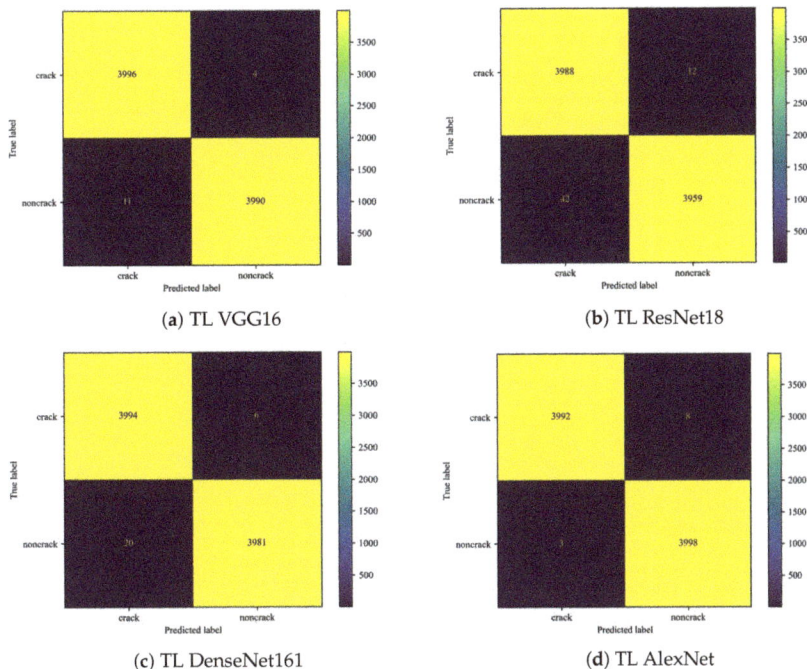

Figure 12. Confusion matrix of TL VGG16, TL ResNet18, TL DenseNet161, and TL AlexNet.

The TL ResNet18, on the other hand, predicts 3988 (TP) cracks and 3959 (TN) non-cracks images correctly, as well as 12 (FN) cracks images predicted as non-crack and 42 (FP) non-cracks images predicted as cracks Figure 12b. In this case, the number of FP is the highest among other models.

We can see in the TL DenseNet161 model's confusion matrix Figure 12c, that it predicts 3994 (TP) cracks and 3981 (TN) non-cracks images correctly, as well as 8 (FN) cracks images predicted as non-crack and 20 (FP) non-cracks image predicted as cracks. TL AlexNet Figure 12d shows the balance between FN and FP and shows the minimum number of FP (3 FP) among all other models.

Table 3 displays several standard assessment scores, with the number of samples utilized during the evaluation represented in the Support column which is denoted as Sup.

From Table 3, we can conclude that TL AlexNet achieves the highest 99.86% F1 scores and 99.86% accuracies among other models and precision of 99.92% on cracks and recall of 99.93% on non-cracks. In the case of popular statistical tests named MCC and CK (Cohen's Kappa), AlexNet performs better than others. The values of MCC and CK are almost the same, we took 4 digits after the decimal point. Although, AlexNet achieves the best validation accuracy of 99.90% during the 13th epoch training, shown in Table 4.

As a succinct outline of every TL algorithm throughout training as well as validation, Table 4 displays the highest, lowest, and average accuracy. From the summary, we can conclude that AlexNet models achieve the best train accuracy of 99.85% on the 24th epoch and the best validation accuracy of 99.90% on the 13th epoch among all other models.

Table 5 shows the training duration of each epoch during training on Google Colaboratory GPU runtime. The TL AlexNet achieves 1st place by taking minimum training time among the other models.

Table 3. Various scores were calculated in the test dataset (CCIC) for different TL models after 30 epochs of training where P = Precision, R = Recall, F1 = F1-score, Sup = Support, A = Accuracy, CK = Cohen's Kappa.

Model		P (%)	R (%)	F1 (%)	Sup	A (%)	MCC (%)	CK (%)
TL VGG16	Crack	99.73	99.90	99.81	4000	99.81	99.6252	99.6250
	Non-crack	99.90	99.73	99.81	4001			
TL ResNet18	Crack	98.96	99.70	99.33	4000	99.33	98.6529	98.6502
	Non-crack	99.70	98.95	99.32	4001			
TLDenseNet161	Crack	99.50	99.85	99.68	4000	99.68	99.3507	99.3501
	Non-crack	99.85	99.50	99.67	4001			
TL AlexNet	Crack	99.92	99.80	99.86	4000	99.86	99.7251	99.7250
	Non-crack	99.80	99.93	99.86	4001			

Table 4. Performance measurement of used TL methods during 30 epochs of training where MA_E = Maximum Accuracy at epoch, MinA_E = Minimum Accuracy at epoch, Avg_acc = Average Accuracy.

Model	Train/Test	Max Acc (%)	MA_E	Min Acc (%)	MinA_E	Avg_acc (%)
TL VGG16	Train	99.76	30	98.06	1	99.61
	Test	99.86	29	99.65	17	99.78
TL ResNet18	Train	99.09	29	95.31	1	98.74
	Test	99.41	18	98.09	1	99.22
TL DenseNet161	Train	99.51	25	96.68	1	99.24
	Test	99.68	27	99.29	1	99.60
TL AlexNet	Train	99.85	24	98.34	1	99.72
	Test	99.90	13	99.58	20	99.84
All	Train Max Acc	99.85		TL AlexNet at Epoch 24		
	Test Max Acc	99.90		TL AlexNet at Epoch 13		
	Both Max Acc	99.90		TL AlexNet at Epoch 13		

Table 5. Training time per-epoch of TL models.

Model	Duration Per-Epoch (h:mm:ss)	Remarks
TL VGG16	0:08:46.729322	3rd place
TL ResNet18	0:03:35.636223	2nd place
TL DenseNet161	0:13:39.103467	Lowest place
TL AlexNet	0:02:53.093954	1st place
TL AlexNet takes the 1st position by achieving the least training time		

We also depicted the receiver operating characteristic (ROC) curve for comparing the models in the case of appropriate classification results. It is measured based on the performance of the false positive rate and true positive rate respectively. Figure 13 shows the ROC curve of different TL models in our works. In this figure, we denote four curves of red, green, blue, and orange colored for AlexNet, DenseNet, VGG16, and ResNet18 models. All models' performances are good. On the left side of this figure, all curves are looking together. For understanding better, we observed it as zoom out which is shown in the right portion of the figure. From this figure, we can see that AlexNet places the highest position over other models.

We also presented another way of evaluating the performance of models named the precision-recall (PR) curve. Figure 14 shows the PR curve of different TL models in our works. In this figure, we mark four curves of red, green, blue, and orange colored for AlexNet, DenseNet, VGG16, and ResNet18 models. In the upper side of this figure, all curves are looking together. For understanding better, we observed it as zoom out which is shown in the down portion of the figure. From this figure, we can see that all models' performance is good.

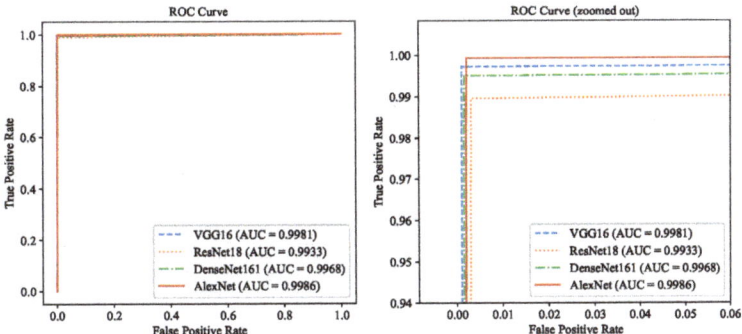

Figure 13. ROC curve of different TL models.

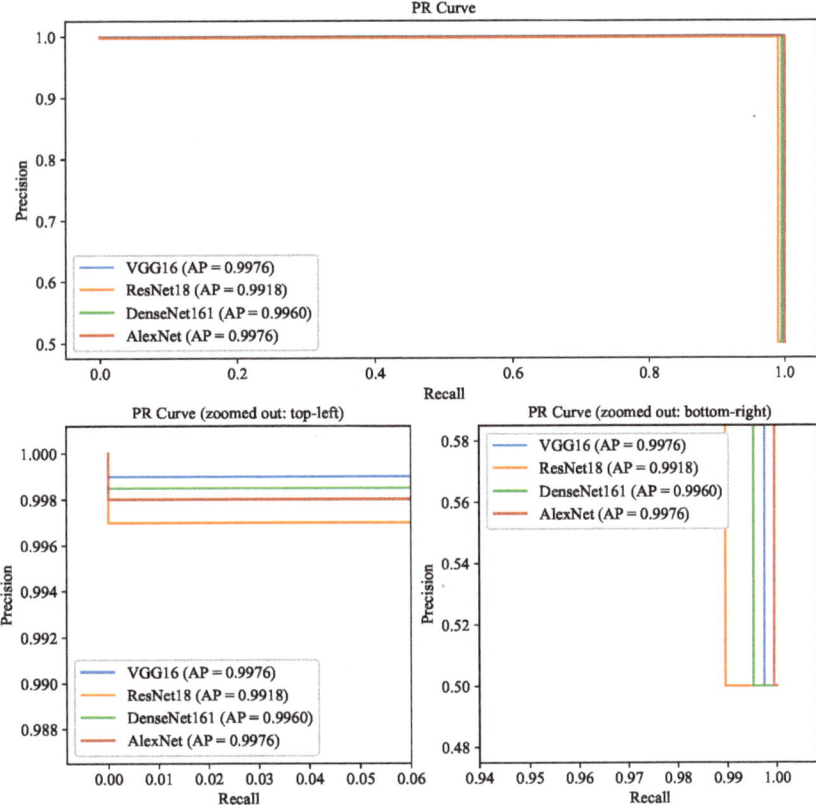

Figure 14. PR curve of different TL models.

In addition, we used the external dataset Building Wall Crack Images (BWCI) from Kaggle to validate our models. This is an open-source dataset. BWCI consists of wall crack images with 27 × 27 pixels. Table 6 shows the description of the dataset and a few samples are shown in Figure 15.

Table 6. Summary of external dataset (BWCI).

Image Folder	No. of Crack Images	No. of Noncrack Images	Total
Test	500	500	1000
Train	1250	1250	2500
Validation	500	500	1000

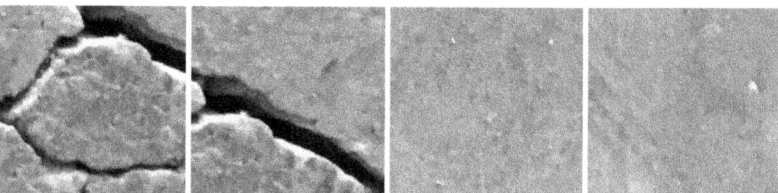

Figure 15. Sample crack and non-crack images of external dataset.

Table 7 represents the result of all models on the external dataset. We used only the test folder dataset to validate the models. It can be seen that the performance for both CCIC and external datasets BWCI are almost same.

Table 7. Performance result of external dataset (BWCI) where P = Precision, R = Recall, F1 = F1-score, A = Accuracy.

Model		P (%)	R(%)	F1 (%)	A (%)	MCC (%)	CK (%)
TL VGG16	Crack	99.80	1.00	99.90	99.90	99.8000	99.7998
	Non-crack	1.00	99.80	99.90			
TL ResNet18	Crack	99.40	99.80	99.60	99.60	99.1999	99.1992
	Non-crack	99.80	99.40	99.60			
TLDenseNet161	Crack	99.60	1.00	99.80	99.80	99.6004	99.5996
	Non-crack	1.00	99.60	99.80			
TL AlexNet	Crack	1.00	99.80	99.90	99.90	99.7999	99.7997
	Non-crack	99.80	1.00	99.90			

Two statistical tests have been carried out, named the Matthews correlation coefficient (MCC) and Cohen's Kappa Statistic [49] for comparing the performance. Matthews correlation coefficient (MCC) is a popular performance metric that is used in the case of an imbalanced dataset. Although the utilized dataset in this paper is a balanced dataset, it is defined by the following mathematical equation number 5.

$$MCC = \frac{TP \times TN - FP \times FN}{\sqrt{(TP + FP) \times (TP + FN) \times (TN + FP) \times (TN + FN)}} \quad (5)$$

The range of MCC is [−1–1]. The value of MCC is near to 1 is better. All of the utilized models perform well. Their values are near to 1. That means, the models classified the crack images accurately.

Cohen's Kappa Statistic is applied to assess the degree of agreement between two raters who categorize objects into mutually exclusive groups which are shown mathematically in Equation (6).

$$CK = \frac{(p_o - p_e)}{(1 - p_e)} \quad (6)$$

Here, p_o is the relative agreement of raters' observation. p_e denotes the theoretical probability of random agreement. we can calculate p_o and p_e between the raters by using the Equations (7)–(10).

$$p_o = \frac{TP + TN}{TP + TN + FP + FN} \quad (7)$$

$$p_e = probability\ of\ Positive + probability\ of\ Negative \qquad (8)$$

Here,

$$Probability\ of\ Positive = \frac{TP+FP}{TP+TN+FP+FN} \times \frac{TP+FN}{TP+TN+FP+FN} \qquad (9)$$

and

$$Probability\ of\ Negative = \frac{FP+TN}{TP+TN+FP+FN} \times \frac{FN+TN}{TP+TN+FP+FN} \qquad (10)$$

Cohen's Kappa is always between 0 and 1, with 0 indicating no agreement as well as 1 showing full agreement between the 2 raters. All models CK is almost full agreement between the actual and predictors. Table 3, shows the performance of the CCIC dataset, and Table 7 shows the performance metrics of the external dataset.

5. Discussion

Noticeable research has been done for detecting concrete surface cracks and researchers concluded different solutions. In this segment, we discuss and liken our presented model to the existing similar study.

Table 8 shows the summary of several publications for cracks detection using CNN. SegNet and MobileNet achieve 99% and 99.59% accuracy, respectively. Other mentioned papers achieve less than 99% accuracy except for our proposed TL AlexNet model, which obtains 1st position by achieving an accuracy of 99.90%. That is why our proposed transfer learning (TL) approach to the AlexNet model is an excellent candidate for concrete surface cracks detection.

Table 8. Summary of publications using CNN-based transfer learning techniques for cracks detection.

SN	Reference	Base Model or Method	Accuracy	Dataset
01	[14]	VGG16	90%	Beam, column, wall and joint brace images of a building
02	[16]	FF-BLS	96.72%	CCIC dataset
03	[17]	VGG16	94%, 98%	Fatigue cracks in gusset plate joints in steel bridges
04	[12]	SegNet	99%	Concrete pavement, asphalt pavement, and bridge deck cracks images
05	[18]	VGG16	92.27%	Concrete surfaces dataset collected from the Danish Technological Institute
06	[21]	DCNN model	97.70%	CCIC dataset
07	[23]	ResNet18	98.80%	Roads and bridges crack images
08	[24]	GoogLeNet Inception V3	97.30%	Wall images at college of environmental resources of Fuzhou University
09	[13]	MobileNet	99.59%	Wall, pavements, bridge deck images
10	[26]	YOLOv5	88.10%	Asphalt crack pavement images
11	Proposed	AlexNet	99.90%	CCIC dataset

6. Conclusions

In this paper, we applied a deep convolutional neural network based on transfer learning models to detect crack images using a popular crack dataset named Concrete Crack Images for Classification (CCIC). We utilized four transfer learning models for the experimental setup containing VGG16, ResNet18, DenseNet161, and AlexNet. As a performance metric, we used four terms named accuracy, recall, precision, and f1-score. Among the utilized models, AlexNet outperforms all the cases of performance metrics by achieving the accuracy of 99.90%, P of 99.92%, R of 99.80%, and F1-score of 99.86%. We also showed the training duration per epoch of all models. In this case, AlexNet achieves the first position in less time. In future work, we will conduct further research to provide a robust description of changing knowledge in our model.

Author Contributions: Conceptualization, M.M.I. and M.B.H.; Methodology and software, M.M.I. and M.B.H.; validation and formal analysis, M.B.H., M.M.I. and K.F.H.; resources, M.M.I. and M.B.H.; data curation, M.M.I. and M.B.H.; writing—original draft preparation, M.M.I., M.B.H. and K.F.H.; writing—review and editing, K.F.H. and M.A.M.; visualization, K.F.H. and M.M.I.; supervision, M.N.A. All authors have read and agreed to the published version of the manuscript.

Funding: This research received no external funding.

Institutional Review Board Statement: Not Applicable.

Informed Consent Statement: Not Applicable.

Data Availability Statement: The source code of this research work available at the GitHub repository (https://github.com/belal-bh/concrete-crack-detection-CNN-TL) (accessed on 11 August 2022).

Conflicts of Interest: The authors declare no conflict of interest.

References

1. Aggelis, D.G.; Alver, N.; Chai, H.K. Health Monitoring of Civil Infrastructure and Materials. *Sci. World J.* **2014**, *2014*, 435238. [CrossRef] [PubMed]
2. Gavilán, M.; Balcones, D.; Marcos, O.; Llorca, D.F.; Sotelo, M.A.; Parra, I.; Ocaña, M.; Aliseda, P.; Yarza, P.; Amírola, A. Adaptive road crack detection system by pavement classification. *Sensors* **2011**, *11*, 9628–9657. [CrossRef] [PubMed]
3. Wang, P.; Hu, Y.; Dai, Y.; Tian, M. Asphalt pavement pothole detection and segmentation based on wavelet energy field. *Math. Probl. Eng.* **2017**, *2017*, 1604130. [CrossRef]
4. Yamaguchi, T.; Nakamura, S.; Saegusa, R.; Hashimoto, S. Image-based crack detection for real concrete surfaces. *IEEJ Trans. Electr. Electron. Eng.* **2008**, *31*, 128–135. [CrossRef]
5. Tsai, Y.C.; Kaul, V.; Mersereau, R.M. Critical assessment of pavement distress segmentation methods. *J. Transp. Eng.* **2010**, *136*, 11–19. [CrossRef]
6. Albert, P.; Nii, A. Evaluating pavement cracks with bidimensional empirical mode decomposition. *EURASIP J. Adv. Signal Process.* **2008**, *2008*, 861701. [CrossRef]
7. Peggy, S.; Jean, D.; Vincent, L.; Dominique, B. Automation of pavement surface crack detection using the continuous wavelet transform. In Proceedings of the 2006 International Conference on Image Processing, Atlanta, GA, USA, 8 October 2006.
8. Yann, L.; Yoshua, B.; Geoffrey, H. Deep learning. *Nature* **2015**, *521*, 436–444. [CrossRef]
9. Valuevaa, M.; Nagornovb, N.; Lyakhovab, P.; Valueva, G.; Chervyakova, N. Application of the residue number system to reduce hardware costs of the convolutional neural network implementation. *Math. Comput. Simul.* **2020**, *177*, 232–243. [CrossRef]
10. Hasan, K.F.; Overall, A.; Ansari, K.; Ramachandran, G.; Jurdak, R. Security, privacy and trust: Cognitive internet of vehicles. *arXiv* **2021**, arXiv:2104.12878.
11. Jinsong, Z.; Song, J. An intelligent classification model for surface defects on cement concrete bridges. *Appl. Sci.* **2020**, *10*, 972. [CrossRef]
12. Chen, T.; Cai, Z.; Zhao, X.; Chen, C.; Liang, X.; Zou, T.; Wang, P. Pavement crack detection and recognition using the architecture of segNet. *J. Ind. Inf. Integr.* **2020**, *18*, 100144. [CrossRef]
13. Sayyed, B.A.; Reshul, W.; Sameer, K.; Anurag, S.; Santosh, K. Wall Crack Detection Using Transfer Learning-based CNN Models. In Proceedings of the 2020 IEEE 17th India Council International Conference (INDICON), New Delhi, India, 10–13 December 2020.
14. Yuqing, G.; Khalid, M.M. Deep transfer learning for image-based structural damage recognition. *Comput. Civ. Infrastruct. Eng.* **2018**, *33*, 748–768. [CrossRef]
15. Zheng, Z.; Qi, H.; Zhuang, L.; Zhang, Z. Automated rail surface crack analytics using deep data-driven models and transfer learning. *Sustain. Cities Soc.* **2021**, *70*, 102898. [CrossRef]
16. Zhang, Y.; Yuen, K.V. Crack detection using fusion features-based broad learning system and image processing. *Comput. Civ. Infrastruct. Eng.* **2021**, *36*, 1568–1584. [CrossRef]
17. Cao, V.D.; Hidehiko, S.; Suichi, H.; Takayuki, O.; Chitoshi, M. A vision-based method for crack detection in gusset plate welded joints of steel bridges using deep convolutional neural networks. *Autom. Constr.* **2019**, *102*, 217–229. [CrossRef]
18. Wilson, R.L.S.; Diogo, S.L. Concrete cracks detection based on deep learning image classification. *Multidiscip. Digit. Publ. Inst. Proc.* **2018**, *2*, 489. [CrossRef]
19. Xiuying, M. Concrete Crack Detection Algorithm Based on Deep Residual Neural Networks. *Sci. Program.* **2021**, *2021*, 3137083. [CrossRef]
20. Ozgenel, Ç.F.; Sorguç, G.A. Performance comparison of pretrained convolutional neural networks on crack detection in buildings. In Proceedings of the 35th International Symposium on Automation and Robotics in Construction (ISARC 2018), Berlin, Germany, 20–25 July 2018.
21. Tien-Thinh, L.; Van-Hai, N.; Minh Vuong, L.E. Development of deep learning model for the recognition of cracks on concrete surfaces. *Appl. Comput. Intell. Soft Comput.* **2021**, *2021*, 18858545. [CrossRef]

22. Ren, Y.; Huang, J.; Hong, Z.; Lu, W.; Yin, J.; Zou, L.; Shen, X. Image-based concrete crack detection in tunnels using deep fully convolutional networks. *Constr. Build. Mater.* **2020**, *234*, 117367. [CrossRef]
23. Yang, C.; Chen, J.; Li, Z.; Huang, Y. Structural Crack Detection and Recognition Based on Deep Learning. *Appl. Sci.* **2021**, *11*, 2868. [CrossRef]
24. Wu, L.; Lin, X.; Chen, Z.; Lin, P.; Cheng, S. Surface crack detection based on image stitching and transfer learning with pretrained convolutional neural network. *Struct. Control Health Monit.* **2021**, *28*, e2766. [CrossRef]
25. Kong, X.; Li, J. Vision-based fatigue crack detection of steel structures using video feature tracking. *Comput. Civ. Infrastruct. Eng.* **2018**, *33*, 783–799. [CrossRef]
26. Guo, X.H.; Bao, L.H.; Zhong, Y.L.; Li, H.; Ping, L. Pavement Crack Detection Method Based on Deep Learning Models. *Wirel. Commun. Mob. Comput.* **2021**, *2021*, 5573590. [CrossRef]
27. Li, W.; Chen, H.; Zhang, Y.; Shi, Y. Track slab crack detection based on full convolutional neural network. In Proceedings of the 2021 4th International Conference on Advanced Algorithms and Control Engineering (ICAACE 2021), Sanya, China, 29–31 January 2021.
28. Gerivan, S.J.; Janderson, F.; Cristian, M.; Ramiro, D.; Alberto, C.J.; Bruno, J.T.F. Ceramic cracks segmentation with deep learning. *Appl. Sci.* **2021**, *11*, 6017. [CrossRef]
29. Wei, Y.; Wei, Z.; Xue, K.; Yao, W.; Wang, C.; Hong, Y. Automated detection and segmentation of concrete air voids using zero-angle light source and deep learning. *Autom. Constr.* **2021**, *130*, 103877. [CrossRef]
30. Diana, A.A.; Anand, N.; Eva, L.; Prince, A.G. Deep Learning based Thermal Crack Detection on Structural Concrete Exposed to Elevated Temperature. *Adv. Struct. Eng.* **2021**, *24*, 1896–1909. [CrossRef]
31. Zhang, Y.; Lu, C.; Wang, J.; Wang, L.; Yue, X.G. Concrete cracks detection based on FCN with dilated convolution. *Appl. Sci.* **2019**, *9*, 2686. [CrossRef]
32. Liu, Z.; Cao, Y.; Wang, Y.; Wang, W. Computer vision-based concrete crack detection using U-net fully convolutional networks. *Autom. Constr.* **2019**, *104*, 129–139. [CrossRef]
33. Lei, Z.; Fan, Y.; Yimin, D.Z.; Ying, J.Z. Road crack detection using deep convolutional neural network. In Proceedings of the 2016 IEEE International Conference on Image Processing (ICIP), Phoenix, AZ, USA, 25–28 September 2016.
34. Connor, S.; Taghi, M.K. A survey on image data augmentation for deep learning. *J. Big Data* **2019**, *6*, 60. [CrossRef]
35. Shin, H.C.; Roth, H.R.; Gao, M.; Lu, L.; Xu, Z.; Nogues, I.; Yao, J.; Mollura, D.; Summers, R.M. Deep convolutional neural networks for computer-aided detection: CNN architectures, dataset characteristics and transfer learning. *IEEE Trans. Med. Imaging* **2016**, *35*, 1285–1298. [CrossRef]
36. Talukder, M.A.; Islam, M.M.; Uddin, M.A.; Akhter, A.; Hasan, K.F.; Moni, M.A. Machine learning-based lung and colon cancer detection using deep feature extraction and ensemble learning. *Expert Syst. Appl.* **2022**, *205*, 117695. [CrossRef]
37. Bala, M.; Ali, M.H.; Satu, M.S.; Hasan, K.F.; Moni, M.A. Efficient Machine Learning Models for Early Stage Detection of Autism Spectrum Disorder. *Algorithms* **2022**, *15*, 166. [CrossRef]
38. Bengio, Y.; Lecun, Y.; Hinton, G. Deep learning for AI. *Commun. ACM* **2021**, *64*, 58–65. [CrossRef]
39. Kim, D.; MacKinnon, T. Artificial intelligence in fracture detection: Transfer learning from deep convolutional neural networks. *Clin. Radiol.* **2018**, *73*, 439–445. [CrossRef]
40. Karen, S.; Andrew, Z. Very deep convolutional networks for large-scale image recognition. *arXiv* **2015**, arXiv:1409.1556.
41. He, K.; Zhang, X.; Ren, S.; Sun, J. Deep residual learning for image recognition. In Proceedings of the IEEE Conference on Computer Vision and Pattern Recognition (CVPR), Las Vegas, NV, USA, 27–30 June 2016.
42. Huang, G.; Liu, Z.; Van Der Maaten, L.; Weinberger, K.Q. Densely connected convolutional networks. In Proceedings of the IEEE Conference on Computer Vision and Pattern Recognition, Honolulu, HI, USA, 21–26 July 2017.
43. Alex, K. One weird trick for parallelizing convolutional neural networks. *arXiv* **2014**, arXiv:1404.5997.
44. Christian, S.; Vincent, V.; Sergey, I.; Jon, S.; Zbigniew, W. Rethinking the inception architecture for computer vision. In Proceedings of the IEEE Conference on Computer Vision and Pattern Recognition(CVPR), Las Vegas, NV, USA, 27–30 June 2016.
45. Szegedy, C.; Liu, W.; Jia, Y.; Sermanet, P.; Reed, S.; Anguelov, D.; Erhan, D.; Vanhoucke, V.; Rabinovich, A. Going Deeper with Convolutions. In Proceedings of the IEEE Conference on Computer Vision and Pattern Recognition (CVPR), Boston, MA, USA, 7–12 June 2015.
46. Sandler, M.; Howard, A.; Zhu, M.; Zhmoginov, A.; Chen, L.C. Mobilenetv2: Inverted residuals and linear bottlenecks. In Proceedings of the IEEE Conference on Computer Vision and Pattern Recognition (CVPR), Salt Lake City, UT, USA, 18–22 June 2018.
47. Alex, K. Adam: A method for stochastic optimization. *arXiv* **2014**, arXiv:1412.6980.
48. Hossain, M.B.; Iqbal, S.H.S.; Islam, M.M.; Akhtar, M.N.; Sarker, I.H. Transfer learning with fine-tuned deep CNN ResNet50 model for classifying COVID-19 from chest X-ray images. *Inform. Med. Unlocked* **2022**, *30*, 100916. [CrossRef]
49. Chicco, D.; Jurman, G. The advantages of the Matthews correlation coefficient (MCC) over F1 score and accuracy in binary classification evaluation. *BMC Genom.* **2020**, *21*, 6. [CrossRef]

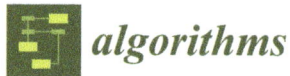

Article

Comparing Activation Functions in Machine Learning for Finite Element Simulations in Thermomechanical Forming

Olivier Pantalé

Laboratoire Génie de Production, Institut National Polytechnique/Ecole Nationale d'Ingénieurs de Tarbes, Université de Toulouse, 47 Av d'Azereix, F-65016 Tarbes, France; olivier.pantale@enit.fr; Tel.: +33-562-442-933

Abstract: Finite element (FE) simulations have been effective in simulating thermomechanical forming processes, yet challenges arise when applying them to new materials due to nonlinear behaviors. To address this, machine learning techniques and artificial neural networks play an increasingly vital role in developing complex models. This paper presents an innovative approach to parameter identification in flow laws, utilizing an artificial neural network that learns directly from test data and automatically generates a Fortran subroutine for the Abaqus standard or explicit FE codes. We investigate the impact of activation functions on prediction and computational efficiency by comparing Sigmoid, Tanh, ReLU, Swish, Softplus, and the less common Exponential function. Despite its infrequent use, the Exponential function demonstrates noteworthy performance and reduced computation times. Model validation involves comparing predictive capabilities with experimental data from compression tests, and numerical simulations confirm the numerical implementation in the Abaqus explicit FE code.

Keywords: constitutive behavior; ANN flow law; numerical implementation; user hardening; activation functions; abaqus

Citation: Pantalé, O. Comparing Activation Functions in Machine Learning for Finite Element Simulations in Thermomechanical Forming. *Algorithms* 2023, 16, 537. https://doi.org/10.3390/a16120537

Academic Editors: Nuno Fachada and Nuno David

Received: 27 October 2023
Revised: 21 November 2023
Accepted: 24 November 2023
Published: 25 November 2023

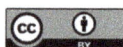

Copyright: © 2023 by the author. Licensee MDPI, Basel, Switzerland. This article is an open access article distributed under the terms and conditions of the Creative Commons Attribution (CC BY) license (https://creativecommons.org/licenses/by/4.0/).

1. Introduction

In industry and research, numerical simulations are commonly employed to predict the behavior of structures under severe thermomechanical conditions, such as high-temperature forming of metallic materials. These simulations rely on finite element (FE) codes, like Abaqus [1], or academic codes. The accuracy of these simulations is heavily influenced by constitutive equations and the identification of their parameters through experimental tests. These tests, conducted under conditions similar to the actual service loading, involve quasi-static or dynamic tensile/compression tests, thermomechanical simulators (e.g., Gleeble [2–5]), or impact tests using gas guns or Hopkinson bars [6]. The choice and formulation of behavior laws and the accurate identification of coefficients from experiments are crucial for obtaining reliable simulation results.

1.1. Constitutive Behavior and Material Flow Law

Thermomechanical behavior laws used in numerical integration algorithms such as the radial-return method [7] involve nonlinear flow law functions due to the complex nature of materials and associated phenomena like work hardening, dislocation movement, structural hardening, and phase transformations. The applicability of these flow laws is confined to specific ranges of deformations, strain rates, and temperatures. In the context of simulating forming processes, these behavior laws dictate how the material's flow stress σ depends on three key input variables: strain ε, strain rate $\dot{\varepsilon}$, and temperature T. The general form of the flow law is expressed through a mathematical equation:

$$\sigma = \sigma(\varepsilon, \dot{\varepsilon}, T). \tag{1}$$

The historical development of behavior laws for simulating hot forming processes, beginning in the 1950s, involved the use of power laws to describe strain/stress relationships, later adapted to incorporate temperature effects. In the 1970s, thermomechanical models evolved to include time dependence, linking flow laws to strain rate and time. Notable models like the Johnson–Cook [8], Zerilli–Armstrong [9], and Arrhenius [10] flow laws emerged and are commonly used in forming process simulations. The selection of a flow law for simulating material behavior in finite element analysis is crucial, and it should be based on experimental tests conducted under conditions resembling real-world applications. Researchers face a challenge in choosing the appropriate flow law after characterizing experimental behavior. This decision is influenced by the availability of flow laws within the finite element analysis software being used. For instance, users of Abaqus FE code [1] may prefer the native implementation of the Johnson–Cook flow law. Opting for alternative flow laws like Zerilli–Armstrong or Arrhenius requires users to personally compute material yield stress σ through a VUMAT subroutine in Fortran, which is time-consuming, demands expertise in flow law formulations, numerical integration, Fortran programming, and model development and testing [11–13].

Developing and implementing a user behavior law on the Abaqus code involves calculating σ, defined by Equation (1), and its three derivatives with respect to ε, $\dot{\varepsilon}$, and T. This process becomes complex and time-consuming with increasing flow law complexity. The choice of a flow law for simulating thermomechanical forming is influenced by both material behavior and process physics, but primarily by the flow laws available in the FE code. The decision often prioritizes the availability of a flow law over the quality of the model, making the choice of flow law a critical factor in the simulation process. In Tize Mha et al. [14], several flow laws were investigated through experimental compression tests on a Gleeble-3800 thermomechanical simulator for P20 medium-carbon steel used in foundry mold production. The examined flow laws included Johnson–Cook, Modified Zerilli–Armstrong, Arrhenius, Hensel–Spittle, and PTM. The findings revealed that, among the tested strain rates and temperatures, only the Arrhenius flow law accurately replicated the compression behavior of the material with a fidelity suitable for industrial applications.

Based on all these considerations, we have presented a novel approach, as outlined in Pantalé et al. [15,16], for formulating flow laws. This approach leverages the capacity of artificial neural networks (ANNs) to act as universal approximators, a concept established by Minsky et al. [17] and Hornik et al. [18]. With this innovative method, there is no longer a prerequisite to predefine a mathematical form for the constitutive equation before its use in a finite element simulation.

Artificial neural networks have been investigated in the field of thermomechanical plasticity modeling as reported by Gorji et al. [19] or Jamli et al. [20]. These studies explore the application of ANNs in FE investigation of metal forming processes and their characterization of meta-materials. Lin et al. [21] successfully applied an ANN to predict the yield stress of 42CrMo4 steel in hot compression, and ANNs have demonstrated success in predicting the flow stress behavior under hot working conditions [22,23]. They have also been applied recently in micromechanics for polycrystalline metals by Ali et al. [24]. The domain of application has been extended to dynamic recrystallization of metal alloys by Wang et al. [25]. Some approaches mix analytical and ANN flow laws such as, for example, the work proposed by Cheng et al. [26], where the authors use a combination of an ANN with the Arrhenius equation to model the behavior of a GH4169 superalloy. ANN behavior laws can also include chemical composition of materials in their formulation to increase the performance during simulation hot deformation for high-Mn steels with different concentrations, as proposed by Churyumov et al. [27].

In the majority of the works presented in the previous paragraph, the authors work either on the proposal of a neural network model and its identification in relation to experimental tests, or on the use of ANNs within the framework of a numerical simulation of a process. The approach proposed here is more complete in that we identify a neural network from experimental tests (in our case, cylinder compression tests performed on a

Gleeble device), then identify the network parameters. We then implement this ANN in Abaqus as a user subroutine in Fortran, and subsequently validate and use this network in numerical simulations. This can be performed for either Abaqus explicit or Abaqus standard since we can generate the Fortran subroutines for both versions of the code. We therefore work on the entire calculation chain, from experimental data acquisition, through network formulation and learning, to implementation and use.

In this study, we will focus only on the use of the explicit version of Abaqus, since the computation of the flow stress in an explicit integration scheme becomes very CPU intensive due to the integration method, and variations in the performance of this implementation have a significant impact on the total CPU time. On the other hand, in an implicit integration scheme, as used in the Abaqus standard, most of the time is spent in inverting the linear system of equations, therefore variations in the performance of the stress computation has no influence on the final result, hoping that the stress is calculated correctly.

1.2. Experimental Tests and Data

This study uses a medium-carbon steel, type P20, with the chemical composition presented in Table 1.

Table 1. Chemical composition of medium-carbon steel. Fe = balance.

Element	C	Mn	Mo	Si	Ni	Cr	Cu
Wt %	0.30	0.89	0.52	0.34	0.68	1.86	0.17

The experiments used in this study mirror those previously conducted by Tize Mha et al. [14]. These tests involve hot compression on a Gleeble-3800 of P20 steel cylinders with initial dimensions of $\phi_0 = 10$ mm and $h_0 = 15$ mm. Only the most relevant information about those experiments is reported hereafter. In order to have a more complete knowledge about the compression tests conducted during this study, we refer to Tize Mha et al. [14]. Hot compression tests were performed for five temperatures, $[1050, 1100, 1150, 1200, 1250]$ °C and six strain rates $[0.001, 0.01, 0.1, 1, 2, 5]$ s^{-1}. Figure 1 reports a plot of all 30 strain/stress curves extracted from the experiments.

The experimental database is composed of all strain/stress data for all 30 couples of strain rate and temperature. Each strain/stress curve contains 701 equidistant strains $\varepsilon = [0.0, 0.7]$ in $\Delta\varepsilon = 0.001$ increments. The complete database contains 21,030 quadruplets ($\varepsilon, \dot{\varepsilon}, T$ and σ). This dataset will be used here after to identify the ANN flow law parameters depending on the selected hyperparameters of the ANNs.

Section 2 is dedicated to the presentation of the ANN based flow law. The first part is dedicated to a reminder of the basic notions on ANNs, with a section on the choice of activation functions to be used in the formulation. The architecture chosen for the formulation of the flow laws based on a two-hidden-layer network will then be presented, together with the formulation of the derivatives of the output with regard to the input variables. The learning methodology and the results in terms of network performance as a function of the activation functions selected will then be presented. Section 3 is dedicated to the FE simulation of a compression test using the explicit version of Abaqus, integrating the ANN implemented as a user routine in Fortran. The quality of the numerical solution obtained and its performance in terms of computational cost will be analyzed as a function of the network structure. Finally, the last section concerns conclusions and recommendations.

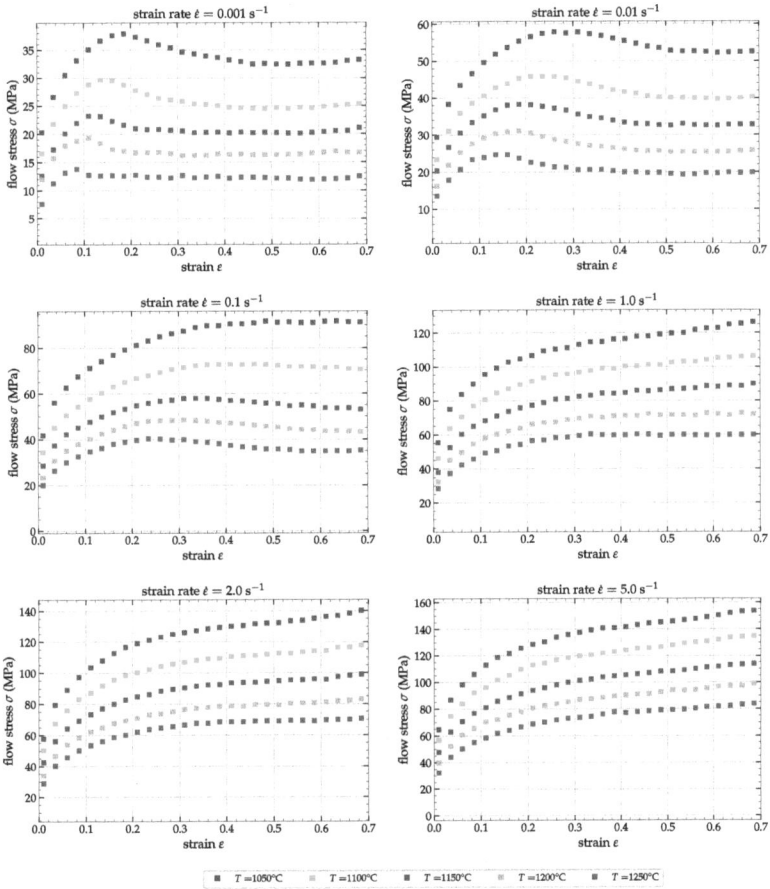

Figure 1. Stress/strain curves of P20 alloy extracted from the Gleeble device for the five temperatures (T) and six strain rates ($\dot{\varepsilon}$).

2. Artificial Neural Network Flow Law

As previously proposed by Pantalé et al. [15,16], the employed methodology involves embedding the flow law, defined by a trained ANN, into the Abaqus code as a Fortran subroutine. The ANN is trained using the experiments, as introduced in Section 1, to compute the flow stress σ as a function of ε, $\dot{\varepsilon}$ and T. Following the training phase, the ANN's weights and biases are transcribed into a Fortran subroutine, which is then compiled and linked with Abaqus libraries. This integration enables Abaqus to incorporate the thermomechanical behavior by computing the flow stress and its derivatives ($\partial\sigma/\partial\varepsilon$, $\partial\sigma/\partial\dot{\varepsilon}$, and $\partial\sigma/\partial T$) essential for the radial-return algorithm within the FE code.

2.1. Artificial Neural Network Equations
2.1.1. Network Architecture

As illustrated in Figure 2, the ANN used for computing σ from ε, $\dot{\varepsilon}$ and T is a two hidden layers network.

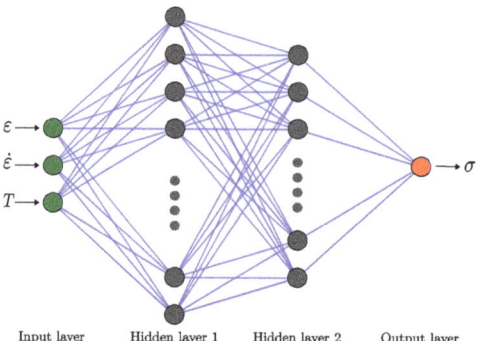

Figure 2. Two hidden layers ANN architecture with 3 inputs (ε, $\dot{\varepsilon}$ and T) and 1 output (σ).

The input of the neural network is a three component vector noted $\vec{x}$. Layer $[k]$, composed of n neurons, computes the weighted sum of the outputs $\vec{y}_{[k-1]}$ of previous layer $[k-1]$, composed of m neurons, according the equation:

$$\vec{y}_{[k]} = \mathsf{w}_{[k]} \cdot \vec{y}_{[k-1]} + \vec{b}_{[k]}, \tag{2}$$

where $\vec{y}_{[k]}$ are the internal values of the neurons resulting the summation at the layer level $[k]$, $\mathsf{w}_{[k]}$ is the weights matrix $[n \times m]$ linking layer $[k]$ and layer $[k-1]$, $\vec{b}_{[k]}$ is the bias vector of layer $[k]$ and $\vec{y}_{[k-1]}$ is the output vector of layer $[k-1]$ result of the activation function defined hereafter.

The number of learning parameters N for any layer $[k]$ is the sum of the weights and biases in that layer, expressed as $N = n(m+1)$. Following the summation operation outlined in Equation (2), each hidden layer $[k]$ produces an output vector $\vec{y}_{[k]}$ computed through an activation function $f_{[k]}$, as defined by the subsequent equation:

$$\vec{y}_{[k]} = f_{[k]}(\vec{y}_{[k]}). \tag{3}$$

This process is repeated for each hidden layer of the ANN until we reach the output layer where the formulation differ, so that the output s of the neural network is given by:

$$s = \vec{w}^T \cdot \vec{y}_{[2]} + b, \tag{4}$$

where $\vec{w}$ is the vector of the output weights of the ANN and b is the bias associated with the output neuron. As usually done in a regression approach, there is no activation function associated with the output neuron of the network (or some authors consider here a linear activation function).

2.1.2. Activation Functions

At the heart of ANNs lies the concept of activation functions, pivotal elements that determine how information is transformed within the neurons. Choosing activation functions is a critical design decision, as these functions greatly influence the network's capacity to learn and represent complex patterns in data. The selection of activation functions is guided by their distinct properties, including non-linearity, differentiability, and computational efficiency.

In regression ANNs, the choice of activation functions is typically driven by the need to approximate continuous output values rather than class labels. Many studies have been proposed concerning the right activation function to use depending on the physical problem to solve, such as the reviews proposed by Dubey et al. [28] or Jagtap et al. [29]. The activation function is essential for introducing non-linearity into a neural network, allowing it to capture non-linear features. Without this non-linearity, the network would behave like a linear regression model, as emphasized by Hornik et al. [18]. A number of activation functions can be used in neural networks.

In our previous published work [15,16], we have mostly used the Sigmoid activation function for the ANN flow laws. In the present paper, we are going to explore other activation functions and their influence on the final results, up-to the implementation into a FE software. Among the number of activation functions available in the literature, we have selected the six ones reported in Figure 3.

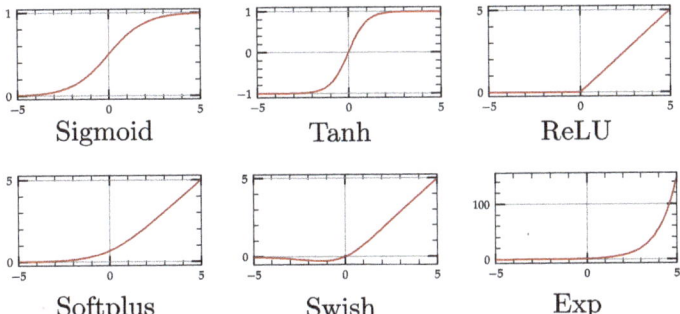

Figure 3. Activation functions used in ANNs.

The Sigmoid activation function [30], also known as the logistic activation function, is widely used in ANNs. It was originally developed in the field of logistic regression and later adapted for use in neural networks. It maps any input to an output in the range $[0,1]$, making it suitable for tasks where the network's output needs to represent probabilities or values between 0 and 1. The Sigmoid activation function $f(x)$ and its derivative $f'(x)$ are defined by:

$$f(x) = \frac{1}{1+e^{-x}} \quad \text{and} \quad f'(x) = f(x) \cdot [1 - f(x)]. \tag{5}$$

This function has been widely used until the early 1990s. Its main advantage is that it is bounded, while its main drawbacks are the problem of vanishing gradient, a non-centered on zero output and saturation for large input values.

From the 1990s to 2000s, the hyperbolic tangent activation function has been introduced and was preferred to the Sigmoid function for the training of ANNs. The hyperbolic tangent function squashes the output within the range $[-1,+1]$, and its formulation is given by the following equations:

$$f(x) = \frac{e^x - e^{-x}}{e^x + e^{-x}} \quad \text{and} \quad f'(x) = 1 - f(x)^2. \tag{6}$$

This function is useful when the network needs to model data with mean-centered features, as it can capture both positive and negative correlations. The Tanh activation function and the Sigmoid activation function are closely related in the sense that they both introduce non-linearity and squash their inputs into bounded ranges. The evaluation of this activation function requires more CPU time than the Sigmoid function, since we need to compute two exponential functions (e^x and e^{-x}) to evaluate $f(x)$.

ReLU is a classic function in classification ANNs due to its simplicity and computational efficiency, as it involves simple thresholding. It introduces non-linearity and is computationally efficient. It outputs the input if it is positive and zero if it is negative:

$$f(x) = \max(0, x) \quad \text{and} \quad f'(x) = \begin{cases} 1 & x > 0 \\ 0 & x \leq 0 \end{cases}. \tag{7}$$

ReLU mitigates the vanishing gradient problem better than Sigmoid and Tanh, making it suitable for deep networks. It often leads to faster convergence in training deep neural networks. The vanishing gradient for all negative input is the major drawback of the ReLU function.

The Softplus function [31] approximates the ReLU activation function smoothly. It is defined as the primitive of the Sigmoid function and is written:

$$f(x) = \log(1 + e^x) \quad \text{and} \quad f'(x) = \frac{1}{1 + e^{-x}}. \tag{8}$$

Softplus activation function enhances a more gradual transition from zero than ReLU, and can model positive and negative values. The main drawback is that its computational efficiency is low, since we need to compute two exponential and one logarithmic functions to evaluate $f(x)$ and its derivative.

Swish [32] is a smooth and differentiable activation function defined as:

$$f(x) = \frac{x}{1 + e^{-x}} \quad \text{and} \quad f'(x) = f(x) + \frac{1 - f(x)}{1 + e^{-x}}. \tag{9}$$

Swish demonstrates enhanced performance in certain network architectures, particularly when employed as an activation function in deep learning models, and its simplicity and similarity to ReLU facilitate straightforward substitution in neural networks by practitioners. Even if the expression of the Swish function and its derivative seems more complex that the Softplus function presented earlier, the CPU time is lower.

Looking at the shape of the ReLU and Swish functions, apart from those classic activation functions already widely used in ANNs, we propose hereafter to add an extra one, based on the exponential function and simply defined by:

$$f(x) = e^x \quad \text{and} \quad f'(x) = f(x). \tag{10}$$

We found very few papers about the use of the exponential activation function in ANNs, but it has been reported that in specific domains and mathematical modeling tasks, exponential activations can be highly relevant and effective. The idea here is to use the property so that the derivative expression is defined only by the function itself, as well as for the Sigmoid and Tanh, but with the simplest formulation. This will reduce the CPU cost since we need to compute both the function and its derivative for our implementation in the FE code into a very CPU intensive subroutine, due to the explicit integration.

Of course, there is no limitation to the use of alternative activation functions in ANNs, and there exist some much more complicated, such as the one proposed by Shen et al. [33], which is a combination of a floor, an exponential and a step function. Those authors have proven that a three hidden layer with this activation function can approximate any Hölder continuous function with an exponential approximation rate.

In order to compare the different activation functions, all six activation functions presented earlier will be used in the rest of this paper and efficiency, precision of the models and computational cost will be analyzed.

2.1.3. Pre- and Post-Processing Architecture

As we are using activation functions that mitigate vanishing gradients for large values, it is essential to normalize the three inputs and the output within the range of $[0, 1]$ to prevent ill-conditioning of the neural network. This range has been chosen because we will use the Sigmoid activation function as one of the six proposed formulations, while this later squashed the output to the lowest range $[0, 1]$.

Concerning the inputs, the range $\Delta[\ ]$ and minimum $[\ ]_0$ values of the input quantities are very different according to the data presented in Section 1. In our case, the range and minimum values of the strain are $\Delta \varepsilon = 0.7$ and $\varepsilon_0 = 0$, respectively. Concerning the strain rate $\Delta\dot{\varepsilon} = 4.999\ \mathrm{s}^{-1}$ and $\dot{\varepsilon}_0 = 0.001\ \mathrm{s}^{-1}$ and concerning the temperature $\Delta T = 200\ °\mathrm{C}$ and $T_0 = 1050\ °\mathrm{C}$.

As introduced in Pantalé et al. [15], and with regard to considerations concerning the influence of the strain rate over the evolution of the stress, we first substitute $\log(\dot{\varepsilon}/\dot{\varepsilon}_0)$ for $\dot{\varepsilon}$. Then, in a second time, we remap the inputs x_i within the range $[0, 1]$, so that the input vector $\vec{x}$ is calculated from ε, $\dot{\varepsilon}$ and T using the following expressions:

$$\vec{x} = \begin{cases} x_1 = (\varepsilon - \varepsilon_0)/\Delta\varepsilon \\ x_2 = (\log(\dot{\varepsilon}/\dot{\varepsilon}_0) - [\log(\dot{\varepsilon}/\dot{\varepsilon}_0)]_0)/\Delta[\log(\dot{\varepsilon}/\dot{\varepsilon}_0)] \\ x_3 = (T - T_0)/\Delta T \end{cases}, \quad (11)$$

where $[\ ]_0$ and $\Delta[\ ]$ are the minimum and range values of the corresponding field.

The flow stress σ enhances the same behavior with $\Delta\sigma = 153.7$ MPa and $\sigma_0 = 0$ MPa. Therefore, we apply the same procedure as previously presented and the flow stress σ is related to the output s according to the expression:

$$\sigma = \Delta\sigma \cdot s + \sigma_0. \quad (12)$$

2.1.4. Derivatives of the Neural Network

As presented in Section 1, in order to implement the ANN as a Fortran routine in Abaqus, we need to compute the three derivatives of σ with respect to $t\varepsilon$, $\dot{\varepsilon}$ and T. We can compute those derivatives using differentiation of the output with respect to the inputs. As illustrated in Figure 2, we are using here a two hidden layers neural network. Therefore, as Equations (2)–(4) are used to compute $\vec{y}_{[k]}$ and $\vec{\hat{y}}_{[k]}$ for each hidden layer and the output s from the input vector $\vec{x}$ of the ANN, we can write the derivative $\vec{s}'$ of a two hidden layers network as follows:

$$\vec{s}' = \mathbf{w}_{[1]}^T \cdot \left[\left(\mathbf{w}_{[2]}^T \cdot \left(\vec{w}^T \circ f'(\vec{y}_{[2]}) \right) \right) \circ f'(\vec{y}_{[1]}) \right], \quad (13)$$

where $f'(\square)$ is the activation function's derivative introduced by Equations (5)–(10) and $\circ$ is the Hadamard product (the so-called element-wise product). Because of the pre and post processing of the values introduced in Section 2.1.3, the derivative of the flow stress σ with respect to the inputs ε, $\dot{\varepsilon}$ and T is then given by:

$$\begin{cases} \partial\sigma/\partial\varepsilon = s'_1 \cdot \Delta\sigma/\Delta\varepsilon \\ \partial\sigma/\partial\dot{\varepsilon} = s'_2 \cdot \Delta\sigma/(\dot{\varepsilon} \cdot \Delta\dot{\varepsilon}) \\ \partial\sigma/\partial T = s'_3 \cdot \Delta\sigma/\Delta T \end{cases}, \quad (14)$$

where s'_i is one of the three components of the vector $\vec{s}'$ defined by Equation (13).

Finally, Equations (2)–(4), (11)–(14) and the requested activation function defined by one of Equations (5)–(10) will be used to implement the ANN as a Fortran subroutine for the Abaqus FE software, as it will be presented in Section 3.1.

2.2. Training of the ANN on Experimental Data

The Python program, developed with the dedicated library Tensorflow [34], utilized the Adaptive Moment Estimation (ADAM) optimizer [35] and the Mean Square Error for assessing the loss function during the training phase. With regard to our previous publications about ANN constitutive flow law [15], we have made the choice to arbitrarily fix some hyper-parameters of the ANNs, so to use a two hidden layers ANN with 15 neurons for the first hidden layer and 7 neurons for the second hidden layer. There is a total number of 180 trainable parameters to optimize. As we have three inputs and one output, we reference each of the ANNs using the notation 3-15-7-1-act, where act refers the activation function used for the model. All six models underwent parallel training for a consistent number of iterations (6000 iterations, lasting around 1 h), on a Dell PowerEdge R730 server running Ubuntu 22.04 LTS 64-bit, equipped with 96 GB of RAM and 2 Intel Xeon CPU E5-2650 2.20 GHz processors.

Concerning the dataset used for the training of the ANN, as already introduced in the previous sections, this dataset is composed of 21,030 quadruplets (ε, $\dot{\varepsilon}$, T and σ) acquired during the Gleeble experiments described in Section 1.2. A chunk of 75% of the dataset is used for training while the rest is used for the test during the training of the ANN. All details about this procedure can be found in Pantalé [36] where the interested reader can download the source, data and results of this training program. Regarding the training procedure, specifically the starting point, all models are initialized with precisely identical weights and biases. However, due to different activation functions, the initial solution varies from one model to another.

Error evaluation of the models uses the Mean Square Error (E_{MS}), the Root Mean Square Error (E_{RMS}) and the Mean Absolute Relative Error (E_{MAR}) given by the following equations:

$$\begin{cases} E_{MS} = \frac{1}{N} \sum_{i=1}^{N} (\sigma_i^e - \sigma_i)^2 \\ E_{RMS}(MPa) = \sqrt{E_{MS}} \\ E_{MAR}(\%) = \frac{1}{N} \sum_{i=1}^{N} \left| \frac{\sigma_i - \sigma_i^e}{\sigma_i^e} \right| \times 100 \end{cases}, \quad (15)$$

where N is the total number of points for the computation of those errors, σ_i is the ith output value of the ANN, and σ_i^e is the corresponding experimental value.

Figure 4 shows the evolution of the common logarithm of the Mean Square Error, i.e., $\log_{10}(E_{MS})$, of the output s of the ANN during the training, evaluated using only the test data (25% of the dataset).

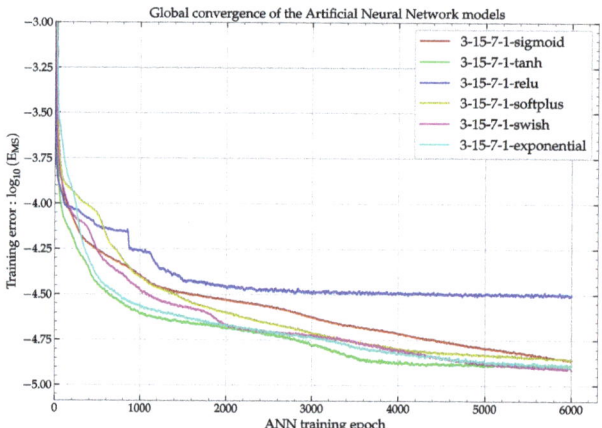

Figure 4. Global convergence of the six ANN models.

By examining this figure, we can assess and compare the convergence rates of various ANNs, concluding that a stable state was more-or-less achieved for all analyzed ANNs after 6000 iterations. As expected, the ReLU activation function gives the worst results with a final value of $E_{MS} = 32 \times 10^{-6}$, mainly due to the low number of neurons and the fact that this function is a piecewise linear function and not able to efficiently approximate the nonlinear behavior of the material. The other five activation functions enhance more or less the same behavior. The final value of the E_{MS} is pretty much the same for all of them, and around $E_{MS} = 12 \times 10^{-6}$. Table 2 reports the results of the training phase, the errors reported in this Table are computed using the whole dataset (both train and test parts).

Table 2. Comparison of the models' error depending on the activation function used.

Activation	CPU	$E_{MS} \times 10^{-6}$	E_{RMS} (MPa)	ΔE_{RMS} (%)	E_{MAR}	ΔE_{MAR}	ΔE	Rank
Sigmoid	1:04	13.853	0.604	1.007	1.412	1.201	1.536	2
Tanh	1:03	12.890	0.621	1.035	1.634	1.390	1.748	5
ReLU	1:03	31.537	0.860	1.434	2.750	2.339	2.881	6
Softplus	1:04	13.968	0.600	/	1.617	1.375	1.724	4
Swish	1:04	12.434	0.619	1.417	0.720	1.205	1.546	3
Exp	1:03	12.843	0.688	1.147	1.176	/	1.362	1

From the data, it is evident that all models require approximately the same training time to complete the specified number of iterations, with the complexity of activation functions influencing this duration; notably, the training time is a bit greater for Swish and Softplus functions compared to ReLU. We also reported in this table the real values of the E_{RMS} and E_{MAR} concerning the flow stress σ using the whole experimental database. From the latter, we can see that the E_{RMS} is about 0.6 MPa for all activation functions except the ReLU one, where the value is above 0.8 MPa. Concerning the E_{MAR}, the value of all models is around 1%, while it is more than 2% for the ReLU function. Of the six activation functions, the Exponential function gives the best results in terms of solution quality, while the ReLU function gives the worst, as reported by computing the global error using the following expression $\Delta E = \sqrt{E_{RMS}^2 + E_{MAR}^2}$. But we must note that the results of all models, except the ReLU one are very close at the end of the training stage, as illustrated in Figure 4 and Table 2. Depending on when the train is stopped, a particular model may yield the best performance due to the varying slopes of convergence among the models.

Figure 5 reports a comparison of the experimental stress acquired during the Gleeble compression tests (reported as dots in Figure 5) and the predicted stress σ using the ANN for the strain rate $\dot{\varepsilon} = 1\ \text{s}^{-1}$.

From this observation, we can infer that all ANNs effectively replicate the experimental results, except for the ReLU activation function. In the case of ReLU, as depicted in Figure 5, the predicted flow stress exhibits a piecewise linear behavior.

Of the six activation functions introduced, as detailed in Section 2.1.2, the exponential function stands out due to its unique features. The computation of the function and its derivative in a single step necessitates only one evaluation of the exponential function, as indicated by $f'(x) = f(x)$ in Equation (10). If we analyze the results reported in Table 2 and Figure 5 concerning the exponential activation function, we can see that this one has a $E_{RMS} = 0.688$ MPa, $E_{MAR} = 1.176\%$ and the global behavior of the flow stress for $\dot{\varepsilon} = 1\ \text{s}^{-1}$ is similar to the Sigmoid, Tanh, Swish or Softplus functions.

In terms of the global performance of the 3-15-7-1-exp ANN, Figure 6 reports the comparison of the experimental data (dots) and the ANN flow stress for all strain rates and temperatures defined in Section 1.2.

We can see that over the whole temperatures T and strain rates $\dot{\varepsilon}$, the performance of the model based on an exponential function is very good overall. This model will therefore be retained for the remainder of the comparative study.

It is well known that artificial neural networks are able to interpolate data correctly within their learning domain, but behave unsatisfactorily when we wish to evaluate results outside the boundaries of this learning domain. The ANNs developed in this study follow this general rule, but with different degrees of progress depending on the nature of the activation function used. In order to test the extreme limits of the proposed networks, Figure 7 shows the comparison of predicted values according to the nature of the network for conditions globally outside the learning limits.

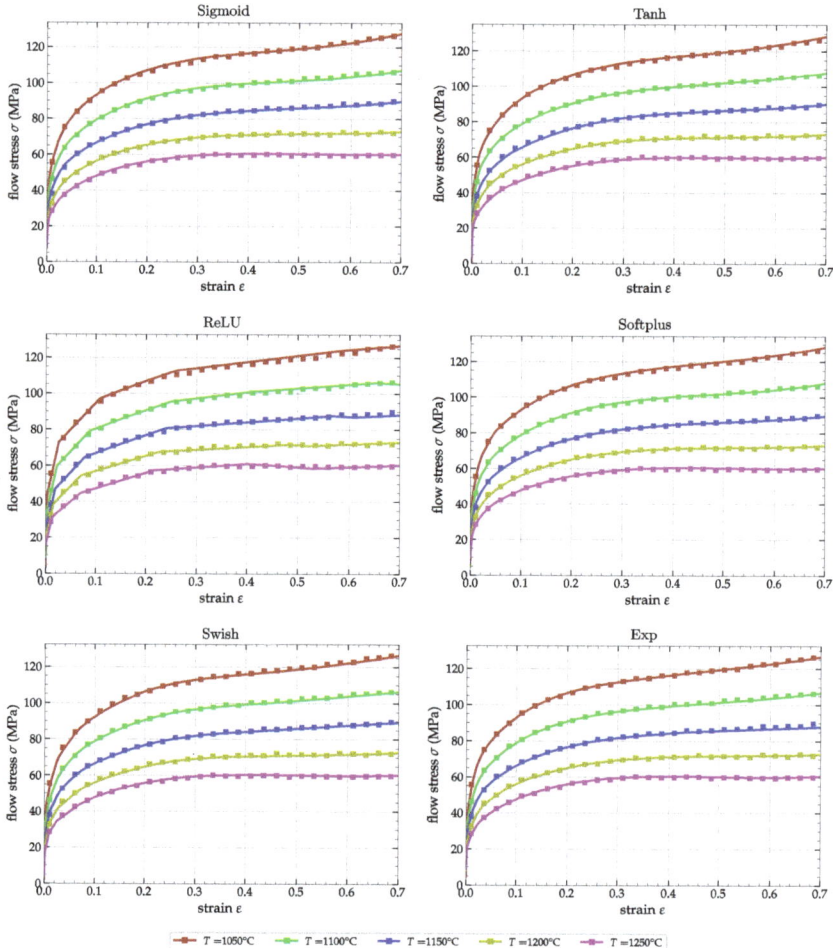

Figure 5. Comparison of experimental (dots) and the flow stress σ predicted by the ANN (continuous line) for $\dot{\varepsilon} = 1 \text{ s}^{-1}$.

We selected the worst case, multiplied the strain range by 2 (up to $\varepsilon = 1.4$), multiplied the strain rate by 2 ($\dot{\varepsilon} = 10$) and lowered the temperature to $T = 1000$ °C. Figure 7 shows the evolution of the flow stress predicted by the six models. In Figure 7, top left, when deformation alone is extended, we can see that all six models correctly predict the flow stress evolution over the interval $\varepsilon = [0, 0.7]$, whereas they diverge beyond a deformation of $\varepsilon = 0.7$. The behavior of the different models is highly variable, and overall, only the Sigmoid and Tanh models show a physically consistent trend. The model with an exponential activation function behaves catastrophically outside the learning range, due to the very nature of the exponential function. When deformation and temperature are out of range (top right), behavior is consistent below $\varepsilon = 0.7$ and divergent beyond. Again, only the Sigmoid and Tanh models show a physically consistent trend above $\varepsilon = 0.7$. When strain and strain rate are out of range (bottom left in Figure 7), the behavior is consistent below $\varepsilon = 0.7$, while diverging above $\varepsilon = 0.7$. The values given by the exponential model are out of range for all strain values. Finally, when all inputs are out of range (bottom right), the behavior is consistent and identical, except for the ReLU model below $\varepsilon = 0.7$. It is divergent above $\varepsilon = 0.7$, and consistent only for the Sigmoid and Tanh models.

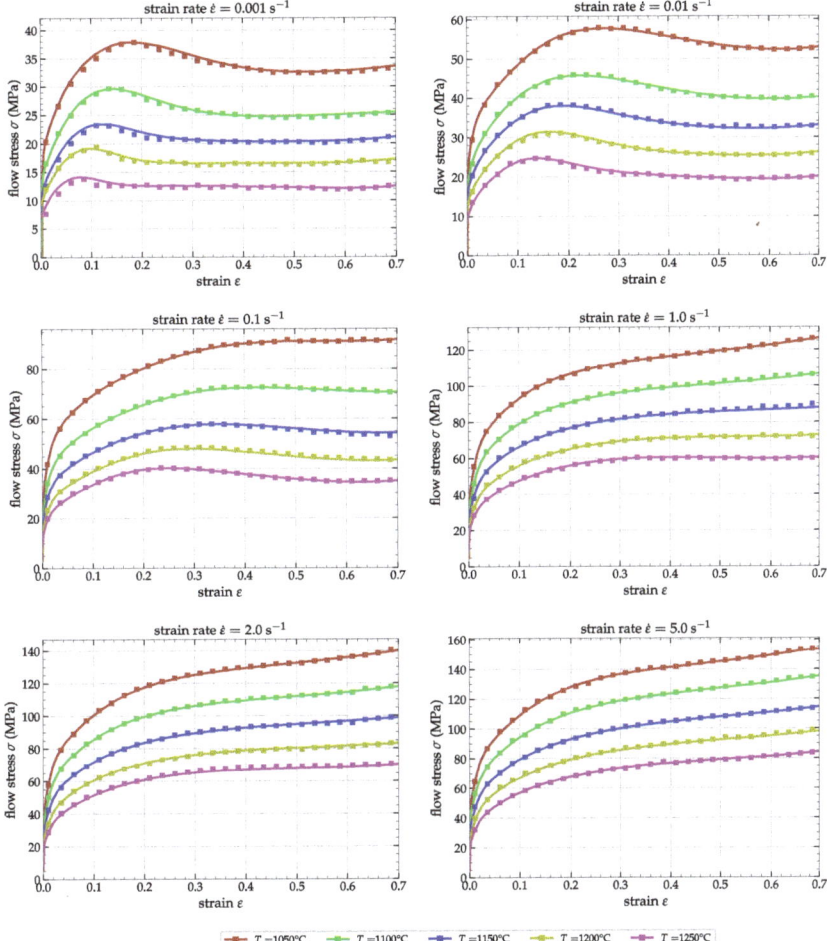

Figure 6. Comparison of experimental (dots) and ANN predicted flow stresses (continuous line) using the Exponential activation function.

We can therefore conclude from this extrapolation study that it is important to remain as far as possible within the limits of the neural network's learning domain if the results are to be physically admissible. Furthermore, from these analyses, it appears that only the Sigmoid and Tanh models are capable of physically admissible prediction of the flow stress values outside the learning domain. This is due in particular to the double saturation of the tanh and sigmoid functions, as illustrated in Figure 3, when the input values are outside the usual limits.

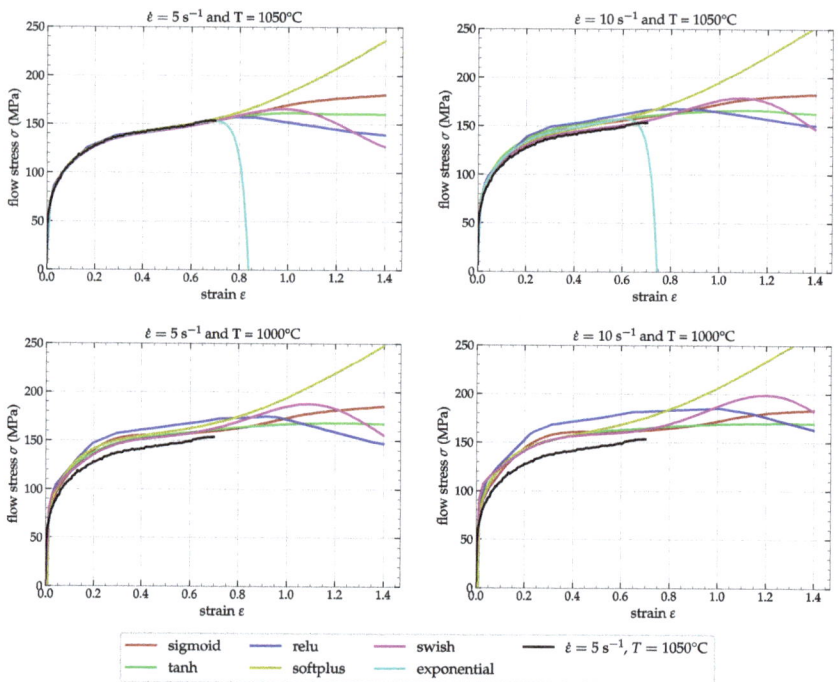

Figure 7. Comparison of the provided ANN results during an out of range computation.

3. Numerical Simulations Using the ANN Flow Law

Now that the flow stress models have been defined, trained and the results analyzed in terms of their relative performance in reproducing the experimental behavior recorded during compression tests on Gleeble, we will now numerically implement these models in Abaqus as a user routine in Fortran in order to perform numerical simulations. Following training, the optimized internal parameters of the ANNs are saved in HDF5 [37] files. Subsequently, a Python program is responsible for reading these files and generating the Fortran 77 subroutine for Abaqus.

The implementation of a user flow law in Abaqus FE code, specifically using the Explicit version, involves programming the computation of the stress tensor σ_1 based on the stress tensor at the beginning of the increment σ_0 and the strain increment $\Delta \varepsilon$. A predictor/corrector algorithm, such as the radial-return integration scheme [7], is typically employed. For detailed implementations, Ming et al. [12] discusses the Safe Newton integration scheme, and Liang et al. [13] focuses on an application related to the Arrhenius flow law. During the corrector phase, the flow stress σ must be evaluated at the current integration point as a function of ε, $\dot{\varepsilon}$, and T. This process involves solving a non-linear equation defining the plastic corrector expression and computing three derivatives of the flow stress: $\partial\sigma/\partial\varepsilon$, $\partial\sigma/\partial\dot{\varepsilon}$, and $\partial\sigma/\partial T$. Typically, the subroutine VUHARD in the Abaqus explicit is responsible for computing these quantities, and its implementation depends on the structure and activation functions of the ANN.

3.1. Numerical Implementation of the ANN Flow Law

In order to have a better understanding of the implementation of the VUHARD subroutine, we are going to detail the computation of the flow stress and the three derivatives in one step as a function of the triplet of input values ε, $\dot{\varepsilon}$, T. We suppose that the current input is stored in a three components vector $\vec{\zeta}^T = [\varepsilon, \log(\dot{\varepsilon}/\dot{\varepsilon}_0), T]$. We also suppose that the minimum and range values of the inputs, used during the learning phase, are stored in two vectors $\vec{\zeta}_0$ and $\Delta\vec{\zeta}$, respectively.

- We first use Equation (11) to compute the vector $\vec{x}$ where all components of $\vec{\zeta}$ will be remapped within the range $[0, 1]$:

$$\vec{x} = \left(\vec{\zeta} - \vec{\zeta}_0\right) \oslash \Delta\vec{\zeta}, \tag{16}$$

where $\oslash$ is the Hadamard division operator.

- Conforming to Equation (2), we compute the vector:

$$\vec{y}_{[1]} = \mathsf{w}_{[1]} \cdot \vec{x} + \vec{b}_{[1]}. \tag{17}$$

- Then, from Equation (3) and the expression of the activation function in the first layer and defined by one of the Equations (5)–(10), we compute the vector:

$$\vec{\bar{y}}_{[1]} = f_{[1]}(\vec{y}_{[1]}). \tag{18}$$

- We repeat the process for the second layer, so that we compute the vectors:

$$\vec{y}_{[2]} = \mathsf{w}_{[2]} \cdot \vec{\bar{y}}_{[1]} + \vec{b}_{[2]}, \tag{19}$$

and:

$$\vec{\bar{y}}_{[2]} = f_{[2]}(\vec{y}_{[2]}). \tag{20}$$

- From Equations (4) and (12), we compute the flow stress σ using the following equation:

$$\sigma = \Delta\sigma \cdot \left(\vec{w}^T \cdot \vec{\bar{y}}_{[2]} + b\right) + \sigma_0. \tag{21}$$

- Then, we can compute in a single step the three derivatives $\vec{\sigma}'$ from Equation (13) with the following expression:

$$\vec{\sigma}' = \Delta\sigma \cdot \mathsf{w}_{[1]}^T \cdot \left[\left(\mathsf{w}_{[2]}^T \cdot \left(\vec{w}^T \circ f'(\vec{y}_{[2]})\right)\right) \circ f'(\vec{y}_{[1]})\right] \oslash \Delta\vec{\zeta},$$
$$\sigma_2' := \sigma_2'/\dot{\varepsilon} \tag{22}$$

where the expression used for $f'()$ changes depending on the activation function used.

As an illustration the corresponding implementation using Python of those equations is proposed in Appendix A. A dedicated Python program is used to translate those equations into a Fortran 77 subroutine. During the translation phase, all functions corresponding to array operators, as matrix–matrix multiplications or element-wise operations, are converted into unrolled loops (explicitly written), all values of the ANNs parameters are explicitly written as data at the beginning of the subroutine, so that the a 3-15-7-1-exp Fortran routine consist of more than 400 lines of code. A small extract of the corresponding VUHARD subroutine is presented in Figure A2 in Appendix B. All full source files of the six VUHARD subroutines is available in the Software Heritage Archive [36].

The Fortran subroutine is compiled with double precision directive using the Intel Fortran 14.0.2 compiler on a Ubuntu 22.04 server and linked to the main Abaqus explicit executable.

3.2. Numerical Simulations and Comparisons

To compare the influence of choosing different activation functions on the numerical results using Abaqus explicit, we have made the choice to model the compression test presented earlier in Section 1.2. We consider therefore a medium-carbon steel, type P20 cylinder in compression with the initial dimensions $\phi_0 = 10$ mm and $h_0 = 15$ mm as reported in Figure 8, where only the superior half part of cylinder is represented, as the solution is symmetrical on either side of a cutting plane located halfway up the cylinder.

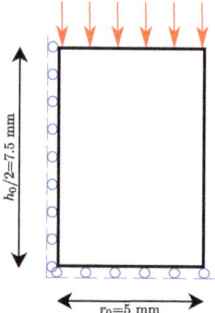

Figure 8. Half axis-symmetric model for the numerical simulation of the compression of a cylinder.

At the end of the process, the height of the cylinder is $h_f = 9$ mm, i.e., the top edge displacement is $d = 6$ mm and the reduction is 40% of the total height. The displacement is applied with a constant speed and the simulation time is fixed to $t = 1$ s, i.e., the strain rate is in the range $\dot{\varepsilon} = [0.5, 1.0]$ s^{-1} at the center of the specimen. The mesh comprises 600 axis-symmetric thermomechanical quadrilateral finite elements (CAX4RT) featuring four nodes and reduced integration. It includes 20 elements along the radial direction and 30 elements along the axis. The element size is 0.25×0.25 mm^2. Only reduced integration is available in Abaqus explicit for an axis-symmetric structure. The anvils are modeled as two rigid surfaces and a Coulomb friction law with $\mu = 0.15$ is used. To reduce the computing time, a global mass scaling with a value of $M_s = 1000$ is used. The initial temperature of the material is set to $T_0 = 1150$ °C, and we use an explicit adiabatic solver for the simulation of the compression process. All simulations are performed using the 2022 version of the Abaqus explicit solver on the same computer as the one used for the learning of the ANNs in Section 2.2. Simulations are performed with the double precision version of the solver without any parallelization directive to better compare the CPU times.

Figure 9 shows, at the end of the simulation (when the displacement of the top edge is $d = 6$ mm), a comparison of the equivalent plastic strain $\bar{\varepsilon}^p$ contourplot for the six activation functions.

From the latter, we can clearly see that all activation functions gives almost the exact same results and the choice of any of the available ANN has no influence on the values and isovalues contourplot reported in Figure 9.

Figure 10 shows a comparison of the von Mises equivalent stress $\bar{\sigma}$ contourplot.

In this figure, we can see that the solutions differ slightly both in terms of maximum stress value and stress isovalues distribution.

In order to compare the different models quantitatively, Table 3 reports the values of the plastic strain $\bar{\varepsilon}^p$, the von Mises equivalent stress $\bar{\sigma}$ and the temperature T for the element located at the center of the specimen at the end of the simulation.

Table 3. Comparison of quantitative results concerning the six activation functions analyzed.

Activation	CPU (s)	N_{inc}	N_{inc}/s	$\bar{\varepsilon}^p$ (MPa)	$\bar{\sigma}$	T (°C)
Sigmoid	574	1,092,001	1902	0.762	87.6	1164.3
Tanh	648	1,096,099	1691	0.761	88.3	1164.4
ReLU	460	1,082,453	2353	0.750	85.6	1163.9
Softplus	906	1,087,812	1200	0.753	87.4	1164.1
Swish	738	1,082,832	1467	0.753	86.6	1164.0
Exp	540	1,077,954	1996	0.757	85.6	1164.1

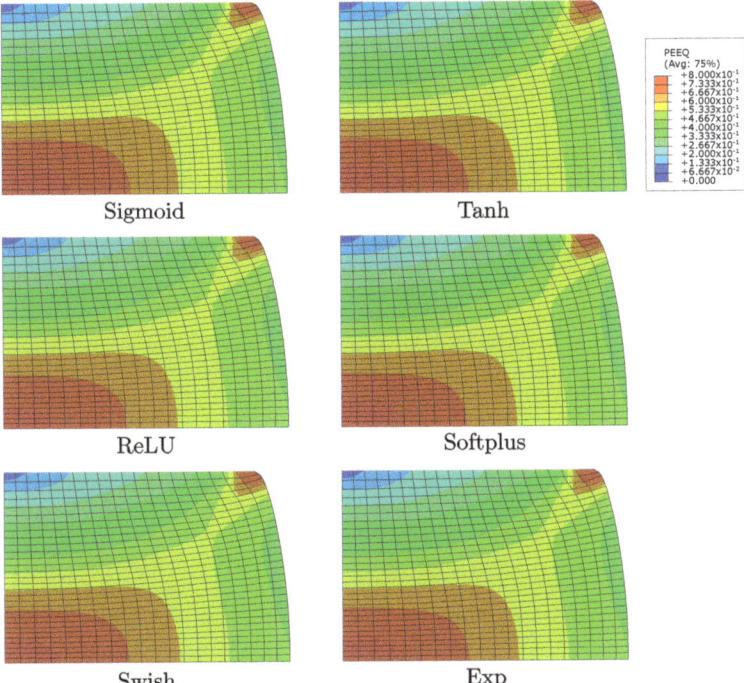

Figure 9. Equivalent plastic strain $\bar{\varepsilon}$ contourplot for the six activation functions.

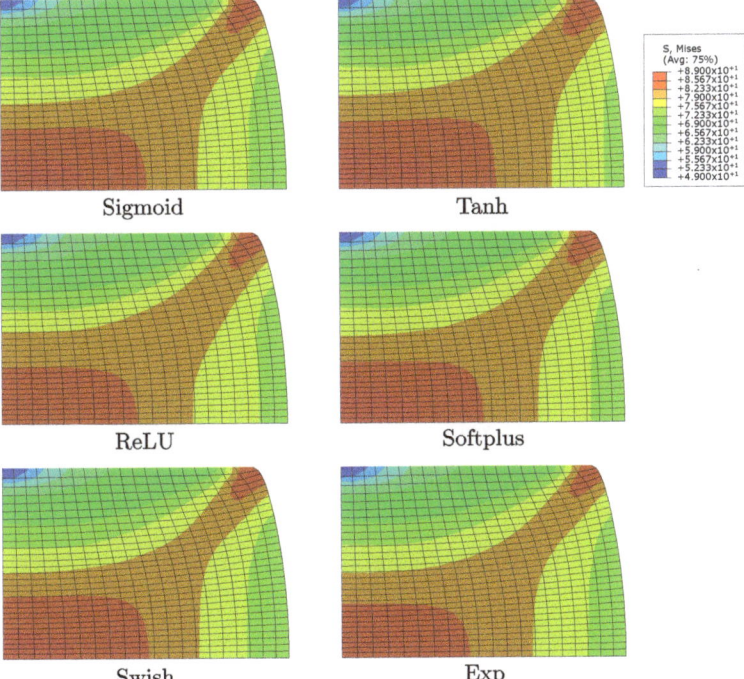

Figure 10. Von Mises equivalent stress $\bar{\sigma}$ contourplot for the six activation functions.

From the values reported in this table, we can see that the models differ a little concerning the equivalent stress (below 1%), the equivalent plastic strain (below 1%) and the temperature (below 0.02%). It is important to note that one origin of the differences between the models comes from the fact that in the end of the simulation, the plastic strain $\bar{\varepsilon}^p$ is greater than 0.7, so the model has to extrapolate the yield stress with respect to the data used for the training phase. This increases the discrepancy between the models, since each extrapolates the results from the training domain differently with respect to its internal formulation.

In Table 3, we also have reported the number of increments N_{inc} needed to complete the simulation along with the total CPU time. We remark that the number of increment varies from one activation function to another one, since the convergence of the model differ because it takes into account the stress in the computation of the stable time increment. From these two, we can calculate the number of increments performed per second and propose a classification from the fastest to the slowest ANN, where ReLU is the fastest (with 2353 iteration per second) and Softplus is the slowest (with 1200 iteration per second) of the proposed models (two times slower than the ReLU one). Those results are directly linked to the complexity of the expression of the activation function and its derivative as introduced in Section 2.1.2. For example, we can note that a simulation using the Sigmoid activation function requires 1,092,001 increments and the model contains 400 under integrated CAX4RT elements; therefore, we will have 436,800,400 computations of the code presented in Figure A3. From those results, we can note that, as expected, the Exp activation function is very efficient in terms of CPU computation time (with 1996 iteration per second) as it is just second after the very light ReLU function, but gives quite good results as reported in Table 3, which is not the case for the ReLU function.

Figure 11 shows the evolution of the von Mises stress vs. displacement of the top edge for the center of the cylinder for all activation functions.

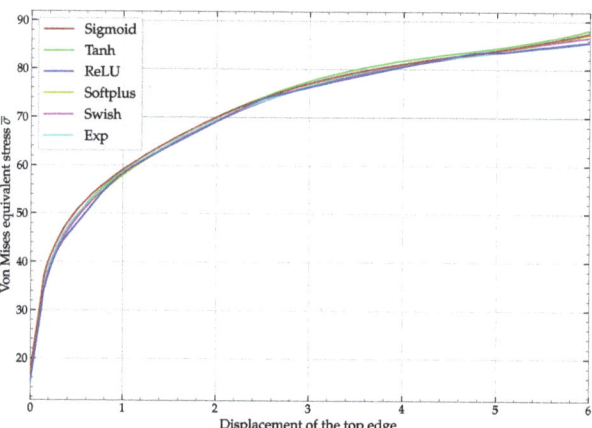

Figure 11. Von Mises stress vs. displacement of the top edge of the cylinder for all activation functions.

From this later, we can see that all activation functions give almost the same results, while the ReLU enhances a piecewise behavior due to its formulation and the low number of neurons used for the ANN. This behavior has an influence on the precision of the ANN flow law, and we suggest avoiding the use of the ReLU activation function in this kind of application. Any other type of activation function give quite good results for this application, while among them, the use of the Exp activation function gives accurate results and minimum computation time for numerical applications.

4. Conclusions and Major Remarks

In this paper, several ANN-based flow laws for thermomechanical simulation of the behavior of a P20 medium-alloy steel have been identified. These six laws exhibit distinctions solely in the choice of their activation functions, while maintaining a uniform architectural framework characterized by consistent specifications regarding the quantity of hidden layers and the number of neurons present on each of these hidden layers. In addition to the five classic activation functions (Sigmoid, Tanh, ReLU, Softplus and Swift), in this paper, we proposed the use of the Exp (exponential) function as an activation function, although this is almost never used in neural network formulations. The expressions of the activation functions and their derivatives were used in the neural network writing formalism to calculate the derivatives of σ with respect to ε, $\dot{\varepsilon}$ and T.

Comparison of the ANNs results (in terms of flow stress σ) with experiments have shown that all five activation functions, with the exception of the ReLU function, give very good results, far superior to those obtained conventionally using formalisms based on analytical flow laws from the literature, such as the Johnson–Cook, Arrhenius or Zerilli–Armstrong models [14]. To improve the extrapolation ability of the models, it is recommended to use the Sigmoid and Tanh activation functions. These functions can effectively squash out of bounds values, giving the artificial neural network a more realistic behavior beyond the training bounds.

Based on the equations describing the mathematical formulation of an ANN with two hidden layers, and depending on the nature of these activation functions, we have implemented these constitutive laws in the form of a Fortran 77 subroutine for Abaqus explicit. The same approach can also be used to write a UHARD routine enabling the same flow laws to be used in Abaqus standard.

Numerical results obtained from a compression test on a metal cylinder using the Abaqus explicit code have shown that neural network behavior models give very satisfactory results, in line with experimental tests. The Exp activation function, which is rarely used in the formulation of artificial neural networks, showed very good results (in agreement with more complex models such as Tanh), while enabling the code user to benefit from the efficiency and ease of implementation of an exponential function. These results are satisfactory insofar as the inputs remain entirely within the model's learning domain, since the extrapolation capabilities of the network based on the exponential function are very limited. We then obtain results equivalent in terms of solution quality to sigmoid or tanh-type formulations, while having computation times comparable to a ReLU function.

Overall, this study concludes by recommending the use of the sigmoid activation function for the development of flow laws, since it gives very good results in the identification domain, allows us to leave the learning domain with a behavior that is certainly biased, but physically admissible, and offers very good performance in terms of simulation time when implemented in a finite element code. This study emphasizes the valuable impact of neural network-derived flow laws for numerical finite element simulation executed with a commercial FE code like Abaqus.

Funding: This research received no external funding.

Data Availability Statement: Source files of the numerical simulations and the ANN flow laws are available from [36].

Acknowledgments: The author thanks the team of Mohammad Jahazi from the Ecole Technique Supérieure de Montréal, Canada, for providing the experimental data used in Section 1.2.

Conflicts of Interest: The author declares no conflict of interest.

Abbreviations

The following abbreviations are used in this manuscript:

ANN	Artificial Neural Network
CAX4RT	Abaqus 4 nodes axis-symmetric thermomechanical element
CPU	Central processing unit
FE	Finite Element
UHARD	Abaqus standard user subroutine
VUHARD	Abaqus explicit user subroutine

Appendix A. Python Code to Compute Stress and Derivatives

The implementation using Python of Equations (16) to (22) is proposed in Figure A1, where the arguments of the function stressAndDerivatives are xi for the $\vec{\zeta}$ vector, deps for $\dot{\varepsilon}$, Act for the activation function and dAct for its derivative.

```
1   def stressAndDerivatives(xi, deps, Act, dAct):
2       x = (xi - xi0) / Dxi
3       y1 = w1.dot(x) + b1
4       yf1 = Act(y1)
5       y2 = w2.dot(yf1) + b2
6       yf2 = Act(y2)
7       Sig = Dsig*(w.dot(yf2) + b) + sig0
8       dSig = Dsig*((w1.T).dot((w2.T).dot(w.T*dAct(y2))*dAct(y1))) / Dxi
9       dSig[1] = dSig[1] / deps
10      return Sig, dSig
```

Figure A1. Python function to compute the flow stress and the derivative vector.

The network architecture is defined by the numpy arrays w1, w2, w, b1, b2 and b, which are global variables in the proposed piece of code. The other variables xi0, Dxi, sig0 and Dsig correspond to the quantities $\vec{\zeta}_0$, $\Delta\vec{\zeta}$, σ_0 and $\Delta\sigma$, respectively.

Line 2 in Figure A1 corresponds to Equation (16). Lines 3 and 4 correspond to Equations (17) and (18) and concern the first hidden layer, while lines 5 and 6 correspond to Equations (19) and (20) and concern the second hidden layer. Finally, line 7 computes the flow stress σ conforming to Equation (21) and lines 8 and 9 compute the three derivatives of the flow stress conforming to Equation (22). The stress Sig and the three derivatives array dSig are returned as a tuple at line 10.

Appendix B. Fortran 77 Subroutines to Implement the ANN Flow Law

A portion of the Fortran 77 code defining the numerical implementation of the VUHARD routine for Abaqus Explicit is presented in Figure A2. The complete source codes for the flow laws corresponding to the six activation functions can be found in the Software Heritage archive [36]. In Figure A2, the '...' symbols denote a continuation of the code that is not transcribed here due to space constraints in the figure for the sake of conciseness.

Depending on the kind of activation function used, some lines differ from one version to the other one, such as the definitions of the activation functions (see line 16 in Figure A2) and the expressions of the internal variables xa and xb (see lines 26 and 28 in Figure A2).

Figure A3 shows the declaration of the Sigmoid activation function and its derivative as defined by Equation (5), while Figure A4 shows the same part of the code with the use of the Softplus activation function as defined by Equation (8).

```
1         subroutine vuhard (... Heading of VUHARD routine ...)
2         ...
3   c Block of Data
4         double precision w1(15, 3)
5         data w1/-0.480648012140D0, 1.20722861399D0, -0.024459252119D0,
6       + -0.088911109397D0,
7         ...
8   c Preprocessing of the variables
9         xeps  = (eqps(k) - xml(1))/xrl(1)
10        xdeps = (log(eqpsRate(k)/xdeps0) - xml(2))/xrl(2)
11        xtemp = (tempNew(k) - xml(3))/xrl(3)
12  c Hidden layer #1 (y11 to y115)
13        y11 = w1(1,1)*xeps + w1(1,2)*xdeps + w1(1,3)*xtemp + b1(1)
14        ...
15  c exponential activation function (yf11 to yf115)
16        yf11 = exp(y11)
17        ...
18  c Hidden layer #2 (y21 to y27)
19        y21 = w2(1,1)*yf11 + w2(1,2)*yf12 + w2(1,3)*yf13
20      + +w2(1,4)*yf14 + ... + b2(1)
21        ...
22  c exponential activation function (yf21 to yf27)
23        yf21 = exp(y21)
24        ...
25  c Derivatives terms (xa1 to xa7), (xb1 to xb15)
26        xa1 = w3(1)*yf21
27        ...
28        xb1 = (w2(1,1)*xa1 + w2(2,1)*xa2 + w2(3,1)*xa3
29      + +w2(4,1)*xa4 + ... + w2(7,1)*xa7)*yf11
30        ...
31  c Outputs of the subroutine
32        Yield(k) = xr0*(w3(1)*yf21 + w3(2)*yf22
33      + +w3(3)*yf23 + ... + b3) + xm0
34        dyieldDeqps(k,1) = xr0*(w1(1,1)*xb1 + w1(2,1)*xb2
35      + +w1(3,1)*xb3 + ... + w1(15,1)*xb15) / xrl(1)
36        dyieldDeqps(k,2) = xr0*(w1(1,2)*xb1 + w1(2,2)*xb2
37      + +w1(3,2)*xb3 + ... + w1(15,2)*xb15)/(xrl(2)*eqpsRate(k))
38        dyieldDtemp(k) = xr0*(w1(1,3)*xb1 + w1(2,3)*xb2
39      + +w1(3,3)*xb3 + ... + w1(15,3)*xb15) / xrl(3)
40  c Return from the VUHARD subroutine
41        return
42        end
```

Figure A2. Part of the VUHARD Fortran 77 subroutine for the ANN flow law and the exponential activation function.

```
1   c sigmoid activation function (yf11 to yf115)
2         yf11 = 1/(1 + exp(-y11))
3         ...
4   c Derivatives terms (xa1 to xa7), (xb1 to xb15)
5         xa1 = w3(1)*(yf21*(1 - yf21))
6         ...
7         xb1 = (w2(1,1)*xa1 + w2(2,1)*xa2 + w2(3,1)*xa3
8       + +w2(4,1)*xa4 + ... + w2(7,1)*xa7)*(yf11*(1 - yf11))
9         ...
```

Figure A3. Part of the VUHARD Fortran 77 subroutine with the Sigmoid activation function.

```fortran
1  c softplus activation function (yf11 to yf115)
2       yf11 = log(1 + exp(y11))
3       ...
4  c Derivatives terms (xa1 to xa7), (xb1 to xb15)
5       xa1 = w3(1)*(1/(1 + exp(-y21)))
6       ...
7       xb1 = (w2(1,1)*xa1 + w2(2,1)*xa2 + w2(3,1)*xa3
8       + +w2(4,1)*xa4 + ... + w2(7,1)*xa7)*(1/(1 + exp(-y11)))
9       ...
```

Figure A4. Part of the VUHARD Fortran 77 subroutine with the Softplus activation function.

References

1. Abaqus. *Reference Manual*; Hibbitt, Karlsson and Sorensen Inc.: Providence, RI, USA, 1989.
2. Lin, Y.C.; Chen, M.S.; Zhang, J. Modeling of flow stress of 42CrMo steel under hot compression. *Mater. Sci. Eng. A* **2009**, *499*, 88–92. [CrossRef]
3. Bennett, C.J.; Leen, S.B.; Williams, E.J.; Shipway, P.H.; Hyde, T.H. A critical analysis of plastic flow behaviour in axisymmetric isothermal and Gleeble compression testing. *Comput. Mater. Sci.* **2010**, *50*, 125–137. [CrossRef]
4. Kumar, V. Thermo-mechanical simulation using gleeble system-advantages and limitations. *J. Metall. Mater. Sci.* **2016**, *58*, 81–88.
5. Yu, D.J.; Xu, D.S.; Wang, H.; Zhao, Z.B.; Wei, G.Z.; Yang, R. Refining constitutive relation by integration of finite element simulations and Gleeble experiments. *J. Mater. Sci. Technol.* **2019**, *35*, 1039–1043. [CrossRef]
6. Kolsky, H. An Investigation of the Mechanical Properties of Materials at very High Rates of Loading. *Proc. Phys. Soc. Sect. B* **1949**, *62*, 676–700. [CrossRef]
7. Ponthot, J.P. Unified Stress Update Algorithms for the Numerical Simulation of Large Deformation Elasto-Plastic and Elasto-Viscoplastic Processes. *Int. J. Plast.* **2002**, *18*, 36. [CrossRef]
8. Johnson, G.R.; Cook, W.H. A Constitutive Model and Data for Metals Subjected to Large Strains, High Strain Rates and High Temperatures. In Proceedings of the Proceedings 7th International Symposium on Ballistics, The Hague, The Netherlands, 19–21 April 1983; pp. 541–547.
9. Zerilli, F.J.; Armstrong, R.W. Dislocation-mechanics-based constitutive relations for material dynamics calculations. *J. Appl. Phys.* **1987**, *61*, 1816–1825. [CrossRef]
10. Jonas, J.; Sellars, C.; Tegart, W.M. Strength and structure under hot-working conditions. *Metall. Rev.* **1969**, *14*, 1–24. [CrossRef]
11. Gao, C.Y. FE Realization of a Thermo-Visco-Plastic Constitutive Model Using VUMAT in Abaqus/Explicit Program. In *Computational Mechanics*; Springer: Berlin/Heidelberg, Germany, 2007; pp. 301–301.
12. Ming, L.; Pantalé, O. An Efficient and Robust VUMAT Implementation of Elastoplastic Constitutive Laws in Abaqus/Explicit Finite Element Code. *Mech. Ind.* **2018**, *19*, 308. [CrossRef]
13. Liang, P.; Kong, N.; Zhang, J.; Li, H. A Modified Arrhenius-Type Constitutive Model and its Implementation by Means of the Safe Version of Newton–Raphson Method. *Steel Res. Int.* **2022**, *94*, 2200443. [CrossRef]
14. Tize Mha, P.; Dhondapure, P.; Jahazi, M.; Tongne, A.; Pantalé, O. Interpolation and extrapolation performance measurement of analytical and ANN-based flow laws for hot deformation behavior of medium carbon steel. *Metals* **2023**, *13*, 633. [CrossRef]
15. Pantalé, O.; Tize Mha, P.; Tongne, A. Efficient implementation of non-linear flow law using neural network into the Abaqus Explicit FEM code. *Finite Elem. Anal. Des.* **2022**, *198*, 103647. [CrossRef]
16. Pantalé, O. Development and Implementation of an ANN Based Flow Law for Numerical Simulations of Thermo-Mechanical Processes at High Temperatures in FEM Software. *Algorithms* **2023**, *16*, 56. [CrossRef]
17. Minsky, M.L.; Papert, S. *Perceptrons; An Introduction to Computational Geometry*; MIT Press: Cambridge, UK, 1969.
18. Hornik, K.; Stinchcombe, M.; White, H. Multilayer Feedforward Networks Are Universal Approximators. *Neural Net.* **1989**, *2*, 359–366. [CrossRef]
19. Gorji, M.B.; Mozaffar, M.; Heidenreich, J.N.; Cao, J.; Mohr, D. On the Potential of Recurrent Neural Networks for Modeling Path Dependent Plasticity. *J. Mech. Phys. Solids* **2020**, *143*, 103972. [CrossRef]
20. Jamli, M.; Farid, N. The Sustainability of Neural Network Applications within Finite Element Analysis in Sheet Metal Forming: A Review. *Measurement* **2019**, *138*, 446–460. [CrossRef]
21. Lin, Y.; Zhang, J.; Zhong, J. Application of Neural Networks to Predict the Elevated Temperature Flow Behavior of a Low Alloy Steel. *Comput. Mater. Sci.* **2008**, *43*, 752–758. [CrossRef]
22. Stoffel, M.; Bamer, F.; Markert, B. Artificial Neural Networks and Intelligent Finite Elements in Non-Linear Structural Mechanics. *Thin-Walled Struct.* **2018**, *131*, 102–106. [CrossRef]
23. Stoffel, M.; Bamer, F.; Markert, B. Neural Network Based Constitutive Modeling of Nonlinear Viscoplastic Structural Response. *Mech. Res. Commun.* **2019**, *95*, 85–88. [CrossRef]
24. Ali, U.; Muhammad, W.; Brahme, A.; Skiba, O.; Inal, K. Application of Artificial Neural Networks in Micromechanics for Polycrystalline Metals. *Int. J. Plast.* **2019**, *120*, 205–219. [CrossRef]

25. Wang, T.; Chen, Y.; Ouyang, B.; Zhou, X.; Hu, J.; Le, Q. Artificial neural network modified constitutive descriptions for hot deformation and kinetic models for dynamic recrystallization of novel AZE311 and AZX311 alloys. *Mater. Sci. Eng. A* **2021**, *816*, 141259. [CrossRef]
26. Cheng, P.; Wang, D.; Zhou, J.; Zuo, S.; Zhang, P. Comparison of the Warm Deformation Constitutive Model of GH4169 Alloy Based on Neural Network and the Arrhenius Model. *Metals* **2022**, *12*, 1429. [CrossRef]
27. Churyumov, A.Y.; Kazakova, A.A. Prediction of True Stress at Hot Deformation of High Manganese Steel by Artificial Neural Network Modeling. *Materials* **2023**, *16*, 1083. [CrossRef] [PubMed]
28. Dubey, S.R.; Singh, S.K.; Chaudhuri, B.B. Activation functions in deep learning: A comprehensive survey and benchmark. *Neurocomputing* **2022**, *503*, 92–108. [CrossRef]
29. Jagtap, A.D.; Karniadakis, G.E. How important are activation functions in regression and classification? A survey, performance comparison, and future directions. *J. Mach. Learn. Model. Comput.* **2023**, *4*, 21–75. [CrossRef]
30. Han, J.; Moraga, C. The influence of the sigmoid function parameters on the speed of backpropagation learning. In *From Natural to Artificial Neural Computation*; Mira, J., Sandoval, F., Eds.; Springer: Berlin/Heidelberg, Germany, 1995; pp. 195–201.
31. Dugas, C.; Bengio, Y.; Bélisle, F.; Nadeau, C.; Garcia, R. Incorporating Second-Order Functional Knowledge for Better Option Pricing. In *Advances in Neural Information Processing Systems*; Leen, T., Dietterich, T., Tresp, V., Eds.; MIT Press: Cambridge, UK, 2000; Volume 13.
32. Ramachandran, P.; Zoph, B.; Le, Q.V. Searching for Activation Functions. *arXiv* **2018**, arXiv:1710.05941
33. Shen, Z.; Yang, H.; Zhang, S. Neural network approximation: Three hidden layers are enough. *Neural Net.* **2021**, *141*, 160–173. [CrossRef]
34. Abadi, M.; Agarwal, A.; Barham, P.; Brevdo, E.; Chen, Z.; Citro, C.; Corrado, G.S. TensorFlow: Large-Scale Machine Learning on Heterogeneous Systems. 2015. Software. Available online: tensorflow.org (accessed on 5 July 2023).
35. Kingma, D.P.; Lei, J. Adam: A Method for Stochastic Optimization. *arXiv* **2014**, arXiv:1412.6980.
36. Pantalé, O. Comparing Activation Functions in Machine Learning for Finite Element Simulations in Thermomechanical Forming: Software Source Files. Software Heritage. 2023. Available online: https://archive.softwareheritage.org/swh:1:dir:b418ca8e27d05941c826b78a3d8a13b07989baf6 (accessed on 15 November 2023).
37. Koranne, S. Hierarchical data format 5: HDF5. In *Handbook of Open Source Tools*; Springer: Berlin/Heidelberg, Germany, 2011; pp. 191–200.

Disclaimer/Publisher's Note: The statements, opinions and data contained in all publications are solely those of the individual author(s) and contributor(s) and not of MDPI and/or the editor(s). MDPI and/or the editor(s) disclaim responsibility for any injury to people or property resulting from any ideas, methods, instructions or products referred to in the content.

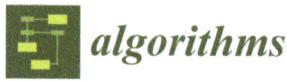 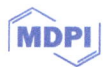

Review

A Literature Review on Some Trends in Artificial Neural Networks for Modeling and Simulation with Time Series

Angel E. Muñoz-Zavala [1], Jorge E. Macías-Díaz [2,3,*], Daniel Alba-Cuéllar [4] and José A. Guerrero-Díaz-de-León [1]

1. Departamento de Estadística, Universidad Autónoma de Aguascalientes, Aguascalientes 20100, Mexico; aemz@correo.uaa.mx (A.E.M.-Z.); antonio.guerrero@edu.uaa.mx (J.A.G.-D.-d.-L.)
2. Department of Mathematics and Didactics of Mathematics, Tallinn University, 10120 Tallinn, Estonia
3. Departamento de Matemáticas y Física, Universidad Autónoma de Aguascalientes, Aguascalientes 20131, Mexico
4. Instituto Nacional de Estadística y Geografía, Aguascalientes 20276, Mexico; daniel.alba@inegi.org.mx
* Correspondence: jorge.macias_diaz@tlu.ee or jemacias@correo.uaa.mx

Abstract: This paper reviews the application of artificial neural network (ANN) models to time series prediction tasks. We begin by briefly introducing some basic concepts and terms related to time series analysis, and by outlining some of the most popular ANN architectures considered in the literature for time series forecasting purposes: feedforward neural networks, radial basis function networks, recurrent neural networks, and self-organizing maps. We analyze the strengths and weaknesses of these architectures in the context of time series modeling. We then summarize some recent time series ANN modeling applications found in the literature, focusing mainly on the previously outlined architectures. In our opinion, these summarized techniques constitute a representative sample of the research and development efforts made in this field. We aim to provide the general reader with a good perspective on how ANNs have been employed for time series modeling and forecasting tasks. Finally, we comment on possible new research directions in this area.

Keywords: time series forecasting; artificial neural network architectures; machine learning; dynamical systems; time series statistical modeling techniques

Citation: Muñoz-Zavala, A.E.; Macías-Díaz, J.E.; Alba-Cuellar, D.; Guerrero-Díaz-de-León, J.A. A Literature Review on Some Trends in Artificial Neural Networks for Modeling and Simulation with Time Series. *Algorithms* **2024**, *17*, 76. https://doi.org/10.3390/a17020076

Academic Editors: Nuno Fachada and Nuno David

Received: 15 December 2023
Revised: 18 January 2024
Accepted: 2 February 2024
Published: 7 February 2024

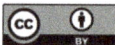

Copyright: © 2024 by the authors. Licensee MDPI, Basel, Switzerland. This article is an open access article distributed under the terms and conditions of the Creative Commons Attribution (CC BY) license (https:// creativecommons.org/licenses/by/ 4.0/).

1. Introduction

Predictions can have great importance on various topics, like birthrates, unemployment rates, school enrollments, the number of detected influenza cases, rainfall, individual blood pressure, etc. For example, predictions can guide people, organizations, and governments to choose the best options or strategies to achieve their goals or solve their problems. Another example of the application of predictions can be found in the consumption of electrical energy to guarantee the optimal operating conditions of an energy network that supplies electrical energy to its customers [1–5]. A time series is a set of records about a phenomenon that is ordered equidistantly with respect to time; this is also called a forecast. Time series are used in a wide variety of areas, including science, technology, economics, health, the environment, etc. [6]. Initially, statistical models were used to forecast the future values of the time series. These models are based on historical values of the time series to extract information about patterns (trend, seasonality, cycle, etc.) that allow the extrapolation of the behavior of the time series [1].

We can identify in the literature two main classes of methodologies for time series analysis:

- **Parametric statistical models.** Among the traditional parametric modeling techniques, we have the autoregressive integrated moving average (ARIMA) linear models [7]. The 1970s and 1980s were dominated by linear regression models [8].
- **Nonparametric statistical models.** Some of these techniques include the following: self-exciting threshold autoregressive (SETAR) models [9], which are a nonlinear extension to the parametric autoregressive linear models; autoregressive conditional

heteroskedasticity (ARCH) models [10], which assume that the variance of the current error term or innovation depends on the sizes of previous error terms; and bilinear models [11], which are similar to ARIMA models, but include nonlinear interactions between AR and MA terms.

The main difference between both classes is that the parametric model has a fixed number of parameters, while the nonparametric model increases the number of parameters with the amount of training data [12].

Although nonlinear parametric models represent an advance over linear approaches, they are still limited because an explicit relational function must be hypothesized for the available time series data. In general, fitting a nonlinear parametric model to a time series is a complex task since there is a wide possible set of nonlinear patterns. However, technological advancements have allowed researchers to consider more flexible modeling techniques, such as support vector machines (SVMs) adapted to regression [13], artificial neural networks (ANNs), and wavelet methods [14].

McCulloch and Pitts [15] and Rosenblatt [16] established the mathematical and conceptual foundations of ANNs, but these nonparametric models really took off in the late 1980s, when computers were powerful enough to allow people to program simulations of very complex situations observed in real life, generated by simple and easy-to-understand stochastic algorithms that nevertheless demanded intensive computing power. ANNs belong to this class of simulations since they are capable of modeling brain activity in classification and pattern recognition problems. It was demonstrated that ANNs are a good alternative to time series forecasting. In 1987, Lapedes and Farber [17] reported the first approach to modeling nonlinear time series with an ANN. ANNs are an attractive and promising alternative for several reasons:

- ANNs are data-driven methods. They use historical data to build a system that can give the desired result [18].
- ANNs are flexible and self-adaptive. It is not necessary to make many prior assumptions about the data generation process for the problem under study [18].
- ANNs are able to generalize (robustly). They can accurately infer the invisible part of a population even if there is noise in the sample data [19].
- ANNs can approximate any continuous linear or nonlinear function with the desired accuracy [20].

The aim of this review is to provide the general reader with a good perspective on how ANNs have been employed to model and forecast time series data. Through this exposition, we explore the reasons why ANNs have not been widely adopted by the statistical community as standard time series analysis tools. Time series modeling, specifically in the field of macroeconomics, is limited almost exclusively to methodologies and techniques typical of the linear model paradigm, ignoring completely machine learning and artificial neural network techniques, which have effectively produced time series forecasts that are more accurate in comparison to what linear modeling has to offer. This paper (a) introduces ANNs to readers familiar with traditional time series techniques who want to explore more flexible and accurate modeling alternatives, and (b) illustrates recent techniques involving several ANN architectures chiefly employed with the goal of improving time series prediction accuracy.

The rest of this document is organized as follows: Section 2 introduces basic time series analysis concepts. In Section 3, we outline some of the most popular ANN architectures considered in the state-of-the-art for time series forecasting; we also analyze the strengths and weaknesses of these architectures in the context of time series modeling. In Section 4, we provide a brief survey on relevant time series ANN modeling techniques, discussing and summarizing recent research and implementations. Section 5 provides a discussion on the application of ANN in time series forecasting. Finally, in Section 6, we discuss possible new research directions in the application of ANN for time series forecasting.

2. Basic Principles and Concepts in Time Series Analysis

In this section, we define, more or less formally, what a time series is (Section 2.1); then, we discuss how a time series forecast can be analyzed as a functional approximation problem (Section 2.2). This approach will enable us to construct mathematical models aimed at predicting future time series values. We close this section by briefly describing what an ARIMA model is, how ARIMA models are employed for time series predictions, and why they are popular among statisticians and practitioners (Section 2.3).

2.1. What Is a Time Series?

A time series can be represented as a sequence of scalar (or vector) values $y_1, y_2, \ldots, y_n$ corresponding to contiguous, equally spaced points in time labeled $t = 1, 2, \ldots, n$ (e.g., we could measure one y_t value each second, or each hour, or each week, or each month, etc., depending on the nature of the process, on the available technology to measure and store data, and on how we plan to use the collected data); this labeling convention does not depend on the frequency at which y_t values are sampled from a real-world process.

Nowadays, time series have an impact in various fields. For example, they occur daily in economics, where currency quotes are recorded in time periods of minutes, hours, or days. Governments publish unemployment, inflation, or investment figures monthly. Educational institutions maintain annual records of school enrolment, dropout rates, or graduation rates [21]. Recently, international health organizations published the number of people who were infected by or deceased due to the COVID-19 pandemic daily. Several industries record the number of failures that occur per shift in production lines to determine the quality of their processes.

Time series forecasting involves several problems that complicate the task of generating an accurate prediction; for example, missing values, noise, capture errors, etc. Therefore, the challenge is to isolate useful information from the time series, eliminating the aforementioned problems to achieve a forecast [22].

2.2. Time Series Modeling

As mentioned above, time series analysis focuses on modeling a phenomenon y from time t backwards $\{y_t, y_{t-1}, y_{t-2}, ldots\}$, with the objective of forecasting the following values of y up to a *prediction horizon* s. For predicting y_{t+s}, one can assume a functional model f based on the historical records $y_t, y_{t-1}, y_{t-2}, \ldots, y_{t-d+1}$:

$$y_{t+s} = f(y_t, y_{t-1}, y_{t-2}, \ldots, y_{t-d+1}) \qquad (1)$$

Equation (1) is a function approximation problem, and it can be solved by applying the following steps (see [23]):

1. **Functional model f**: Suppose a function f that represents the dependence of y_t related to $y_{t-1}, y_{t-2}, \ldots, y_{t-d+1}$;
2. **Training phase**: For each past value y_{t_k}, train f using as *inputs* the values y_{t_k-1}, y_{t_k-2} and $\ldots, y_{t_k-d+1}$, and as *target* y_{t_k};
3. **Predict value $\hat{y}_{t+1}$**: Apply the trained functional model f to predict y_{t+1} from $y_t, y_{t-1}, y_{t-2}, \ldots, y_{t-d+1}$.

The training phase step should be repeated until all predictions $\hat{y}_{t_k+1}$ are close enough to their corresponding target values y_{t_k+1}. If the functional model f is properly trained, it will produce accurate forecasts, $\hat{y}_{t+1} \approx y_{t+1}$. The above steps can be applied to forecast any horizon s, replacing y_{t_k} with y_{t_k+s} as the target. The three-step procedure presented above is known as an *autoregressive* (AR) model.

2.3. ARIMA Time Series Modeling

In 1970, Box and Jenkins [7] popularized the *autoregressive integrated moving average* (ARIMA) model, which is based on the general *autoregressive integrated moving average* (ARMA) model described by Whittle [24].

$$y_t = \sum_{i=1}^{p} \phi_i y_{t-i} + \sum_{j=1}^{q} \theta_j w_{t-j} + w_t \tag{2}$$

In Equation (2), the first term represents the autoregressive (AR) part, and the second term represents the moving average (MA) part. The w_k terms represent white noise. Typically, w_k are assumed to be random variables that come from a normal distribution $N(0, \sigma_w^2)$. The parameters ϕ_i and θ_j are estimated from the historical values of the time series. We can estimate w_t at time t_k as $\hat{w}_{t_k} = y_{t_k} - \hat{y}_{t_k}$.

The ARIMA model is an improvement on the ARMA model for dealing with non-stationary time series with trends. The SARIMA model is an extension of the ARIMA model for dealing with data with seasonal patterns; for more information, please consult Shumway and Stoffer [21].

Models from the ARIMA family suppose that the time series is generated from linear, time-invariant processes; this assumption is not valid for many situations. Nevertheless, up to now, the ARIMA model and its variants have continued to be very popular; for instance, they are used by most official statistical agencies around the world as an essential part of their modeling strategy when working with macroeconomic or ecological/environmental temporal data. The popularity of ARIMA modeling stems from the following facts:

1. Linear modeling is always at the forefront of the literature;
2. Linear models are easy to learn and implement;
3. Interpretation of results coming from linear models relies on well-defined, well-developed, standardized, mechanized procedures with solid theoretical foundations (e.g., there are established procedures that help us build confidence intervals associated with point forecasts, founded on statistical and probabilistic theory centered around the normal distribution).

On the other hand, when phenomena require the investigation of alternative nonlinear time series models, it is useful to consider the following comment by George E. P. Box:

Since all models are wrong, the scientist cannot obtain a "correct" one by excessive elaboration; on the contrary, following William of Occam, he should seek an economical description of natural phenomena. Just as the ability to devise simple but evocative models is the signature of the great scientist, so over-elaboration and over-parametrization is often the mark of mediocrity.

(Box [25], 1976)

Occam's razor (a principle also known as parsimony) is often used to avoid the danger of overfitting the training data, that is, to choose a model that perfectly fits the time series data but is very complex and hence often does not generalize well. Time series analysis sometimes follows this principle in that many ARIMA or SARIMA models perform increasingly worse as the number of historical values used to forecast y_{t+1} increases [26].

3. Popular ANN Architectures Employed for Time Series Forecasting Purposes

As mentioned previously in Section 1, artificial neural networks (ANNs) belong to the class of nonlinear, nonparametric models; they can be applied to several pattern recognition, classification, and regression problems. An ANN is a set of mathematical functions inspired by the flow of electrical and chemical information within real biological neural networks.

Biological neural networks are made up of special cells called neurons. Each neuron within the biological network is connected to other neurons through dendrites and axons (neurons transmit electrical impulses through their axons to the dendrites of other neurons; the connections between axons and dendrites are called synapses). An ANN consists of a set of interconnected artificial neurons. Figure 1 shows a graphical representation of a set of neurons interconnected by arrows, which helps us see how information is processed within an ANN.

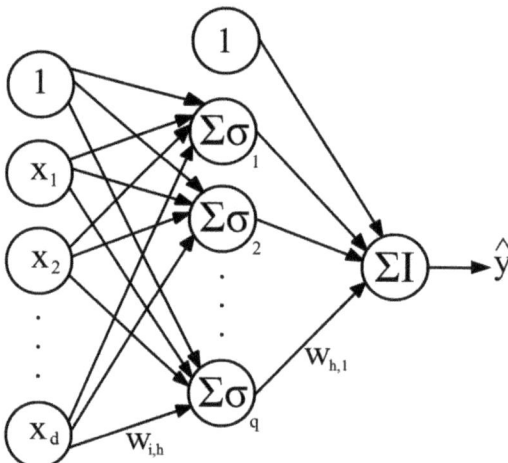

Figure 1. Single hidden layer feedforward neural network.

In this section, we are going to briefly describe the basic aspects of some popular ANN architectures commonly employed for time series forecasting: feedforward neural networks (FFNNs), radial basis function networks (RBFNs), recurrent neural networks (RNNs), and self-organizing maps (SOMs). As we advance in our discussion of FFNNs, occasionally we will encounter some specific concepts needed to transform an FFNN into a time series forecasting model; most of these additional concepts are also applicable to the remaining ANN architectures considered in this section. Comments in Sections 3.2, 3.4, and 3.5 are based on material found in an online course prepared by Bullinaria [27]. In turn, this online material is based on the following textbooks: Beale and Jackson [28], Bishop [29], Callan [30], Fausett [31], Gurney [32], Ham and Kostanic [33], Haykin [34], and Hertz [35].

3.1. Feedforward Neural Networks

3.1.1. Basic Model

Also known in the state of the art by the name of multilayer perceptron (MLP), a feedforward neural network (FFNN), is an ANN architecture where information flows in one direction only, from one layer to the next. Typically, an FFNN is composed of an input layer, one or more hidden layers, and an output layer. In each hidden layer and the output layer, there are neurons (nodes) that are usually connected to all the neurons in the next layer. Figure 1 shows a single FFNN hidden layer with inputs $x_1, x_2, \ldots, x_d$ and output $\hat{y}$.

In the structure shown in Figure 1, information is transmitted from left to right; the inputs $x_1, x_2, \ldots, x_d$ are transformed into the output $\hat{y}$. In the context of time series modeling, focusing on the AR model, FFNN inputs $x_1, x_2, \ldots, x_d$ correspond to time series values $y_t, y_{t-1}, y_{t-2}, \ldots, y_{t-d+1}$, while FFNN output $\hat{y}$ typically corresponds to a prediction value $\hat{y}_{t+1}$, which attempts to approximate future time series value y_{t+1} (see Section 2.2).

Each arrow in the FFNN structure in Figure 1 represents a weight w for the input value x that enters on the left of the arrow, and exits on the right side with the value $w \cdot x$. The input layer is formed by the independent variables $x_1, x_2, \ldots, x_d$ and a constant value known as the *intercept*. For each neuron, all its inputs are summed, and then this sum Σ is transformed by applying a nonlinear activation function σ. One of the most-used activation functions in ANNs is the logistic (sigmoid) function $\sigma(s) = \dfrac{1}{1+e^{-s}}$. The hyperbolic tangent is another frequently used activation function $\sigma(s) = \dfrac{e^{2s}-1}{e^{2s}+1}$. The functionality of each neuron in the hidden layer h ($h = 1, 2, \ldots, q$) is described by

$$\sigma\left(\sum_{i=0}^{d} w_{i,h} \cdot x_i\right), \tag{3}$$

where each $w_{i,h}$ represents the weight that corresponds to the arrow that connects the input node x_i with the neuron h. In Figure 1, the output layer contains only one neuron; this is the number of output units needed if we are interested in predicting a single scalar time series value, but we can employ more output units if we need multiple prediction horizons (scalar or vector). Neurons in an output layer have identical functionality to those in hidden layers, although output neurons sometimes employ the identity function $I(z) = z$ as an activation function (especially for time series forecasting tasks). It is also possible, however, to use as an activation function for output units the same sigmoidal activation functions employed by hidden units (i.e., logistic or hyperbolic tangent). It is even possible to employ different activation functions for units in the same layer. The output layer functionality for our FFNN, depicted in Figure 1, assuming an identity activation function, is described by

$$\hat{y} = w_{0,1} + \sum_{h=1}^{q} w_{h,1} \cdot \sigma\left(\sum_{i=0}^{d} w_{i,h} \cdot x_i\right), \tag{4}$$

3.1.2. FFNN Training

In summary, the ANN has a set of parameters that must be set to determine how the input data are processed and the output generated: weights and biases. The weights are related to the control of the connection between two neurons. The weight value determines the magnitude and direction of the impact of a given input on the output. Biases can be defined as the constant that is added to the product of features and weights. It helps models change the activation function to the positive or negative side [36].

FFNNs are trained, or "taught", with the help of supervised machine learning algorithms. *Backpropagation* (BP) is probably the most popular machine learning algorithm employed to train FFNN models. Next, we describe briefly how BP works. The idea is to adjust all weights and biases in the FFNN model so that, in principle, they minimize some fitting criterion E; for example, the mean squared error:

$$E = \frac{1}{n}\sum_{p=1}^{n}\left(y^{(p)} - \hat{y}^{(p)}\right)^2, \tag{5}$$

where n is the number of example input patterns available for training our model, $y^{(p)}$ is the target (desired value) for the pth example input pattern, and $\hat{y}^{(p)}$ is the FFNN output also for the pth example input pattern, $p = 1, 2, \ldots, n$. FFNN weights are adjusted according to the backpropagation rule: $\Delta w = -\eta \dfrac{\partial E(\vec{W})}{\partial w}$, where meta-parameter η is a small positive number called "learning rate", $\vec{W}$ is a vector containing all FFNN weights, and w is a single FFNN weight (i.e., w can be any single component of $\vec{W}$). Basically, the BP algorithm consists of the following steps:

1. Initialize $\vec{W}$ randomly;
2. Repeat (a) and (b) until $E(\vec{W})$ is below a given threshold T or a pre-established maximum number of iterations M has been reached:

(a) $\vec{W}_{old} \leftarrow \vec{W}$;

(b) Update all network weights: $w \leftarrow w + \left[-\eta \dfrac{\partial E(\vec{W}_{old})}{\partial w}\right]$;

3. Return $\vec{W}$.

From this algorithm outline, we see that BP starts from a random point $\vec{W}_0$ in search space W and looks for the global minimum of the error surface $E(\vec{W})$, say $\vec{W}^*$, by taking small steps, each towards a direction opposite to the derivative (gradient) of the multivariate error function E, evaluated at the current location in the search space W where BP has advanced so far. If $E(\vec{W})$ is smooth enough, BP will descend monotonically when moving from one step to the next; this is why BP is said to be a stochastic gradient descent procedure.

In summary, the goal of BP is to iteratively adjust $\vec{W}$, applying the gradient descent technique, so that the output of the FFNN is close enough to the target values in the training data [29]. For convex error surfaces, BP would do a nice job; unfortunately, $E(\vec{W})$ often contains local minima, and in such situations, BP can easily become stuck into one of those minima. A heuristic approach to facing this issue is to run BP several times, keeping all FFNN settings fixed (e.g., set of training data, number of inputs d, number of hidden neurons q, and BP meta-parameters).

Another important issue we face when training FFNNs with BP is that of *overfitting*. This condition occurs when a model adapts too well to the local stochastic structure of (noisy) training examples but produces poor predictions for inputs not in the training examples. If we strictly aim for $E(\vec{W})$ global minimum, then we focus only on *interpolating exactly* all training data examples. In most situations, however, we would like to use our FFNN model for predicting, as accurately as possible, y values corresponding to unseen (although fairly similar to training examples) inputs $x_1, x_2, \ldots, x_d$, i.e., we would like our FFNN model to have small prediction error (prediction error can be measured much like training error E using, for example, the mean squared error once the unseen future values become available). Note that the true prediction error cannot be measured simultaneously with the training error during the BP process, but we can estimate the former if we reserve some training examples as if they were future inputs (see Section 3.1.5).

From all of this, we conclude that reaching $E(\vec{W})$ global minimum, in fact, should not be our main objective when training an FFNN for prediction purposes; we should instead employ heuristic techniques in order to improve the prediction (generalization) ability of our FFNN model. A simple heuristic approach is to use *early stopping*, so that BP becomes close, but not too close, to the global minimum $E(\vec{W})$. Another possibility is to employ *regularization*. In this technique, we would incorporate, for instance, the term $\vec{W}^T \cdot \vec{W}$ to our error function $E(\vec{W})$ and run BP as usual. This would force BP to produce a smoother, non-oscillating output $\hat{y}$, thereby reducing the risk of over-fitting. Regularization penalizes FFNN models with large weights w and establishes a balance between bias and variance for the output $\hat{y}$.

3.1.3. Time Series Training Examples for FFNNs

The above description of FFNN training is very general, and thus, many questions arise. Specifically, when we attempt to teach an FFNN how to forecast future time series values, we face an obvious question: how do we arrange our available time series values into a set of training examples so that we are able to use BP or some other supervised machine learning algorithm? Suppose that we have N time series values $y_1, y_2, \ldots, y_N$ at our disposal to train our FFNN model and we want to produce one-step-ahead forecasts. According to the autoregressive approach, the inputs to the FFNN model are the time series values $y_t, y_{t-1}, \ldots, y_{t-d+1}$, while the time series value y_{t+1} is the target value. From our available time series data, we see that t can take values $d, d+1, \ldots, N-1$. Thus, a very simple way to build a training dataset for FFNN models intended to produce one-step-ahead univariate time series forecasts consists of rearranging available time series values $y_1, y_2, \ldots, y_N$ in a rectangular array (see Table 1), where we fixed the number of inputs in our FFNN model to $d = 12$, so the first twelve columns contain values for predictor variables $y_{t-11}, y_{t-10}, \ldots, y_t$ and the right column contains values for the (target) response variable y_{t+1}. Each row in Table 1 represents an example of training that can be applied in conjunction with a supervised machine learning algorithm, such as BP.

Table 1. Training dataset for one-step-ahead FFNN time series models.

Example	y_{t-11}	y_{t-10}	...	y_t	y_{t+1}
1	y_1	y_2	...	y_{12}	y_{13}
2	y_2	y_3	...	y_{13}	y_{14}
3	y_3	y_4	...	y_{15}	y_{16}
⋮	⋮	⋮	...	⋮	⋮
$N-12$	y_{N-12}	y_{N-11}	...	y_{N-1}	y_N

3.1.4. FFNN Time Series Predictions

Now, suppose we want to predict still unavailable time series values $y_{N+1}, y_{N+2}, \ldots, y_{N+k}$ using an FFNN model trained with the examples in Table 1 and designed to produce one-step-ahead forecasts. How do we achieve this task? To generate predicted values $\hat{y}_{N+1}, \hat{y}_{N+2}, \ldots, \hat{y}_{N+k}$, first, we estimate $\hat{y}_{N+1}$ using values $y_{N-11}, y_{N-10}, \ldots, y_N$ as inputs to our FFNN model. Next, we predict $\hat{y}_{N+2}$ using the values $y_{N-10}, y_{N-9}, \ldots, y_N, \hat{y}_{N+1}$ as inputs. Note that the most recently calculated model forecast is used as one of the inputs. To predict $\hat{y}_{N+3}$, the two most recently calculated forecasts are used as two of the model inputs. This iterative process continues until the forecast value $\hat{y}_{N+k}$ is obtained.

3.1.5. Cross-Validation

Cross-validation (CV) is a statistical technique for estimating the prediction (or forecasting) accuracy of any model using only available training examples. CV can be helpful when deciding which model to select from a list of properly trained models; we would of course select the model that exhibits the smallest prediction error, as estimated by the CV procedure. CV can also serve as a training framework for ANNs; in fact, CV is often regarded as an integral part of the FFNN model construction process. In general, when training FFNNs for prediction purposes, CV is employed to fine-tune FFNN meta-parameters (such as d, the number of input nodes, and q, the number of hidden units), aiming at reducing over-fitting risk and at the same time improving generalization ability (i.e., prediction accuracy). The idea here is to regard a combination of meta-parameters, say $(d = 12, q = 3)$, as a unique FFNN model. Following this idea, we would apply CV, for example, to each element in the combination set $\{(d, q) | d = 3, 6, 12; q = 2, 3, 4, 5\}$, generating an estimated CV prediction error for each one of the 12 possible combinations. We would finally keep the combination (i.e., FFNN model) that generates the smallest CV prediction error. So, how does CV work? Typically, we randomly split our set of available training examples into two complementary sets: one set, containing approximately 80% of all training examples, is used exclusively for training the considered model, while the other set, containing the remaining 20% of all training examples, is used exclusively for measuring prediction accuracy by comparing target values and their corresponding model outputs via an error function similar to that employed in BP to quantify training error, e.g., mean squared error. The former of these two complementary sets is obviously called the *training set* and the latter is called the *validation set*. The 80% and 20% sizes are just a rule of thumb, and other sizes for these two sets could be chosen. So, we use the training set to obtain a fully trained FFNN model via BP, for example, and then feed to this trained FFNN model the input values contained in the examples from the validation set, thus obtaining outputs that are compared against their corresponding target values from the validation set, producing a prediction error measure, PEM. This is the basic CV iteration. We repeat many times the basic CV iteration (random generation computation) in order to generate many PEM measures, and finally, we average all generated PEMs. This final average would be the estimated prediction error produced by the CV procedure. As we can see, this is a procedure that makes intensive use of available computational resources but produces robust results. We can combine CV with regularization for even better results. For more information about CV, early stopping, regularization, and other techniques to improve FFNN performance, see Bishop [29].

It is important to keep in mind that to obtain valid results from the CV procedure, we must make sure that our training data examples are independent and come from the same population. Unfortunately, the condition of independence does not hold with time series data, as chronologically ordered observations are almost always serially correlated in time (one exception is white noise). To our knowledge, there is not currently a standard way of performing CV for time series data, but two useful CV procedures that deal with the issue of serial dependence in temporal data can be found in Arlot, Celisse, et al. [37,38]. Essentially, the modified CV procedure proposed by Arlot, Celisse, et al. [37] chooses the training and validation sets in such a way that the effects of serial correlation are minimized, while [38] proposes a procedure called *forward validation*, which exclusively uses the most recent training examples as validation data. CV error produced by the forward validation procedure would be a good approximation to unknown prediction error since the short-term future behavior of a time series tends to be similar to that of its most recently recorded observations.

3.1.6. FFNN Ensembles for Time Series Forecasting

FFNN models can be trained with stochastic optimization algorithms like BP, PSO, GA, etc. Because of this, FFNN models for time series prediction produce forecasts $\hat{y}_t$ that depend on the result of the optimization that is being carried out. That is, the optimization process conditions the random variable $\hat{y}_t$. The above is true even when the optimization process always has the same initial conditions (the same training dataset and the same initial parameters). This stochastic prediction property of FFNN models, combined with their conceptual simplicity and their ease of training and implementation (relative to other ANN architectures), allows us to easily construct, from a fixed set of training examples, n independent FFNN models, collectively known as an *FFNN ensemble*. This FFNN ensemble model constructed produces, for a fixed time point t, a set of individual predictions $\{\hat{y}_{s,t} | s = 1, \ldots, n\}$ in response to a single input pattern. Such individual predictions can then be combined in some way, e.g., by averaging, to produce an aggregate prediction that is hopefully more robust, stable, and accurate when compared against their individual counterparts. This basic averaging technique is similar to that found in Makridakis and Winkler [39]. It is important to emphasize here that prediction errors from individual ensemble components need to be independent, i.e., non-correlated or at least only weakly correlated, in order to guarantee a decreasing total ensemble error with an increasing number of ensemble members. FFNN ensemble models in particular fulfill this precondition, given the stochastic nature of their individual outputs. Additionally, all individual predictions could be used to estimate prediction intervals since the distribution of individual forecasts already contains valuable information about the model uncertainty and robustness. Barrow and Crone [40] average the individual predictions from several FFNN models that are generated during a cross-validation process, thus constructing an FFNN ensemble model aimed at producing robust time series forecasts. They compare their proposed strategy (called "crogging") against conventional FFNN ensembles and individual FFNN models. They conclude that their crogging strategy produces the most accurate forecasts. From this, it could be argued that FFNN ensembles whose individual components are trained with different sets of training examples (all coming from the same population) have superior performance with respect to conventional FFNN ensembles whose individual components are all trained with a single fixed set of training examples. Another recent work related to ANN ensembles consists of a comparative study by Lahmiri [41] in which four types of ANN ensembles are compared when using them for predicting stock market returns. The compared ensembles are as follows: an FFNN ensemble, an RNN ensemble, an RBFN ensemble, and a NARX ensemble. The results in this particular study confirm that any ensemble of ANNs performs better than single ANNs. It was also found in this case that the RBFN ensemble produced the best performance. Finally, also note that the Bayesian learning framework involves the construction of FFNN ensembles (also known as committees in the literature).

3.2. Radial Basis Function Networks

Radial basis function networks (RBFNs) are based on function approximation theory. RBFNs were first formulated by Broomhead and Lowe [42]. We outlined in Section 3.1 how FFNNs with sigmoid activation functions (one hidden layer) can approximate functions. RBFNs are slightly different from FFNNs, but they are also capable of universal approximation [43]. In principle, FFNNs arise from the need to classify data points (clustering), while RBFNs rely on the idea of interpolating data points (similarity analysis). An RBFN has a three-layer structure, similar to the structure of an FFNN. The difference lies in the implementation of a Gaussian function instead of a sigmoid activation function in the hidden layer of the RBFN for every neuron. These Gaussian functions are also called *radial basis functions*, because their output value depends only on the distance between the function's argument and a fixed center.

In order to understand the training process of an RBFN, let us recap the concept of *exact interpolation*, mentioned earlier in Section 3.1.2. Given a multidimensional space D, the exact interpolation of a set of N data points requires that the dimensional input vectors $\vec{x}^{(p)} = \langle x_1^{(p)}, \ldots, x_D^{(p)} \rangle$ will be mapped to the corresponding target output $t^{(p)}$ $\forall p = 1, \ldots, N$. The objective is to propose a function $f(x)$ such that $f(\vec{x}^{(p)}) = t^{(p)}$. The *naïve* radial basis function method uses a set of basis functions N of the form $\phi(\|\vec{x} - \vec{x}^{(p)}\|)$, where $\phi(\cdot)$ is a nonlinear function. A linear combination of the basis functions $f(\vec{x}) = \sum_{p=1}^{N} w_p \phi(\|\vec{x} - \vec{x}^{(p)}\|)$ can be obtained as a result of the mapping, for which it is required to find the "weights" w_p such that the function passes through the data points. The most famous and recommended basis function is the Gaussian function:

$$\phi(r) = \exp\left(-\frac{r^2}{2\sigma^2}\right) \tag{6}$$

with width parameter $\sigma > 0$. Figure 2 shows an RBFN under this naïve approach. Please observe that, in this architecture, the N input patterns $\{\vec{x}^{(p)}, p = 1, \ldots, N\}$ determine the input to the hidden layer weights directly.

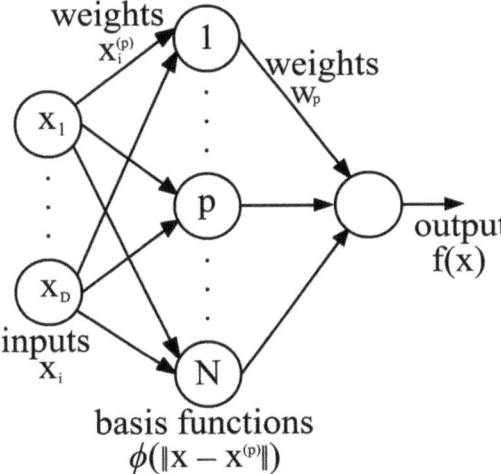

Figure 2. Radial basis function network under the naïve radial basis function approach.

There are problems with the exact interpolation (naïve radial basis function) approach. First, when the data are noisy, it is not desirable for the network outputs to pass through all data points because the resulting function could be highly oscillatory and would not provide adequate generalization. Second, if the training dataset is very large, the RBFN will not be computationally efficient to evaluate if we employ one basis function for every training data point.

3.3. How Do We Improve Radial Basis Function Networks?

The RBFN can be improved by the following strategies when applying exact interpolation [42]:

1. The number of basis functions M must be much smaller than the number of data points N, $(M < N)$;
2. Determine the centers of the basic functions using a training algorithm; they should not be defined as training data input vectors;
3. The basis functions should have a different width parameter σ, which could be solved by a training algorithm;
4. To compensate for the difference between the mean value of all basis functions and the corresponding mean value of the targets, bias parameters can be used in the linear sum of activations in the output layer.

Notwithstanding the above, proposing the ideal value for M is an open problem. By applying the cross-validation technique discussed in Section 3.1.5, a feasible value M could be obtained by comparing results for a range of different values.

So, how do we find the parameters of an RBFN? The input to hidden "weights" (i.e., radial basis function parameters $\{\mu_{ij}, \sigma_j\}$ for $i = 1, \ldots, D; j = 1, \ldots, M$) can be trained using unsupervised learning techniques, such as fixed training data points selected at random and k-means clustering of training data. Supervised learning techniques can also be used, albeit with a higher computational cost. Then, the input-to-hidden "weights" are preserved at a constant while the hidden-to-output "weights" are learned. These weights can be easily found by solving a system of linear equations because this second training stage has only one layer of weights $\{w_{jk}\}, k = 1, \ldots, O$ and O linear output activation functions. For more information on RBFN training, please refer to Bishop [29] and Haykin [34].

RBFNs, applied to time series prediction tasks, require inputs of the same form as those used by FFNNs; for instance, we would rearrange our time series data as shown in Table 1 in order to teach an RBFN how to predict one-step-ahead scalar time series values. Recent research on RBFN modeling applied to time series prediction can be found, for instance, in the work of Chang [44], where RBFN models are used to produce short-term forecasts for wind power generation. Other recent examples include the following: in Sermpinis, Theofilatos, Karathanasopoulos, Georgopoulos, and Dunis [45], RBFN-PSO hybrid models are employed for financial time series prediction; Yin, Zou, and Xu [46] use RBFN models to predict tidal waves on Canada's west coast; Niu and Wang [47] employ gradient-descent-trained RBFNs for financial time series forecasting; Mai, Chung, Wu, and Huang [48] use RBFNs to forecast electric load in office buildings; and Zhu, Cao, and Zhu [49] employ RBFNs to predict traffic flow at some street intersections.

3.4. Recurrent Neural Networks

The main characteristic of a recurrent neural network (RNN) is that it has at least one *feedback connection*, where the output of the previous step is fed as input to the current step. This recurrent connection system makes RNNs ideal for sequential or time series data, "remembering" past information. Another distinctive feature of an RNN is that each layer shares the same weight parameter. RNNs are not easy to train, but very accurate forecasts for time series can be obtained when trained correctly. There are several RNN architectures; however, they all have the following characteristics in common:

1. RNNs contain a subsystem similar to a static FFNN;

2. RNNs can take advantage of the nonlinear mapping abilities of an FFNN, with an added memory capacity for past information.

RNN's learning can be performed by using the gradient descent method, similar to how it is used in the BP algorithm. Specifically, RNNs can be trained by using an algorithm called *backpropagation through time* (BPTT). BPTT trains the network by computing errors from the output layer to the input layer, but unlike BP, it adds errors at each time step because it shares parameters at each layer.

A basic RNN architecture, called the Elman network [50], has the inputs of the next time step together with its hidden unit activations that feed back on the network. Figure 3a shows the Elman network architecture. It is observed that it is necessary to discretize the time and update the activations step by step. In real neurons, this could correspond to the time scale on which they operate, and for artificial neurons, it could be any time step size related to the prediction to be made. In particular, for time series modeling applications, it seems like a natural choice to make the time-step size in an RNN equal to the time separation between any two consecutive time series values. A delay unit is introduced, which simply delays the signal/activation until the next time step. This delay unit can be regarded as a short-term memory unit. Suppose the vectors $\vec{x}(t)$ and $\vec{y}(t)$ are the inputs and outputs, $\vec{W}_{IH}$, $\vec{W}_{HH}$, and $\vec{W}_{HO}$ are the three connection weight matrices, and f and g are the output and hidden unit activation functions of an Elman network; then, the operation of the said RNN can be described as a dynamic system characterized by the pair of nonlinear matrix equations:

$$\begin{aligned} \vec{h}(t) &= f\left(\vec{W}_{IH}\vec{x}(t) + \vec{W}_{HH}\vec{h}(t-1)\right) & \text{State transition} \\ \vec{y}(t) &= g\left(\vec{W}_{HO}\vec{h}(t)\right) & \text{Output equation} \end{aligned} \quad (7)$$

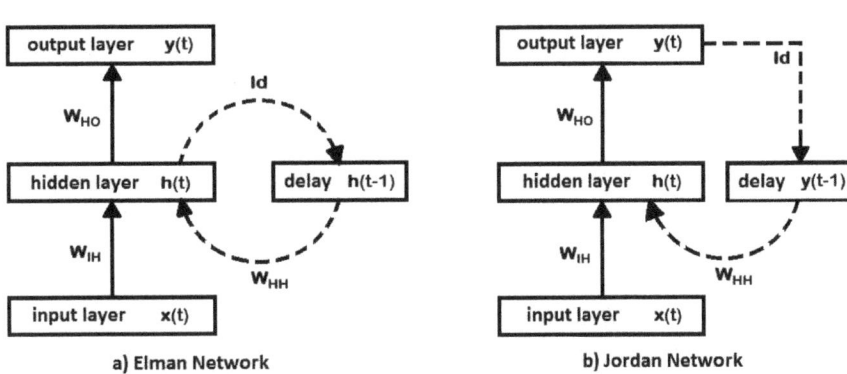

a) Elman Network   b) Jordan Network

Figure 3. Two simple types of recurrent neural networks. Each rectangle contains input units, artificial neurons or delay/memory units; their outputs being indicated by vector quantities $\vec{x}(t)$, $\vec{y}(t)$, $\vec{h}(t)$, etc. A solid arrow connecting two rectangles represents the full set of connection weights among all involved units, which are encoded as matrices $\vec{W}_{IH}$ and $\vec{W}_{HO}$. Dashed arrows represent one-to-one connections between involved units; this means $\vec{Id}$ (identity matrix) and $\vec{W}_{HH}$ are diagonal matrices.

In a dynamical system, its state can be represented as a set of values that recapitulates all the information from the past about the system. The hidden unit activations $\vec{h}(t)$ define the state of the dynamical system. Elman networks are useful in modeling chaotic time series, which are more closely related to chaos theory and dynamical systems. For further information on chaotic time series, see Sprott [51]. Some recent applications of Elman networks in time series forecasting can be found in Ardalani-Farsa and Zolfaghari [52], Chandra and Zhang [53], and Zhao, Zhu, Wang, and Liu [54].

Another simple recurrent neural network architecture, similar to an Elman network, is the Jordan network [55]. In this type of recurrent network, it is the output of the network itself that feeds back into the network along with the inputs of the next time step (see Figure 3b). Jordan networks show dynamical properties and are useful for modeling chaotic time series and nonlinear auto regressive moving average (NARMA) processes. Some examples of models based on the Jordan neural network architecture and applied to time series forecasting can be found in Tabuse, Kinouchi, and Hagiwara [56], Song [57] and Song [58].

Another variant of RNN, called *nonlinear autoregressive modeling with exogenous inputs (NARX)*, has feedback connections that enclose several layers of the network, which can be used by including present and lagged values of k exogenous variables $x^{(1)}$, $x^{(2)}$, ..., $x^{(k)}$. The full performance of the NARX neural network is obtained using its memory capacity [59].

There are two different architectures of NARX neural network model:

- **Open-loop**. Also known as the series-parallel architecture, in this NARX variant, the present and past values of x_t and the true past values of the time series y_t are used to predict the future value of the time series y_{t+1}.
- **Close-loop**. Also known as the parallel architecture, in this NARX variant, the present and past values of x_t and the past predicted values of the time series $\hat{y}_t$ are used to predict the future value of the time series y_{t+1}.

3.5. Self-Organizing Maps

Self-organizing maps (SOMs) learn to form their classifications of the training data without external help. To achieve this, in SOMs, it is assumed that membership in each class is determined by input patterns that share similar characteristics and that the network will be able to identify such features in a wide range of input patterns. A particular class of unsupervised systems is based on competitive learning, where output neurons must compete with each other to activate, but under the condition that only one is activated at a time, called a winner-takes-all neuron. To apply this competition, negative feedback pathways must be used, which are lateral inhibitory connections between neurons. As a result, neurons must organize themselves.

The main objective of an SOM is to convert, in a topologically ordered manner, an incoming multidimensional signal into a discrete one- or two-dimensional map. This is like a nonlinear generalization of principal component analysis (PCA).

3.5.1. Essential Characteristics and Training of an SOM

An SOM is organized as follows: we have points $\vec{x}$ in the input space that are mapped to points $I(\vec{x})$ in the output space. There is a set of points $\vec{x}$ living in the input space, and we suppose that there is a function to assign $\vec{x}$ to points $I(\vec{x})$ in the output space. In turn, there is another function to assign to each point I in the output space a corresponding point $\vec{w}(I)$ in the input space (see Figure 4).

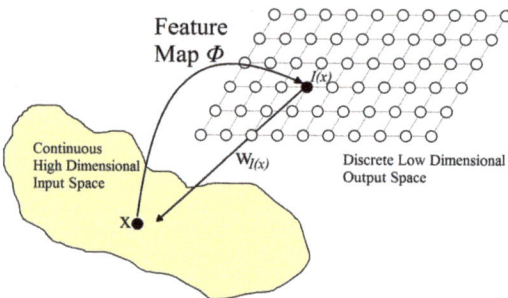

Figure 4. Organization of an SOM.

Kohonen networks [60] are a particular and important kind of SOM. The proposed network has a feedforward structure with a single computational layer, where the neurons are arranged in rows and columns. Nodes in the input layer connect to each of the neurons in the computational layer (see Figure 5).

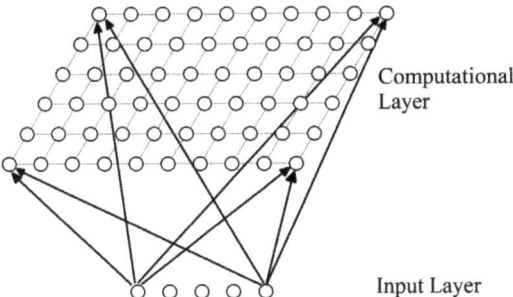

Figure 5. Kohonen network.

$$d_j(\vec{x}) = \sum_{i=1}^{D} (x_i - w_{ji})^2 \tag{8}$$

The self-organization process consists of the following components:

1. *Initialization.* At first, the connection weights are set to small random values.
2. *Competition.* For a D dimensionality input space, $\vec{x} = \langle x_1, \ldots, x_D \rangle$ represents the input patterns and $\vec{w}_j = \langle w_{j1}, \ldots, w_{jD} \rangle$ represents the connection weights between the input units x_i and the neuron j in the computational layer; $j = 1, \ldots, N$, where N is the total number of neurons. The difference $\vec{x}$ between $\vec{w}_j$ for each neuron can be calculated as the Euclidean distance squared, which will represent the discriminant function $d(\vec{x})$.
   The neuron with the lowest discriminant function $d(\vec{x})$ is declared the winner-takes-all neuron. Competition between neurons allows mapping the continuous input space to the discrete output space.
3. *Cooperation.* In neurobiological studies, it was observed that, within a set of excited neurons, there can be lateral interaction. When a neuron is activated, the neurons in its surroundings tend to become more excited than those further away. A similar topological neighborhood that decays with distance exists for neurons in an SOM. Let S_{ij} be the lateral distance between any pair of neurons i and j, then $T_{j,I(\vec{x})} = \exp(-S_{j,I(vecx)}^2 / 2\sigma^2)$ defines our topological neighborhood, where $I(\vec{x})$ is the index of the winner-takes-all neuron. A special quality of the SOM is that the size of the neighborhood σ should decrease over time. An exponential reduction is a commonly used time dependence: $\sigma(t) = \sigma_0 \exp(-t/\tau_\sigma)$.
4. *Adaptation.* SOM has an adaptive (learning) process through which the feature map between inputs and outputs is formed through the self-organization of the latter. Due to the topographic neighborhood, when the weights of the winner-takes-all neuron are updated, the weights of its neighbors are also updated, although to a lesser extent. To update the weight, we define $\Delta w_{ji} = \eta(t) \cdot T_{j,I(\vec{x})}(t) \cdot (x_i - w_{ji})$, in which we have a time-dependent learning rate t $\eta(t) = \eta_0 exp(-t/\tau_\eta)$. These updates are applied to all training patterns $\vec{x}$ for various periods. The goal of each learning weight update is to move the weight vectors $\vec{w}_j$ of the winner-takes-all neuron and its neighbors closer to the input vector $\vec{x}$.

When the SOM training algorithm has converged, important statistical properties of the feature map are displayed. As shown in Figure 4, the set of weight vectors $\{\vec{w}_j\}$ in the output space integrates the feature map Φ, which provides an approximation to the input space. Derived from the above, Φ represents the statistical variations in the input distribution: the largest domains of the output space are allocated to sample training vectors $\vec{x}$ with high probability of occurrence, which are drawn from the regions in the input space; the opposite is the case for training vectors with low probability. In other words, a properly trained self-organizing map is able to choose the best features to approximate the underlying distribution of the input space. For further details on SOM statistical properties, please refer to Haykin [34].

3.5.2. Application of Self-Organizing Maps to Time Series Forecasting

If SOMs are mainly employed to solve unsupervised classification problems, how can they be applied to time series forecasting tasks, which in essence are, as we saw in Section 2.2, function approximation (regression) problems? A simple approach to the univariate time series case is as follows: as training examples for our SOM model, we can use vectors of the form $\vec{x} = \langle y_{t+1}, y_t, y_{t-1}, \ldots, y_{t-d+1} \rangle$, where the first component corresponds to the one-step-ahead target output in our basic FFNN model discussed in Section 3.1. The rest of the components in $\vec{x}$ correspond to the autoregressive inputs also employed by our FFNN model. Thus, any single row in Table 1, which corresponds to a training example for FFNN models, also serves as a training example for SOM models. The computational layer in our SOM model for univariate time series consists of a one-dimensional lattice of neurons. When forecasting, our SOM model utilizes all of the components from input vector $\vec{x}$, except for the first, in a competition process among all neurons in the computational layer, just as described in Section 3.5.1. The winning neuron $I(\vec{x})$ determines our one-step-ahead forecast value $\hat{y}_{t+1}$ by simply extracting the first component from weight vector $\vec{w}_{I(\vec{x})}$ associated to winning neuron $I(\vec{x})$, i.e., $\hat{y}_{t+1} = w_{I(\vec{x}),1}$. Thus, the number of neurons in the computational layer determines how many possible discrete values can assume our one-step-ahead forecast value $\hat{y}_{t+1}$. One disadvantage to this simple approach is the large prediction error due to the step-like output of our SOM model trying to approximate a "smooth" time series. SOMs may require too many neurons if we want to reduce their associated prediction error. This alternative, however, would be accompanied by a prohibitively high computational cost. A more sensible solution to this problem would be using RBFNs in conjunction with SOMs: first, we train a univariate time series SOM model just as described above; then, the resulting SOM weights $\{\vec{w}_j\}$, which define mapping Φ, are used to directly build an RBFN with N Gaussian basis functions and one output unit. SOM weights $w_{j,1}$ would be used as RBFN hidden-to-output weights, while the remaining components in vector $\vec{w}_j$ would play the role of the RBF center for the jth hidden unit. No further RBFN training is required, although we still need to determine the σ_j parameters for each radial basis function in the network; refer to Section 3.2 for more details on RBFNs. Thus, a reduction in prediction error is achieved, at least in places where there are not extreme values in the time series. In these particular locations where extreme values occur, prediction errors are still high for both SOM and SOM–RBFN models. For more details, see Barreto [61], where a comprehensive survey on SOMs applied to time series prediction can also be found. Relatively recent work on model refinements based on the classical SOM and applied to time series prediction can be found in Burguillo [62] and Valero, Aparicio, Senabre, Ortiz, Sancho, and Gabaldon [63]. In Section 4.4, we summarize the work of Simon, Lendasse, Cottrell, Fort, Verleysen, et al. [64], where a double SOM model is proposed to generate long-term time series trend predictions.

3.5.3. Comparison between FFNN and SOM Models Applied to Time Series Prediction

An SOM-based model adapted to time series prediction basically performs local function approximation, i.e., acts on localized regions of the input space. On the other hand, FFNNs are global models, making use of highly distributed representations of the input space. This contrast between global and local models implies that FFNN weights are difficult to interpret in the context of time series modeling. Essentially, FFNNs are black boxes that produce forecasts in response to certain stimuli. The components of a weight vector associated to each neuron in an SOM model fitted to a univariate time series can have a clearer meaning to the user, given the local nature of the model. Specifically, they can be viewed as the mean values for lagged versions of response variable y when we expect a one-step-ahead future value close to the first component on such a weight vector [61].

3.5.4. SOM Models Combined with Autoregressive Models

Another possible approach involving the application of SOM models to time series prediction tasks is a direct extension of the procedure described in Section 3.5.2. We can build a hybrid two-stage predictor based on SOM and autoregressive (AR) models. In the first stage, we train an SOM model so as to produce discrete one-step-ahead time series forecasts. This SOM model is then employed to split the available set of training examples into N clusters, one for each SOM neuron, by simply presenting training example $\vec{x}$ to trained SOM and assigning a cluster label to $\vec{x}$ based on the winning neuron. In the second stage, a local linear AR model is fitted to each cluster defined in the first stage. Now, this fully trained hybrid model can be employed to produce a one-step-ahead forecast for any future input $\vec{x}^f$: first, we determine to which cluster $\vec{x}^f$ belongs, by using our trained first-stage SOM model; then, we use the corresponding AR model to produce the desired forecast. This basic approach is similar in spirit to local function linearization (it seems like a sensible strategy to assume that, locally, a real continuous function can be reasonably approximated by a simpler linear function) and can be extended in many ways; for instance, FFNN (or RBFN, or even RNN) ensembles could replace local AR models in the second stage. Although, this would result in a more complex model, requiring extensive computational resources for its construction. AR parameters can be quickly computed, although statistical training on the modeler's side is required (specifically, the modeler must be familiarized with the Box–Jenkins statistical technique). This SOM–AR approach will work well if each data cluster contains enough consecutive time series observations to adequately train an AR model; otherwise, an ANN alternative for the second stage would be preferable. If all goes well, two-stage SOM–AR models will enable users to make plausible statistical inferences about the relative importance of lagged time series values at a local level. Confidence intervals can additionally be computed for each one-step-ahead forecast produced by the SOM–AR model, giving a statistical quantification of forecast uncertainty. Yadav and Srinivasan [65] propose a specific SOM–AR model implementation for predicting electricity demand in Britain and Wales, while Dablemont, Simon, Lendasse, Ruttiens, Blayo, and Verleysen [66] combine an SOM clustering model with local RBFNs to forecast financial data; Cherif, Cardot, and Boné [67] propose an SOM–RNN model to forecast chaotic time series, and Nourani, Baghanam, Adamowski, and Gebremichael [68] propose a sophisticated SOM–FFNN model to forecast rainfall on multi-step-ahead time scales using precipitation satellite data.

3.6. BP Problems in the Context of Time Series Modeling

We have seen in Section 3.1.2 that BP training presents several challenges that must be overcome: over-fitting, convergence to a local minimum, and convergence problems slow convergence speed (η must be small to improve BP convergence properties at the expense of BP processing speed).

3.6.1. Vanishing and Exploding Gradient Problems

One of the main problems encountered when training recurrent neural networks or deep neural networks (FFNNs with many hidden layers) with BP is the vanishing gradient problem. When the gradients become very small relative to the parameters, it can cause the weights in the initial layers not to change noticeably; this is known as the vanishing gradient problem [69]. This problem is commonly attributed to the architecture of the neural network, certain activation functions (sigmoid or hyperbolic tangent), and small initial values of the weights. The exploding gradient problem appears when the weights are greater than 1 and the gradient continues to increase, causing the gradient descent to diverge. Unlike the vanishing gradient problem, the exploding gradient problem is directly related to the weights in the neural network [69].

For instance, a generic recurrent network has hidden states $h_1, h_2, \ldots$, inputs $u_1, u_2, \ldots$, and outputs $x_1, x_2, \ldots$. Let it be parametrized by θ, so that the system evolves as

$$(h_t, x_t) = F(h_{t-1}, u_t, \theta) \tag{9}$$

Often, the output x_t is a function of h_t, as some $x_t = G(h_t)$. The vanishing gradient problem already presents itself clearly when $x_t = h_t$, so we simplify our notation to the special case with

$$x_t = F(x_{t-1}, u_t, \theta) \tag{10}$$

Now, take its differential:

$$\begin{aligned} dx_t &= \nabla_\theta F(x_{t-1}, u_t, \theta) d\theta + \nabla_x F(x_{t-1}, u_t, \theta) dx_{t-1} \\ dx_{t-k} &= \nabla_\theta F(x_{t-k-1}, u_{t-k}, \theta) d\theta + \nabla_x F(x_{t-k-1}, u_{t-k}, \theta) dx_{t-k-1} \\ dx_t &= (\nabla_\theta F(x_{t-1}, u_t, \theta) + \nabla_x F(x_{t-1}, u_t, \theta) \nabla_\theta F(x_{t-2}, u_{t-1}, \theta) + \cdots) d\theta \end{aligned} \tag{11}$$

Training the network requires us to define a loss function to be minimized. Let it be $L(x_T, u_1, \ldots, u_T)$, then minimizing it by gradient descent gives

$$dL = \nabla_x L(x_T, u_1, \ldots, u_T)(\nabla_\theta F(x_{t-1}, u_t, \theta) + \nabla_x F(x_{t-1}, u_t, \theta) \nabla_\theta F(x_{t-2}, u_{t-1}, \theta) + \cdots) d\theta \tag{12}$$

$$\Delta \theta = -\eta \cdot [\nabla_x L(x_T)(\nabla_\theta F(x_{t-1}, u_t, \theta) + \nabla_x F(x_{t-1}, u_t, \theta) \nabla_\theta F(x_{t-2}, u_{t-1}, \theta) + \cdots)]^T \tag{13}$$

where η is the learning rate. The vanishing/exploding gradient problem appears because there are repeated multiplications of the form

$$\nabla_x F(x_{t-1}, u_t, \theta) \nabla_x F(x_{t-2}, u_{t-1}, \theta) \nabla_x F(x_{t-3}, u_{t-2}, \theta) \cdots \tag{14}$$

Specifically, the vanishing gradient problem arises when the neural network adds multiple layers with activation functions whose gradients approach zero. Since each layer contributes to the product of the activation functions and the layer weights, if the number of layers increases, the product quickly turns small [70].

The explosive gradient problem arises when the network weights are multiplied by the activation functions, and as a result, we have a product with values greater than one, causing the values of the gradients to be large [70].

3.6.2. Alternatives to the BP Problems

Attempts have been made to overcome these issues in the context of time series forecasting. See, for example, Hu, Wu, Chen, and Dou [71] and Nunnari [72]. Below is a brief outline of the main alternatives.

Batch normalization. Ioffe and Szegedy [73] described an *internal covariate shift* as the effect of inputs with a corresponding distribution in each layer of a neural network, which is caused by the randomness that exists in the initialization of parameters and in the input data during the training process. They proposed to address the problem by normalizing the layer inputs, recentering and rescaling them, and applying the normalization to each training mini-batch. Batch normalization relaxes the care of parameter initialization, allows the application of much higher learning rates, and, in certain cases, eliminates the need for dropout to mitigate overfitting. Although batch normalization has been proposed to handle gradient explosion or vanishing problems, recently, Yang, Pennington, Rao, Sohl-Dickstein, and Schoenholz [74] showed that, at the initialization time, a deep batch norm network suffers from gradient explosion.

Gradient clipping. In 2013, Pascanu, Mikolov, and Bengio [70] assumed that a cliff-like structure appears on the error surface when gradients explode, and as a solution, they proposed clipping the norm of the exploded gradients. Furthermore, to solve the vanishing gradient problem, they use a regularization term to force the Jacobian matrices to preserve the norm only in relevant directions, keeping the error signal alive while it travels backwards in time.

Backpropagation through time (BPTT). This famous technique was proposed by Werbos [75] in 1990. If the computational graph of an RNN is expanded (unrolled RNN), it is basically an FFNN with the innovative characteristic that, throughout the unrolled RNN, the same parameters are repeated and these appear in each period. Then, the chain rule can be applied to propagate the gradients backward through the unrolled RNN, as would be performed in any FFNN. It should be considered that, in this unrolled RNN, for each parameter, the gradient with respect to itself must be added at all places where the parameter occurs. In summary, BPTT can be explained as using BP to RNN on sequential data, e.g., a time series [75].

The BPTT algorithm can be described as follows:

- Introduce a time-step sequence of input and output pairs to the network.
- Unroll the network.
- For each time step, calculate and accumulate errors.
- Roll-up the network.
- Update weights.
- Repeat.

Long short-term memory (LSTM). In 1997, Hochreiter and Schmidhuber [76] introduced an RNN along with an appropriate gradient-based learning algorithm. Its goal is to introduce a short-term memory for RNN that can last for thousands of time steps, that is, a "long short-term memory". The main feature of LSTM is its *memory cell* made up of three "gates": the input gate, output gate, and forget gate [77]. The flow of information is regulated by gates inside and outside the cell. First, the forget gate assigns a previous state a value between 0 and 1, compared to a current input. Then, it chooses what information to keep from a previous state. A value of 0 means deleting the information, and a value of 1 means keeping it. By applying the same system as the forget gate, the gateway determines the new information that will be stored in the current state. Finally, the output gate controls which pieces of information in the current state are generated by considering the previous and current states and assigning a value from 0 to 1 to the information. The LSTM network maintains useful long-term dependencies, generating relevant information about the current state.

The goal of LSTM is to create an additional module in an ANN that can learn when to forget irrelevant information and when to remember relevant information [77]. Calin [78] shows that RNNs using LSTM diminish the vanishing gradient problem but do not solve the exploding gradient problem.

Reducing complexity. The vanishing gradient problem can be mitigated by reducing the complexity of the ANN. By reducing the number of layers and/or the number of neurons in each layer, a reduction in the complexity of the network can be achieved, affecting the tunability of the model. Therefore, finding a balance between model complexity and gradient flow is critical to creating successful ANNs in deep learning.

Evolutionary algorithms. Alternatively, it is also possible to employ evolutionary algorithms instead of BP for ANN training purposes [79]. For instance, Jha, Thulasiraman, and Thulasiram [80] and Adhikari, Agrawal, and Kant [81] employ particle swarm optimization (PSO) to train ANN models applied to time series modeling; Awan, Aslam, Khan, and Saeed [82] compare short-term forecast performances for FFNN models trained with genetic algorithm (GA), artificial bee colony (ABC), and PSO by using electric load data; Giovanis [83] combines FFNN and GA for predicting economic time series data.

Statistical techniques ANNs can also be trained using probabilistic techniques such as the Bayesian learning framework. This training technique offers some relevant advantages:

no over-fitting occurs, it provides automatic regularization, and forecast uncertainty can be estimated [29]. Some recent applications using this approach in the context of time series forecasting can be found, for example, in Skabar [84], Blonbou [85], van Hinsbergen, Hegyi, van Lint, and van Zuylen [86], and Kocadağlı and Aşıkgil [87]. Another possible alternative is to train an ANN with BP or some other optimization technique and then build a hybrid ANN–ARIMA model; see, for example, Zhang [88], Guo and Deng [89], Otok, Lusia, Faulina, Kuswanto, et al. [90], and Viviani, Di Persio, and Ehrhardt [91].

4. Brief Literature Survey on ANNs Applied to Time Series Modeling

In this section, we discuss, analyze, and summarize a small sample of recently published research articles. In our opinion, these articles are representative of the state of the art and provide useful information that can be used as a starting point for future research. The choice of articles surveyed in this section is based mainly on the architectures outlined previously in Section 3. In Section 4.1, we study some time series forecasting techniques [92,93], which combine feedforward neural network models with particle swarm optimization. The basic idea here is to show how to combine these techniques to produce new hybrid models and how to design experiments in which we compare several time series prediction models. Section 4.2 explores the work of Crone, Guajardo, and Weber [94] on how to assess the ability of support vector regression and feedforward neural network models to predict basic trends and seasonal patterns found in economic time series of monthly frequency. Section 4.3 highlights useful hints suggested by Moody [95] on how to construct ANN models for predicting short-term behavior in macroeconomic indicators. Section 4.4 summarizes the work found in Simon, Lendasse, Cottrell, Fort, Verleysen, et al. [64], which instructs on how to build a model based on a double application of the self-organizing map to predict medium- to long-term time series trends, focusing on the empirical distribution of several forecasts' paths produced by the same double SOM model. Sections 4.5 and 4.6 summarize the works of Zimmermann, Tietz, and Grothmann [96] and Lukoševičius [97], respectively. Both works contain valuable hints and techniques to build recurrent neural network models aimed at predicting temporal data, possibly coming from an underlying dynamical system. Zimmermann, Tietz, and Grothmann [96] focus on a more traditional approach, using back propagation through time as a training algorithm but employing a novel graphical notation to represent recurrent neural network architectures. Lukoševičius [97] focuses on the echo state network approach, which relies more on numerical linear algebra for training purposes. In Sections 4.2–4.6, we replicated, from the respective surveyed articles, important comments that correspond to theoretical concepts, hints, and relevant bibliographic references, as we believe this is the best way to convey and emphasize them. Our intention is to construct useful, short, and clear summaries that will hopefully save some time for readers interested in gaining a full understanding of similar articles to the ones we are surveying here.

4.1. Combining Feedforward Neural Networks and Particle Swarm Optimization for Time Series Forecasting

As we mentioned already briefly in Section 3.6, it is possible to train ANN models via evolutionary algorithms. The objective of evolutionary algorithms is to discover global solutions that are optimal and low cost. Evolutionary algorithms are usually based on various agents, such as chromosomes, particles, bees, ants, etc., searching iteratively to discover the global optimum or the local optimum (population-based algorithms) [36]. In 1975, Holland [98] introduced the genetic algorithm (GA), which is considered the first evolutionary algorithm. As with any evolutionary algorithm, the GA is based on a metaphor from the theory of evolution. In the field of evolutionary computing, good solutions to a problem can be seen as individuals well-adapted to their environment. Although the GA has had many applications, it has been surpassed by other evolutionary algorithms, such as the PSO algorithm [99].

Today, due to its simplicity and ability to be used in a wide range of applications, the PSO algorithm has become one of the most well-known swarm intelligence algorithms [100]. Eberhart and Kennedy performed the first experiment using PSO to train ANN weights instead of using the more traditional backpropagation algorithm [101]. Several approaches have been proposed to apply PSO in ANN, such as the works published by Eberhart and Shi [102], Eberhart and Shi [103], and Yu, Wang, and Xi [104]. In this section, we explore in a little more detail some possible ways we can pair an ANN model with the PSO algorithm to produce time series forecasts, but first, we will briefly describe how PSO works.

In the words of its creators...

PSO is an optimization algorithm inspired by the motion of a bird flock; any member of the flock is called a "particle".

(Kennedy and Eberhart [101], 1995)

In the PSO algorithm, a particle moves through a real-valued dimensionality search space D, guided by three attributes at each time (iteration) t: position $\vec{x}_t$, velocity $\vec{v}_t$, and memory $\vec{P}_{Best}$. In the beginning, the position of the particle is generated by a random variable with a uniform distribution, delimited in each dimension by the search space $\vec{x}_0 = U(lower, upper)$; thereby, its best visited position is set as equal to its initial position $\vec{P}_{Best} = \vec{x}_0$, with an initial velocity $\vec{v}_0 = 0$. After the first iteration, the attribute $\vec{P}_{Best}$ remembers the best position visited by the particle based on an objective function f; the other two attributes, $\vec{v}_t$ and $\vec{x}_t$, are updated according to Equations (15) and (16), respectively.

The best of all the best particle positions $\vec{P}_{Best}$ is called the global best $\vec{G}_{Best}$. In each iteration of the algorithm, the swarm is inspected to update the best member. Whenever a member is found to improve the objective function of the current leader, that member becomes the new global best [105].

The objective of the PSO algorithm is to minimize function $f: \mathbb{R}^D \to \mathbb{R}$; i.e., find $\vec{a} \in \mathbb{R}^D$ such that $f(\vec{a}) \leq f(\vec{x})$ for all $\vec{x}$ in the search space.

In PSO, *variation* (diversity) comes from two sources. The first is the difference between the current position of particle x_t and its memory P_{Best}. The second is the current position of particle x_t and the global best G_{Best} (see Equation (15)).

$$\begin{aligned} v_{t+1} &= \omega \times v_t + c_1 \times U(0,1) \times (P_{Best} - x_t) \\ &+ c_2 \times U(0,1) \times (G_{Best} - x_t) \end{aligned} \quad (15)$$

$$x_{t+1} = x_t + v_{t+1} \quad (16)$$

Equation (15) reflects the three main elements of the PSO algorithm: the inertia path, local interaction, and neighborhood influence [106]. The inertial path is the previous velocity $\omega * v_t$, where ω is the inertial weight. The local interaction is called the cognitive component $c_1 * U(0,1) * (P_{Best} - x_t)$, with c_1 as the cognitive coefficient. The last term is called the social component and represents the neighborhood influence $c_2 * U(0,1) * (G_{Best} - x_t)$, where c_2 is the social coefficient. $U(0,1)$ is a random variable with a uniform distribution [105]. In [107], Clerc and Kennedy proposed a set of standard parameter values for PSO stability and convergence: $\omega = 0.7298$, $c_1 = 1.49618$, and $c_2 = 1.49618$. A leader can be global to the entire swarm or local to a certain neighborhood of a swarm. In the latter case, there will be as many local leaders as there are neighborhoods, resulting in more attractors scattered throughout the search space. The use of multiple neighborhoods is useful to combat the premature convergence problem of the PSO algorithm [105].

4.1.1. Particle Swarm Optimization for Artificial Neural Networks

In Algorithm 1, the basic PSO algorithm proposed by Kennedy and Eberhart [101] is presented.

Algorithm 1 Basic particle swarm optimization (PSO) algorithm
---
for each particle $i = 1, 2, ..., N$ in the swarm **do**
    initialize particle's position: $\vec{x}_i \leftarrow$ uniform random vector in $\mathbb{R}^D$
    initialize particle's best-known position: $\vec{P}_{Best,i} \leftarrow \vec{x}_i$
    if $f(\vec{P}_{Best,i}) < f(\vec{G}_{Best})$ **then**
        update swarm's best-known position: $\vec{G}_{Best} \leftarrow \vec{P}_{Best,i}$
    end if
    initialize particle's velocity: $\vec{v}_i \leftarrow$ uniform random vector in $\mathbb{R}^D$
end for
repeat
    for each particle $i = 1, 2, ..., N$ in the swarm **do**
        for each dimension $d = 1, 2, ..., D$ **do**
            pick random numbers $r_p, r_g \sim U(0,1)$
            update particle's velocity: $v_{i,d} \leftarrow \omega v_{i,d} + c_1 r_p (\vec{P}_{Best,i,d} - x_{i,d}) + c_2 r_g (\vec{G}_{Best,d} - x_{i,d})$
        end for
        update particle's position: $\vec{x}_i \leftarrow \vec{x}_i + \vec{v}_i$
        if $f(\vec{x}_i) < f(\vec{P}_{Best,i})$ **then**
            update particle's best-known position: $\vec{P}_{Best,i} \leftarrow \vec{x}_i$
            if $f(\vec{P}_{Best,i}) < f(\vec{G}_{Best})$ **then**
                update swarm's best-known position: $\vec{G}_{Best} \leftarrow \vec{P}_{Best,i}$
            end if
        end if
    end for
until a termination criterion is met
Now, $\vec{G}_{Best}$ holds the best found solution

The basic PSO algorithm shown in Algorithm 1 can be applied to ANNs as a multilayer perceptron, where each particle's position $\vec{x}_i$ represents the set of weights and biases of the ANN for the current iteration. Each particle moves in the weighting space trying to minimize the learning error during the training phase, and also maintains the historically best position $\vec{p}_i$ in memory along its exploration path. When the particle changes position, it is analogous to updating the weights of the ANN controller to reduce the tracking error [108]. The termination criterion can be defined as the scope of a predefined MSE value condition [109]. Finally, the best position reached by the swarm $\vec{g}$ can be expressed as the optimal solution for the ANN.

Now let us take a look at some FFNN–PSO time series models proposed in the literature. Adhikari, Agrawal, and Kant [81] assess the effectiveness of FFNN and Elman networks when trained with the PSO algorithm for the prediction of univariate seasonal time series. In this context, a PSO particle moves in the search space $\{\vec{W}\}$ defined by the weights of the ANN model to be trained, while the PSO cost function is the same cost function employed in backpropagation; thus, we could say that a PSO particle is structurally identical to an ANN.

de M. Neto, Petry, Aranildo, and Ferreira [92] take a slightly different approach: they propose a basic PSO optimizer in which each particle is a single hidden layer FFNN designed to produce one-step-ahead forecasts for univariate time series, plus some extra meta-parameters. The search space for their proposed hybrid system consists of the following discrete and continuous variables:

- Relevant time lags for autoregressive inputs (the total number of relevant time lags defines the FFNN's input dimension d);
- Number q of hidden units in the FFNN;
- Training algorithm employed: 1. Levenberg–Marquardt [110], 2. RPROP [111], 3. scaled conjugate gradient [112], or 4. one-step secant [113], all refinements of the basic BP algorithm;
- Variant of FFNN architecture employed: 1. An FFNN architecture identical to the one outlined in Section 3.1, with a linear output unit, 2. an FFNN with structural

modifications proposed by Leung, Lam, Ling, and Tam [114], or 3. the same FFNN architecture as in 1, but with a sigmoidal output unit;
- Initial FFNN weights and meta-parameter configuration.

PSO individuals in this combined method are evaluated by a proposed fitness function, which is directly proportional to a metric measuring the degree of synchronization between time series movements in forecasts and corresponding time series movements in validation data. The proposed fitness function is also inversely proportional to the sum of several regression error metrics, among them, mean squared error (MSE) and Theil's U statistic.

We now summarize, in the next few lines, the experiments conducted by de M. Neto, Petry, Aranildo, and Ferreira [92], their observations, and their conclusions. All investigated time series were normalized to lie within the interval [0,1] and were divided into three sets: the training set with 50% of the data, the validation set with 25% of the data, and the test set with 25% of the data. Ten particles were used in the PSO algorithm, with 1000 iterations. The standard PSO optimization routine was employed to find the minimum in the parameter space; in this way, an optimal FFNN model is found for each time series. This optimal FFNN was then compared (via the same regression error metrics employed in the proposed fitness function) against a random walk model and a standalone FFNN model trained with the Levenberg–Marquardt algorithm.

Benchmarking data used in the experiments consist of two natural phenomena time series (daily starshine measures and yearly sunspot measures) and four financial time series of daily frequency (*Dow Jones Industrial Average Index* (DJIA), *National Association of Securities Dealers Automated Quotation Index* (NASDAQ), *Petrobras Stock Values*, and *Dollar-Real Exchange Rate*). From these experiments, it was observed that the proposed model behaved better than the random walk model, the heads or tails experiment, and the standalone FFNN model for the two time series of natural phenomena that were analyzed. Nevertheless, for the four financial time series that were forecast, the proposed model displayed behavior similar to both a random walk model and a heads or tails experiment and behaved slightly better than the standalone FFNN model. It was also observed by the authors that predictions for all analyzed financial series are *dislocated* one-step-ahead with respect to the original values, noting that this observed behavior is consistent with the work of Sitte and Sitte [115] and de Araujo, Madeiro, de Sousa, Pessoa, and Ferreira [116], which have shown that the forecast of financial time series denotes a distinctive one-step shift concerning the original data.

Finally, de M. Neto, Petry, Aranildo, and Ferreira [92] claim that this behavior can be corrected by a phase prediction adjustment, and conclude that their proposed method is a valid option for predicting financial time series values, obtaining satisfactory forecasting results with an admissible computational cost.

Now let us take a look at a similar but more refined approach. Simplified swarm optimization (SSO) [117] is a refinement of PSO, which, of course, can also be employed for adjusting ANN weights. SSO is a swarm intelligence method that also belongs to the evolutionary computation methods. SSO's updating mechanism for particle position is much simpler than that of PSO.

In turn, parameter-free improved simplified swarm optimization [93], or ISSO for short, is a refinement of SSO; ISSO treats SSO's tunable meta-parameters as variables in the search space where particles move. The idea here is to reduce human intervention during the optimization process, i.e., minimize the need for manual tuning of meta-parameters. In Yeh [93], ISSO is employed for adjusting ANN weights. ISSO uses three different position updating mechanisms: one for updating ANN weights, a second one for updating SSO meta-parameters, and a third one for updating the whole position of a particle if its associated fitness value shows no improvement after several iterations in the process. Yeh [93] conducted a couple of experiments to compare ISSO against five other ANN training methods: BP, GA [118], basic PSO, a PSO variant called cooperative random learning PSO [119], and regular SSO.

- Experiment number 1 tests all six training algorithms on a special ANN architecture called *single multiplicative neuron* (SMN), which is similar to an FFNN but consists of an input layer and an output layer with a single processing unit (this single neuron has a logistic activation function but multiplies its inputs instead of adding them; additionally, there is a bias for each input node, in contrast to FFNNs, which contain just one bias in the input layer).
- Experiment number 2 also tests all six training algorithms, but this time on a regular FFNN with one to six hidden neurons.

Time series employed in this experiment were as follows: Mackey–Glass chaotic time series [120], Box–Jenkins gas furnace [121], EEG data [122], laser-generated data, and computer-generated data [123]. All time series values were transformed to be in the interval $[0.1, 0.9]$ in order to avoid saturation of neural activations and improve convergence of training algorithms. In both experiments, each model was trained 50 times for each time series; 30 particles/chromosomes were employed in each training session. The training algorithms were allowed to run for 1000 generations. The measures used to compare the results were the mean square error (MSE), standard deviation of MSE test errors, and CPU processing time. According to the author, the results from both experiments showed that ISSO outperformed the other five training algorithms, with the exception of BP, which performed better in experiment 1 when forecasting the laser-generated data. Additionally, the FFNN models produced forecasts that were more accurate than the ones generated by the SMN model.

4.1.2. Particle Swarm Optimization Convergence

To prevent the basic gradient descent method (applied in BP) from being caught at the local minimum, we can apply PSO to ANN to optimize the values of the weights' and biases' parameters. Although the PSO algorithm has been shown to perform well, researchers have not adequately explained how it works. In 2003, Gudise and Venayagamoorthy [124] made a comparison of the BP and PSO algorithms, analyzing the computational requirements when used in ANN training. They concluded that when the PSO algorithm is used, the FFNN weights converge faster, outperforming the BP algorithm. Liu, Ding, Li, and Yang [125] used a BP–ANN based on the PSO algorithm (PSO–BP). They demonstrated that their proposed PSO–BP algorithm outperforms a BP trained based on the Levenberg–Marquardt (LM) algorithm for training ANNs. Ince, Kiranyaz, and Gabbouj [126] proposed to find not only the weights of an FFNN but also the optimal architecture of the network, applying the MD–PSO algorithm: a modified version of the PSO. Their approach was to find the optimal number of dimensions for the search space simultaneously searching for the optimal solution in that proposed search space. The MD–PSO algorithm chose the global optimal solution among the optimal solutions found for each dimension. Several works have proposed variants of PSO against BP to optimize ANN [127–130]. However, like other evolutionary algorithms, PSO has some disadvantages, such as an imbalance between exploration and exploitation, sensitivity to parameters, and premature convergence [36]. These problems have been mostly solved by including new parameters, modifying the algorithm with additional operators, or creating hybrid versions with other algorithms [131]. Since its original version in 1995, the PSO algorithm has been expanded to solve a variety of different problems [100]. Multimodal, constrained, and multiobjective optimization problems are some of the most prominent applications that have been addressed with the PSO algorithm [132].

But the question is, why does PSO outperform BP? The study of PSO to optimize ANN has had very good results, but there is no in-depth research on theoretical aspects. Nevertheless, there are works that have tried to explain the PSO convergence. In 2002, Clerc and Kennedy [107] analyzed the full stochastic system of a deterministic version of PSO to supply knowledge about its search mechanism. They proposed reducing the particle velocity formula (Equation (15)) by redefining it as follows:

$$v_{t+1} = \omega * v_t + \phi * (P - x_t) \tag{17}$$

where $P = \frac{c_1 * U(0,1) * P_{Best} + c_2 * U(0,1) * G_{Best}}{c_1 * U(0,1) + c_2 * U(0,1)}$ and $\phi = c_1 * U(0,1) + c_2 * U(0,1)$. This is algebraically identical to the standard two-term form [133]. The analysis begins by removing all coverings from a particle, for example, a population of a one-dimensional deterministic particle, with a constant P and a constant ϕ. Kennedy [133] observed that the value of the parameter ϕ controls the trajectory of the particle and recognized that the explosion of the system depended on randomness. In [134], the authors analyzed the same system and concluded that the particle trajectories follow periodic sinusoidal waves. In their work, Clerc and Kennedy [107] analyzed the movement in discrete time of the PSO, advancing to its visualization in continuous time. These analyses lead to a proposal of controlling the convergence tendencies of the system through a set of coefficients, resulting in a generalized model of the algorithm. When they re-introduced randomness into the PSO with constriction coefficients, the deleterious effects of randomness were seen to be controlled. As a result of this study, the velocity equation changes to

$$v_{t+1} = \chi * \{v_t + c_1 * U(0,1) * (P_{Best} - x_t) + c_2 * U(0,1) * (G_{Best} - x_t)\} \quad (18)$$

where χ is the constriction coefficient calculated as

$$\chi = \frac{2 * \kappa}{|2 - \phi - \sqrt{\phi^2 - 4\phi}|} \quad (19)$$

with $\phi \geq 4$ and $0 \leq \kappa \leq 1$. The constant κ controls the rate of convergence. For $\kappa \approx 0$, faster convergence to a stable point is achieved, and for $\kappa \approx 1$, slow convergence to a stable point is obtained [107].

In 2010, van den Bergh and Engelbrecht [135] formally demonstrated that the original PSO is not a local or global optimizer. They identified an imperfection in PSO and addressed it in their approach called guaranteed convergence PSO (GCPSO). The goal of the GCPSO is to update only the speed of the best particle in the swarm (τ) to

$$v_{\tau,t+1} = -x_{\tau,t} + G_{Best} + \omega * v_{\tau,t} + \rho_t * (1 - 2 * \gamma_t) \quad (20)$$

Substituting Equation (20) into Equation (16), we obtain

$$x_{\tau,t+1} = G_{Best} + \omega * v_{\tau,t} + \rho_t * (1 - 2 * \gamma_t) \quad (21)$$

Equation (21) has three terms: the first term introduces a direct relationship with the current global best position, the second term conveys the inertia of the global best particle, and the third term shows a point of a uniform distribution in a hypercube with side lengths $2 * \rho$; ρ is strictly greater than zero. The authors indicate that their proposal ensures that the best global particle never stops moving completely. van den Bergh and Engelbrecht [135] showed that the GCPSO is a local optimizer.

In 2012, Kan and Jihong [136] demonstrated the existence and uniqueness of the convergence position in PSO, using the theorem of Banach space and the contraction mapping principle. They gave the parameter condition that influences the stability of PSO and showed that, if the parameter satisfies this condition, the probability that the particle swarm optimization converges to the best position is one. In 2018, Qian and Li [137] proposed an improved PSO (IPSO) algorithm according to the following strategy. They introduced a Gaussian perturbation in the P_{Best} position to guarantee that IPSO converges to the ϵ-optimum solution with probability one for any ϵ. Also in 2018, Xu and Yu [138] defined the swarm state sequence and examined its Markov properties according to the theory of PSO. Subsequently, from the evolutionary sequence of the particle swarm with the best fitness value, the authors derived a supermartingale. Based on this result, the authors applied the supermartingale convergence theorem to analyze the convergence of the PSO. The results show that PSO reaches the global optimum in probability. Recently, Huang, Qiu, and Riedl [139] established PSO convergence to a global minimizer based on continuous-time modeling for a non-convex and non-smooth objective function of particle dynamics through a system of stochastic differential equations.

In summary, there are several works that prove the convergence of PSO. However, it may be interesting to carry out a study of the convergence properties of PSO to optimize ANNs.

4.2. A Study on the Ability of Support Vector Regression and Feedforward Neural Networks to Forecast Basic Time Series Patterns

According to Crone, Guajardo, and Weber [94], "Support Vector Regression (SVR) and Feed Forward Neural Networks (FFNNs) have found increasing consideration in forecasting theory, leading to successful applications in time series forecasting for various domains, often outperforming conventional statistical approaches of ARIMA -or exponential smoothing- methods. Despite their theoretical and practical capabilities, FFNN and SVR models are not established forecasting methods. Substantial theoretical criticism on FFNNs has raised skepticism regarding their ability to forecast even simple time series patterns of seasonality or trends without prior data preprocessing [140]". In their study, Crone, Guajardo, and Weber [94] propose an empirical comparison between three different models:

1. FFNNs;
2. SVR models using a radial basis function (RBF) kernel;
3. SVR models using a linear function kernel.

This study reflects, for the considered models, their ability to learn and forecast fundamental time series patterns relevant to empirical forecasting tasks. Next, SVR models are briefly described (description based on text in Crone, Guajardo, and Weber [94]).

Support vector regression. For their experiment, Crone, Guajardo, and Weber [94] employed the common support vector regression (SVR) algorithm described in [141], which applies an ϵ-insensitive loss function for predictive regression problems. Let $\{(\vec{x}_1, y_1), \ldots, (\vec{x}_n, y_n)\}$, where $\vec{x}_i \in \mathbb{R}^d$ and $y_i \in \mathbb{R}$ are the training data points available to build a regression model. A transformation function Φ on the initial input space is applied to map the original data points to a higher dimensional feature space $\mathbb{F}$. A linear model is constructed in $\mathbb{F}$ in correspondence with the nonlinear model of the original space:

$$\Phi : \mathbb{R}^d \to \mathbb{F}, \vec{w} \in \mathbb{F} f(\vec{x}) = \langle \vec{w}, \Phi(\vec{x}) \rangle + b \qquad (22)$$

$\langle \vec{w}, \Phi(\vec{x}) \rangle$ is the inner product between $\vec{w}$ and $\Phi(\vec{x})$. The insensitive loss function ϵ allows you to fit a function that is as flat as possible and has a maximum deviation ϵ for the current training data. This means that we are looking for a small weight vector $\vec{w}$. To solve this problem, the authors introduce slack variables ξ_i, ξ_i^* to allow error levels higher than ϵ, obtaining the following:

$$\begin{aligned} &\min \frac{1}{2}\|\vec{w}\|^2 + C \sum_{i=1}^{n}(\xi_i + \xi_i^*) \\ &\text{s.t. } y_i - \langle \vec{w}, \Phi(\vec{x}_i) \rangle - b \leq \epsilon + \xi_i \\ &\quad \langle \vec{w}, \Phi(\vec{x}_i) \rangle + b - y_i \leq \epsilon + \xi_i^* \\ &\quad \xi_i, \xi_i^* \geq 0, i = 1, 2, \ldots, n \end{aligned} \qquad (23)$$

The construction of the objective function considers two key aspects: the precision in the training set and the generalization capacity, which lead to the principle of minimization of structural risk. The balance between generalization ability and accuracy is measured by C in the training data, and the degree of error tolerance is defined by ϵ. It is convenient to represent the problem in its dual form for its resolution, so a Lagrange function is constructed, from which it can be shown that once the saddle point conditions are applied, the following solution is reached:

$$\vec{w} = \sum_{i=1}^{n} (\alpha_i - \alpha_i^*) \Phi(\vec{x}_i) f(\vec{x}) = \sum_{i=1}^{n} (\alpha_i - \alpha_i^*) K(\vec{x}_i, \vec{x}) + b \quad (24)$$

Here, α_i and α_i^* are the dual variables, and the expression $K(\vec{x}_i, \vec{x})$ represents the inner product between $\Phi(\vec{x}_i)$ and $\Phi(\vec{x})$, which is known as the kernel function. It is possible to achieve a solution to the original regression problem, starting from the existence of the kernel function, leaving aside the transformation $\Phi(\vec{x})$ applied to the data. For more information on SVR models, please consult Drucker, Burges, Kaufman, Smola, and Vapnik [13].

Experiments and results. Crone, Guajardo, and Weber [94] employed a set of five artificial time series in their experiments (see Figure 6):

1. Stationary time series (constant level);
2. Stationary time series with additive seasonality;
3. Linear trend;
4. Linear trend with additive seasonality;
5. Linear trend with multiplicative seasonality.

These artificial data emulate the behavior of monthly retail sales and are taken from Pegel and Gardner's original classification. All artificial series contain additive Gaussian white noise, with $\sigma^2 = 25$. Each time series consists of 228 observations. A lag structure of 13 previous observations was established to produce one-step-ahead forecasts (this number of lags should be adequate to capture seasonal patterns present in monthly time series). Thus, 215 examples are available to construct FFNN and SVR models. From these available examples, the first 119 were reserved for model training, the next 48 for model validation, and the last 48 for model testing.

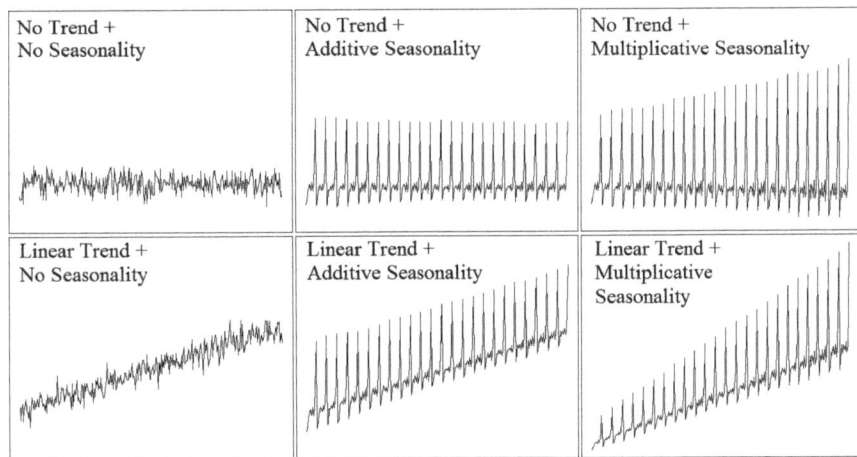

Figure 6. Some basic time series patterns according to Pegel and Gardner's classification. All of these patterns (except for the no trend + multiplicative seasonality) were generated artificially in the experiment of Crone, Guajardo, and Weber [94].

All models were constructed by using training and validation data only, retaining all information in the test suite to ensure valid predicted event testing. To avoid saturation effects, a linear scale in an interval $[-0.5, 0.5]$ was applied in the data transformation, using minimum and maximum values only from the training and validation data. In order to evaluate model performance, mean squared error (MSE), mean absolute error (MAE), and root mean squared error (RMSE) metrics were employed to measure test errors. MAE was employed to fine-tune model meta-parameters (C and ϵ for SVR–linear; C, ϵ, and σ for SVR–RBF; number of hidden nodes and type of activation function for FFNN hidden nodes; available options were sigmoid or hyperbolic tangent). After the construction of all models and test error measuring, Crone, Guajardo, and Weber [94] arrived at the following conclusions:

- The performance of FFNNs and SVRs with linear kernel is similar; they both robustly forecast time series patterns without preprocessing;
- Considering the results obtained in the three error measures of MAE, MSE, and RMSE, the FFNNs outperform the SVR models in the time series forecast of the different patterns tested;
- The results obtained indicate that FFNNs seem to be able to extrapolate seasonal trends and patterns accurately and without preprocessing.

4.3. Forecasting the Economy with Artificial Neural Networks

It is of great interest to economists to forecast the "business cycle". It affects the economic system of any country due to its fluctuations that impact macroeconomic indicators, such as interest rates, housing demand, occupancy rate, demand for manufactured goods, etc. The economic cycle also affects relevant sociopolitical factors, such as the result of a country's presidential elections. Economists use the Gross Domestic Product (GDP) and the Index of Industrial Production (IIP) to track the business cycle [95]. In this contribution, Moody [95] stresses the reasons why macroeconomic modeling and forecasting are challenging tasks:

- **Macroeconomics is a non-experimental science**. It is a complicated task to observe the behavior of an economy as a whole, and the possibility of carrying out controlled experiments is very remote;
- **Lack of a priori models**. It is not possible to carry out controlled studies on the effects of the influence that qualitative (non-quantifiable) variables have on economic activity, due to the complexities of the economic system;
- **Noise present in data**. This is due to two main causes: the way in which information is collected and the number of unobserved (non-measurable) variables in economics. The presence of noise in short time series makes it difficult to control the variance of the model, requiring highly complex models to predict this type of phenomena;
- **Nonlinearity**. Due to high levels of noise and limited data, neural network models do not capture the nonlinear characteristics of macroeconomic series.

In our view, the perceived difficulty in modeling macroeconomic data's nonlinear features is one of the main reasons why many practitioners still use traditional statistical linear techniques to model macroeconomic data (for instance, several official statistics agencies around the world rely on X13ARIMA-SEATS [142] to generate ARIMA-based forecasts for macroeconomic time series). On the other hand, there is a growing group of researchers who feel that it is worth continuing with investigations of efficient ANN models that take into account nonlinear features of macroeconomic data since ANNs are capable of achieving universal function approximation. For example, Kiani [143] applied nonlinear regime change models and artificial neural networks to anticipate the impact of monetary policy shocks on GDP.

Neural Network Challenges in Economy

Moody [95] categorizes several heuristics for ANN model selection and construction, aimed at minimizing expected prediction error. Considered categories are the following:

Meta-parameter selection. Adjusting the regularization parameter can compensate for bias and variance in the forecast, while varying the number of input nodes can compensate for noise and non-stationarity [144].

Input variable selection and pruning. The appropriate selection of input variables is essential for the solution of any prediction problem. The set of variables selected must be representative and provide the greatest possible information with the least amount of them [145–147].

Model selection and pruning. Selecting the right size and appropriate network architecture is a key element in controlling the balance between bias and variance. The above involves eliminating unnecessary weights or nodes, choosing the number of hidden units, selecting a connectivity structure, etc. [148–151].

Better regularizers. Regularization of ANNs reduces model variance and minimizes prediction risk, improving model generalization [152,153].

Committee forecasts. Several economic researchers have made forecasts using a forecasting committee. The approach consists of averaging (weighted or unweighted) the predictions of an ensemble of models [144].

Model interpretation and visualization. In general, great importance is placed on obtaining accurate forecasts, leaving aside the understanding of the factors that influence these forecasts. Sensitivity analysis (SBP) [147] and visualization tools [154] can help achieve a better interpretation of the variables that affect the model obtained by ANNs.

Moody [95] explains in detail some of the techniques cited above and illustrates their use with an empirical example, in which IIP monthly values are predicted (12-month prediction horizon) via an FFNN model with three sigmoidal units, a single linear output unit, and a large number of input nodes. Initially, 48 macroeconomic and financial time series variables are considered potential explanatory variables. Use of sensitivity-based pruning (SBP), guided by estimations of prediction errors provided by nonlinear cross-validation (NCV), finally leaves 13 explanatory variables that optimize prediction performance at the same time, with respect to the initial 48-variable FFNN model.

ANN modeling hints proposed by Moody [95] include the following:

- After selecting the number of hidden units, input removal and weight elimination can be carried out in parallel or sequentially;
- In order to avoid an exhaustive search over the exponentially large space of architectures obtained by considering all possible combinations of inputs, we can employ a directed search strategy using the sensitivity-based input pruning (SBP) algorithm;
- We can employ some of the following optimization criteria in order to select competing models: maximum a posteriori probability (MAP), minimum Bayesian information criterion (BIC), minimum description length (MDL), and estimation (from the training data) of generalization ability, also called prediction risk;
- It is easier to over-fit a model to a small training set, so care must be taken to select a model that is not too large;
- The sensitivity analysis provides a global understanding about which inputs are important for predicting quantities of interest, such as the business cycle. Further information can be gained, however, by examining the evolution of sensitivities over time;
- Given the difficulty of macroeconomic forecasting, no single technique for reducing prediction risk is sufficient to obtain optimal performance. Rather, a combination of techniques is required.

4.4. Double SOM for Long-Term Time Series Prediction

In Section 3.5.2, we outlined how to use the basic self-organizing map (SOM) to forecast observations from univariate time series and how to combine an SOM model with a radial basis function network (RBFN) in order to improve forecast accuracy. Additionally, in Section 3.5.4, we outlined a methodology that combines SOM models with local autoregressive models, once again seeking to improve SOM's output accuracy. Simon, Lendasse, Cottrell, Fort, Verleysen, et al. [64] concentrate mainly on forecasting long-term but not-so-accurate time series trends rather than dealing with the more traditional problem of finding accurate short-term time series predictions. Simon, Lendasse, Cottrell, Fort, Verleysen, et al. [64] describe a technique based on a double application of the SOM model and sketch a proof of its stability. They work in the context of global NAR-like models, i.e., nonlinear autoregressive prediction models, without moving average terms (they mention the possibility of adding exogenous variables to their model). Their goal is to build a global model to be used in long-term predictions, with the view of obtaining future trends and their means and confidence intervals. In some forecasting problems, it is interesting to predict several values of the series in one bloc, rather than a single $\hat{y}_{t+1}$ scalar value. In such a case, the prediction problem, from a nonlinear autoregressive approach, has the form

$$\langle \hat{y}_{t+k}, \hat{y}_{t+k-1}, \ldots, \hat{y}_{t+1} \rangle = f(y_t, y_{t-1}, \ldots, y_{t-p+1}) \tag{25}$$

Size p of the regressor vector is not necessarily equal to the forecasting horizon k. However, in many cases, p will be a multiple of k. A key concept, called *series of deformations*, is defined by Simon, Lendasse, Cottrell, Fort, Verleysen, et al. [64] as

$$d_t = y_{t+k} - y_t. \tag{26}$$

Simon, Lendasse, Cottrell, Fort, Verleysen, et al. [64] also define a regressor vector in the deformation space as

$$D_t = \langle d_t, d_{t-1}, \ldots, d_{t-p+1} \rangle. \tag{27}$$

Regressors $Y_t = \langle y_t, y_{t-1}, \ldots, y_{t-p+1} \rangle$ are arranged into classes, using a one-dimensional Kohonen map; this map performs local averages, which helps to reduce over-fitting. A one-dimensional Kohonen map with n_r centroids (or codevectors) A_i is thus organized in the space of regressors; each regressor Y_t is associated with a centroid $A_{i(t)}$ according to the nearest neighbor rule.

A Kohonen map in the deformation space is also formed: a one-dimensional Kohonen map with n_d centroids B_j is thus organized in the space of deformations; each deformation D_t is associated with a centroid $B_{j(t)}$ according to the nearest neighbor rule. After both Kohonen (SOM) maps for the regressor and deformation spaces are formed, Simon, Lendasse, Cottrell, Fort, Verleysen, et al. [64] proceed next to the construction of a *transition table*, whose entries are defined by

$$T_{i,j} = P(B_j | A_i). \tag{28}$$

$T_{i,j}$ is the empirical probability that deformation D_t is associated with centroid B_j when the corresponding regressor Y_t is associated with centroid A_i. All terms on each row i of the table sum to 1; row i, regarded as a vector μ_i, represents the empirical law of deformations conditional to class i.

The modeling of past behavior of the time series is derived from the organization of one-dimensional SOMs in regressor space and warp space constituted by the evaluation of the transition table. To forecast a time series, we can follow these steps:

- Build regressor Y_t at time t;
- Identify centroid $A_{i(t)}$ corresponding to regressor Y_t;
- Draw randomly a deformation D_j, according to the empirical law μ_i of probabilities $T_{i,j}$;
- Y_t and D_j are summed to form vector $\langle y_{t+k}, y_{t+k-1}, \ldots, y_{t+k-p+1} \rangle$;
- The part $\langle y_{t+k}, y_{t+k-1}, \ldots, y_{t+1} \rangle$ extracted from the left side of the vector computed in the previous step constitutes the prediction.

Like other forecasting models we have reviewed in this article, it is possible to recursively include the calculated predictions in the model to make long-term predictions.

Simon, Lendasse, Cottrell, Fort, Verleysen, et al. [64] assert that their proposed method produces predictions that always remain in a limited domain and therefore cannot diverge; they sketch a proof of their method's stability. They first show that a Markov chain adequately describes the series generated by the model. Then, they prove that this Markov chain is stable. Note that when $k > 1$, injecting predictions into the model means adding k forecasted values to obtain another set of k new predictions. The final objective of the method proposed by Simon, Lendasse, Cottrell, Fort, Verleysen, et al. [64] is to identify trends. Due to the random choice of D_j, different forecast curves can be obtained by repeating the entire procedure of the proposed algorithm. These repetitions can be seen as instances of possible forecasts of the different curves obtained, and their trends, means, standard deviations, etc., as global characteristics of the forecasted time series.

Simon, Lendasse, Cottrell, Fort, Verleysen, et al. [64] illustrate their method using two time series: the Santa Fe A series (a laser series), and the hourly electrical load in Poland from 1989 to 1996. In both cases, Simon, Lendasse, Cottrell, Fort, Verleysen, et al. [64] employ cross-validation for choosing an optimal number of nodes in SOM models, and perform Monte-Carlo simulations in order to obtain global measures (mean, 95% confidence intervals) from computed long-term forecasts. They also include graphics of the experimental results (codevectors, transition tables, graphics of global measures, comparisons between true values and forecasts, etc.). No attempt is made to quantify forecast errors; rather, the objective consists of showing that true test values are within the limits defined by all random predictions constructed by the proposed model.

4.5. Time Series Forecasting with Recurrent Neural Networks

Zimmermann, Tietz, and Grothmann [96] propose a series of architectural modifications aimed at improving the performance of recurrent neural networks (RNNs) applied to time series forecasting tasks. Given the universal approximation properties of RNNs, they can be used to forecast time series in the form of nonlinear state space models [155]. Zimmermann, Tietz, and Grothmann [96] rely on this general framework in order to incrementally build their models. They start out with a given RNN architecture, and then propose a refined version, seeking to correct empirically observed deficiencies found in the initial model. The RNN architectures discussed in their work are listed next:

1. Basic time-delay RNNs in state space formulation, which model *open dynamical systems* (i.e., partly autonomous and partly externally driven dynamical systems);
2. Error-correction neural networks (ECNNs), which refine the basic RNN model by adding an error-correction term in order to handle missing information from unknown external drivers of open dynamical systems;
3. Historically consistent neural networks (HCNNs), which refine ECNNs by internally modeling external drivers, thus transforming ECNNs (and basic RNNs) into *closed dynamical systems*;
4. Causal-retro-causal neural networks (CRCNNs), which refine HCNNs by incorporating into their usual information flow from past into future (causal flow) the effects of rational decision-making and planning via an information flow from future into past (retro–causal flow).

Each model in this listing is useful in its own right for particular real-world applications. Zimmermann, Tietz, and Grothmann [96] provide useful hints that facilitate the construction and training of these models. They also point out real-world scenarios where these models are employed; for instance, they mention that ECNNs have been employed successfully to forecast the demand for finished products and raw materials within the context of supply chain management. These architectures and their related algorithms have been implemented in a software system developed by Siemens Corporate Technology called simulation environment for neural networks (SENN). In the remainder of this subsection, we summarize the main points presented in Zimmermann, Tietz, and Grothmann [96].

1. Basic RNN. Zimmermann, Tietz, and Grothmann [96] show that an open dynamical system can be used to create a vector time series $\vec{y}_\tau$, which can be described in discrete time τ using an output equation and a state transition [34]:

$$\begin{aligned} \vec{s}_{\tau+1} &= f(\vec{s}_\tau, \vec{u}_\tau) & \text{State transition} \\ \vec{y}_\tau &= g(\vec{s}_\tau) & \text{Output equation} \end{aligned} \quad (29)$$

$\vec{s}_\tau$ is the current hidden system state, $\vec{s}_{\tau+1}$ is the upcoming system state, and $\vec{u}_\tau$ represents external factors. This is called an open dynamical system. The data-driven system identification is based on the selected parameterized functions $f()$ and $g()$. Parameters in $f()$ and $g()$ are chosen such that an appropriate error function, such as

$\frac{1}{T}\sum_{\tau=1}^{T}\|\vec{y}_\tau - \vec{y}_\tau^d\|^2$, is minimized ($\vec{y}_\tau^d$ are the target observations). Typically, without loss of generality, $f(\vec{s}_\tau, \vec{u}_\tau) = \tanh(\vec{A}\vec{s}_\tau + \vec{B}\vec{u}_\tau)$ and $g(\vec{s}_\tau) = \vec{C}\vec{s}_\tau$; the hyperbolic tangent is the activation function in the network's hidden layer, while the output function is specified as a linear function; $\vec{A}$ (autonomous dynamics or memory), $\vec{B}$ (external factors), and $\vec{C}$ are weight matrices that model the open dynamical system.

The technique of finite unfolding in time [156] is employed in order to solve the selection of appropriate matrices $\vec{A}$, $\vec{B}$, and $\vec{C}$ that minimize the error function. The idea behind this is that if the matrices $\vec{A}$, $\vec{B}$, and $\vec{C}$ are identical at the individual time steps, then any RNN can be reformulated to form an equivalent FFNN. An advantage of this technique is the moderate number of shared weights, which reduces the risk of overfitting [157]. To perform the training, error backpropagation through time (EBTT) is applied along with a stochastic learning rule; see Rumelhart, Hinton, and Williams [156] and Werbos [158].

Overshooting. We can point out that a disadvantage of RNNs is that they tend to focus only on the most recent external inputs. Overshooting extends the autonomous system dynamics (coded matrix $\vec{A}$) into the future [157]; thus, consistent multi-step forecasts can be computed. For the RNN, an input preprocessing $\vec{u}_\tau = \vec{x}_\tau - \vec{x}_{\tau-1}$ is typically employed as the transformation for the raw data $\vec{x}$; this eliminates biases in the input or target variables of the RNN.

2. Error-correction neural networks (ECNNs). In RNNs, modeling can be altered by unknown external influences or shocks, representing a weakness in the network [159]. The error-correcting neural network (ECNN) addresses this weakness by introducing an additional term in the state transition:

$$\begin{aligned} \vec{s}_{\tau+1} &= \tanh(\vec{A}\vec{s}_\tau + \vec{B}\vec{u}_\tau + \vec{D}\tanh(\vec{y}_\tau - \vec{y}_\tau^d)) & \text{State transition} \\ \vec{y}_\tau &= \vec{C}\vec{s}_\tau & \text{Output equation} \end{aligned} \quad (30)$$

The system identification task is once again solved by finite unfolding in time [34]. ECNNs are an appropriate framework for low-dimensional dynamical systems with less than five target variables Zimmermann et al. [96].

3. Historically consistent neural networks (HCNNs) are a model class adequate for modeling large dynamical systems in which various (nonlinear) dynamics interact with one another, but only a small subset of variables can be observed. HCNNs are useful for modeling many real-world economic applications. A HCNN model is characterized by

$$\begin{aligned} \vec{s}_{\tau+1} &= \vec{A}\tanh(\vec{s}_\tau) & \text{State transition} \\ \vec{y}_\tau &= [\vec{Id}, \vec{0}]\vec{s}_\tau & \text{Output equation} \end{aligned} \quad (31)$$

In the HCNN, the joint dynamic of the observable variables is highlighted by the sequence of states $\vec{s}_\tau$. The observables ($i = 1, \ldots, N$) are organized in the first N state neurons $\vec{s}_\tau$ and followed by hidden variables as later neurons. The observables are read by the connector $[\vec{Id}, \vec{0}]$, which is a fixed array. A bias vector can describe the initial state $\vec{s}_0$. The bias $\vec{s}_0$ and matrix $\vec{A}$ contain the only free parameters.

The HCNN states $\vec{s}_\tau$ are hidden layers with tanh squashing. The output layers $\vec{y}_\tau$ provide the predictions. Since the HCNN model has no inputs, it has to be unfolded along the complete data history. This is different to small RNNs, where training data patterns are constructed in the form of sliding windows. From a single training data pattern, the HCNN can learn large dynamics. In this way, the HCNN model provides a means of overcoming an intrinsic problem in RNNs (and ECNNs): the external inputs $\vec{u}_\tau$, which are used when training RNNs and ECNNs, are missing from the one-step-ahead node to the prediction horizon node. This implies that the open system modeled by the RNN (ECNN) outputs dynamical forecasts $\vec{y}_\tau$ while its corresponding inputs remain static, which is clearly an inconsistency within the model framework. By implementing a model in which inputs and forecasts are encoded together into the hidden network states (thereby closing the dynamical system), HCNNs correct this inherent asymmetry found in RNNs and ECNNs.

Sparsity and dimensionality vs. connectivity and memory. It is clear that dynamical systems must have high dimensions. Zimmermann, Tietz, and Grothmann [96] use $dim(\vec{s}) = 300$ in their commodity price models, and they recommend this value as a top limit for dimensionality. There is a risk in iterating a high-dimensional state transition matrix $\vec{A}$ because operations on matrix vectors can produce large numbers that will be distributed recursively in the network, generating an arithmetic explosion. A sparse matrix $\vec{A}$ can be used to avoid this problem. Zimmermann, Grothmann, Schäfer, Tietz, and Georg [160] have observed that connectivity and memory length are directly related to dimensionality and sparsity. The number of non-zero elements in each row of matrix $\vec{A}$ is defined as connectivity. When a state vector contains all the necessary information from the past, it is said to have reached a Markovian state. The number of steps to collect that amount of information is defined as memory length. Using these relationships and their experience with previous experiments, Zimmermann, Tietz, and Grothmann [96] observe that the EBTT algorithm works stably with a connectivity that is equal to or smaller than 50 and a sparsity of 17%. This means that only 17% of the weights in matrix $\vec{A}$ can be different from zero, and their locations inside of $\vec{A}$ are randomly chosen. EBTT training fine tunes $\vec{A}$ non-zero weights.

4. **Causal-retro-causal neural networks (CRCNNs)** introduce the impacts of rational decision-making and planning in dynamic systems modeling. The CRCNN aims to improve the performance of the HCNN by enriching the causal information flow that is directed from the past to the future, introducing a retro–causal information flow, directed from the future to the past. These models can be employed as the basis for commodity price forecasting tasks. CRCNNs also improve the modeling of deterministic chaotic systems. The following set of equations describes the CRCNN model, and Figure 7 shows the corresponding CRCNN model:

$$\begin{aligned} \vec{s}_\tau &= \vec{A}\tanh(\vec{s}_{\tau-1}) & \text{Causal state transition} \\ \vec{s}'_\tau &= \vec{A}'\tanh(\vec{s}'_{\tau+1}) & \text{Retro-causal state transition} \\ \vec{y}_\tau &= [\vec{Id}, \vec{0}]\vec{s}_\tau + [\vec{Id}, \vec{0}]\vec{s}'_\tau & \text{Output equation} \end{aligned} \quad (32)$$

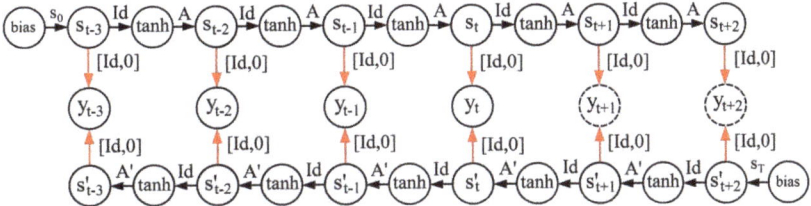

Figure 7. Causal-retro-causal historically consistent neural network (CRCNN).

Architectural teacher forcing (ATF) for CRCNNs. CRCNNs are hard to train because they inherit all the characteristics from HCNNs. This implies that CRCNNs are also unfolded across the entire dataset, so the system has only one opportunity to learn from the whole history of the data. ATF makes the best possible use of the training data, accelerating and stabilizing the EBTT training process for the CRCNN. ATF replaces the outputs $\vec{y}_\tau$, up to time step $\tau = t$, by the desired targets $\vec{y}^d_\tau$, and forces them into the causal network state $\vec{s}_\tau$ and retro-causal network state $\vec{s}'_\tau$.

Stabilizing information flows in dynamical systems. This is analogous to handling the uncertainty of the initial state for a basic RNN model with overshooting. The stability of the CRCNN model is further improved by applying noise in the causal as well as in the retro-causal branch of the network. The noise is injected into the same nodes that receive the biases (see Figure 7).

Uncertainty and risk. Traditional risk management applies diffusion models to interpret risk distributions. The risk can be explained as a random walk, in which, using the observed past error of the underlying model, the diffusion process is calibrated [161]. If the system identification calculation is performed using an HCNN or a CRCNN repeatedly, then solutions will be produced with a prediction error of zero in the past but that differ from each other in the future. If the arithmetic average of the individual ensemble members of the set is taken as the expected value, we will obtain a simplified prediction. Consider the bandwidth of the ensemble in addition to the expected value of Zimmermann, Tietz, and Grothmann [96]. The ensemble average can be taken as the best forecast, assuming that all future trajectories have the same probability and the genuine development of the dynamics is unknown, where the ensemble bandwidth describes the market risk. For any forecast date, all individual forecasts for the ensemble infer the probability distribution over many possible market prices at a single point in time, similar to an empirical density function.

4.6. Applying Echo State Networks to Time Series Forecasting

Training recurrent neural networks (RNNs) is a difficult task; however, they integrate a large dynamic memory and highly flexible computational capabilities, making them a very powerful tool. Error backpropagation (BP) is the standard method to train networks, especially feedforward neural networks (FFNNs), and it has also been extended to RNNs. This extension, however, has not been straightforward: RNNs are dynamical systems, and training them with BP sometimes leads to bifurcations, so chaos (non-convergence) occurs. Echo state networks (ESNs) are an alternative approach for training RNNs, as proposed by Jaeger [162]. In the classical ESN approach, an RNN structure is called a *reservoir*, so ESN methodology is often known in the literature as reservoir computing (RC), which is, at the moment, a prolific research area in RNNs [163]. In Lukoševičius [97], practical techniques and recommendations for successfully applying ESNs are presented, with emphasis on the time series forecasting problem. Lukoševičius [97] points out that ESNs are conceptually simple and easy to implement, but experience and insight are a must for training them successfully. In the remainder of this subsection, we summarize the main points addressed in this important contribution made by Lukoševičius [97].

The basic ESN model. ESNs are used to supervise temporal machine learning tasks where, for a given training input signal $\mathbf{u}(n) \in \mathbb{R}^{N_u}$, a desired target output signal $\mathbf{y}^{\text{target}}(n) \in \mathbb{R}^{N_y}$ is known. The discrete time is $n = 1, \ldots, T$ and the number of data points in the training dataset is T. The task is to learn a model with output $\mathbf{y}(n) \in \mathbb{R}^{N_y}$, where $\mathbf{y}(n)$ matches $\mathbf{y}^{\text{target}}(n)$ as best as possible, minimizing an error measure $E(\mathbf{y}, \mathbf{y}^{\text{target}})$ and, importantly, generalizing well to unseen data. The error measure E is typically a mean-squared error (MSE). The update equations are

$$\tilde{\mathbf{x}}(n) = \tanh\left(\mathbf{W}^{\text{in}}[1; \mathbf{u}(n)] + \mathbf{W}\mathbf{x}(n-1)\right) \tag{33}$$

and

$$\mathbf{x}(n) = (1-\alpha)\mathbf{x}(n-1) + \alpha\tilde{\mathbf{x}}(n), \tag{34}$$

where $\mathbf{x}(n) \in \mathbb{R}^{N_x}$ is a vector of reservoir neuron activations and $\tilde{\mathbf{x}}(n) \in \mathbb{R}^{N_x}$ is its update, all at time step n, $\tanh(\cdot)$ is applied element-wise, $[\cdot;\cdot]$ stands for a vertical vector (or matrix) concatenation, $\mathbf{W}^{\text{in}} \in \mathbb{R}^{N_x \times (1+N_u)}$ and $\mathbf{W} \in \mathbb{R}^{N_x \times N_x}$ are the input and recurrent weight matrices, respectively, and $\alpha \in (0, 1]$ is the leaking rate. It is important to mention here one fundamental difference between regular RNNs and ESNs: while ESN's input and recurrent weight matrices $\mathbf{W}^{\text{in}}$ and $\mathbf{W}$ remain fixed once initialized, the weights in RNN's state transition matrices are updated after each iteration during the learning process. A graphical representation of an ESN is depicted in Figure 8.

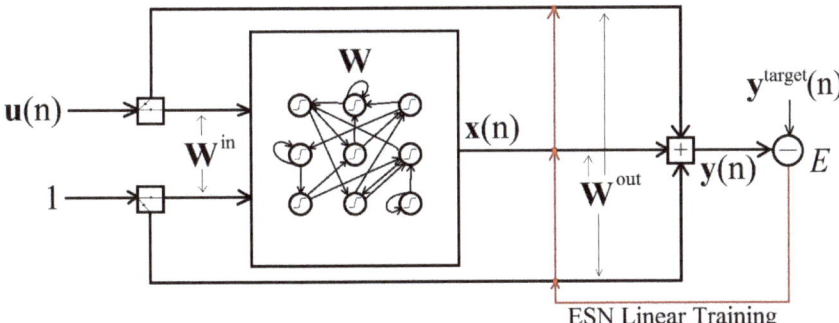

Figure 8. An echo state network (ESN) in schematized form. $\mathbf{u}(n)$ is the training input signal, 1 is a constant input signal (intercept), $\mathbf{W}^{in}$ contains input weights while $\mathbf{W}$ contains recurrent weights (both $\mathbf{W}^{in}$ and $\mathbf{W}$ in the reservoir remain fixed after initialization), $\mathbf{x}(n)$ contains neuronal activations and is the reservoir's output. $\mathbf{W}^{out}$ are trainable output weights, and $\mathbf{y}(n)$ is the ESN's output signal. $\mathbf{W}^{out}$ weights minimize error $E(\mathbf{y}, \mathbf{y}^{target})$ after linear training.

The linear readout layer is defined as

$$\mathbf{y}(n) = \mathbf{W}^{out}[1; \mathbf{u}(n); \mathbf{x}(n)] \tag{35}$$

where $\mathbf{y}(n) \in \mathbb{R}^{N_y}$ is the network output, and $\mathbf{W}^{out} \in \mathbb{R}^{N_y \times (1+N_u+N_x)}$ is the output weight matrix. The RC algorithm introduced with ESNs by Jaeger [162] consists of the following steps:

1. Generate a random reservoir RNN $(\mathbf{W}^{in}, \mathbf{W}, \alpha)$;
2. Run the reservoir using the training input $\mathbf{u}(n)$ and collect the corresponding reservoir activation states $\mathbf{x}(n)$;
3. Compute the linear readout weights $\mathbf{W}^{out}$ from the reservoir, minimizing the MSE between $\mathbf{y}(n)$ and $\mathbf{y}^{target}(n)$;
4. Use the trained network on new input data $\mathbf{u}(n)$ to compute $\mathbf{y}(n)$ by using the trained output weights $\mathbf{W}^{out}$.

Producing a reservoir. At the same time, the reservoir acts as a nonlinear expansion and as a memory of input $\mathbf{u}(n)$. The reservoir can be described as a nonlinear, high-dimensional expansion $\mathbf{x}(n)$ of the input signal $\mathbf{u}(n)$. For classification tasks, input data $\mathbf{u}(n)$ that are not linearly separable in the original space $\mathbb{R}^{N_u}$ often become so in the expanded space $\mathbb{R}^{N_x}$ of $\mathbf{x}(n)$, where they are separated by $\mathbf{W}^{out}$.

Reservoir's global parameters. Given the RNN models (33) and (34), the reservoir is defined by the tuple $(\mathbf{W}^{in}, \mathbf{W}, \alpha)$. The input and recurrent connection matrices $\mathbf{W}^{in}$ and $\mathbf{W}$ are generated randomly. The leaking rate α of the reservoir nodes in (34) can be regarded as the speed of the reservoir update dynamics discretized in time.

Setup for parameter selection. Learning the results is fast in ESNs. This should be leveraged to evaluate how well a reservoir is generated by a particular set of parameters. To evaluate a reservoir, we train the output (35) and measure its error by applying cross-validation or training error. Randomly generated buckets, even with the same parameters, vary slightly in their performance. Keep the random seed fixed and averaged over multiple reservoir samples to eliminate random fluctuations in performance.

ESN ensemble. Training many small ESNs in parallel and averaging their outputs, in some cases, has drastically improved the performance of the basic ESN approach [164,165].

Removing initial transient. Usually $\mathbf{x}(n)$ data from the beginning of a long training sequence are discarded (i.e., not used for learning $\mathbf{W}^{out}$) since they are contaminated by initial transients. The initial transient is a result of an arbitrary setting of $\mathbf{x}(0)$, which is typically $\mathbf{x}(0) = \mathbf{0}$. An unnatural initial state is introduced that is not normally visited once the network has been "prepared" for the task. The number of time steps to discard depends on the network memory, which in turn depends on the reservoir parameters, and are normally at the order of tens or hundreds. From this, we see that regular RNNs (discussed in Section 4.5) and ESNs have differing approaches when dealing with the uncertainty of the initial state in the dynamical system they are trying to identify: RNNs inject noise into the initial state in order to identify a stable dynamical system, while ESNs discard a few initial transient states, relying on their echo state property to achieve stability.

5. Discussion

Statistical techniques, like linear regression, ARIMA, ARCH, and NARX modeling, have been traditionally employed in time series forecasting [166]. Strong assumptions on data are necessary for the construction of such models (e.g., data are generated by linear, time invariant processes, possibly with added Gaussian noise). These assumptions do not hold in many practical situations, and by using these traditional statistical techniques on time series from which we actually know very little about their true data-generating process, we incur the risk of generating inaccurate forecasts. Comparatively, ANN models offer a more flexible modeling strategy, with fewer assumptions on data-generating mechanisms, and produce accurate forecasts.

Generally speaking, the aim of time series forecasting is to predict future values with accuracy and simplicity. However, a large fraction of the ANN architectures reviewed in this article are more complex than others. But this fact seems to contradict the principle of Occam's razor, which maintains that the simplest solution is usually the best. In machine learning literature, Occam's razor is used for two different principles [167]:

1. First razor: Starting from the fact that simplicity is desirable in itself, the simpler model should be preferred between two models with the same generalization error.
2. Second razor: Starting from the fact that you are likely to have a smaller generalization error in the simpler model, it should be preferred between two models with the same error in the training set.

Domingos [167] argued that, in the first razor, simplicity is only a proxy for comprehensibility. Nevertheless, his paper shows that, contrary to the second razor's claim, greater simplicity does not necessarily lead to greater accuracy. *If we accept the fact that the most accurate models will not always be simple or easily understandable, we should allow an explicit trade-off between the two* [167].

Occam's razor is largely controversial. However, a simple and easy-to-understand method is needed to calculate point forecasts from machine learning time series models based on proven techniques.

6. Conclusions

Artificial neural networks (ANNs) have been (and still are) promising modeling techniques with an ever-increasing number of real-world applications. A very wide variety of ANN methods and algorithms are available; in fact, several tens of thousands of articles containing the keywords "time series" and "neural networks" can be found online. In this survey, we covered only a small and (hopefully) not-so-biased sample containing the most representative and popular ANN architectures employed for time series prediction tasks (for a small summary of surveyed studies, see Table 2). All the prototypical ANN architectures reviewed here constitute powerful, appealing machine learning techniques founded on sound mathematical and statistical principles. This is the reason why these methods work so well in many fields of study, including time series modeling and forecasting.

An interesting discussion that attempts to further explain from a theoretical perspective the success and power of ANNs (using concepts from probability and physics) can be found in Lin and Tegmark [168].

Table 2. A small sample of ANN applications to time series forecasting tasks.

Study	Main Model Employed	Time Series Forecasting Application
Adhikari et al. [81]	FFNN–PSO, Elman RNN–PSO	Macroeconomic variables
Alba-Cuéllar et al. [6]	FFNN–PSO ensemble-bootstrap	Monthly transportation data
Barrow and Crone [40]	FFNN ensembles	Transportation data
Blonbou [85]	Bayesian NN	Wind-generated power
Busseti et al. [169]	Deep RNN	Load forecasting
Chandra and Zhang [53]	Elman RNN	Chaotic time series
Chatzis and Demiris [170]	Bayesian ESN	Chaotic time series
Crone et al. [94]	FFNN, SVR	Monthly retail sales
Dablemont et al. [66]	Double SOM–RBFN	German DAX30 index
Giovanis [83]	FFNN–GA	Macroeconomic and financial data
Guo and Deng [89]	Hybrid FFNN–BP–ARIMA	Traffic flow
Jaeger and Haas [164]	ESN	Wireless communication signals
Jha et al. [80]	FFNN–PSO	Financial data
Kocadağlı and Aşıkgil [87]	Bayesian FFNN–GA	Weekly sales of a finance magazine
Lahmiri [41]	RBFN ensemble	NASDAQ returns
Leung et al. [114]	FFNN-improved GA	Natural phenomena (sunspots)
Maciel and Ballini [19]	FFNN	Stock market index forecasting
Mai et al. [48]	RBFN	Electric load
de M. Neto et al. [92]	FFNN–PSO	Financial data
Niu and Wang [47]	Improved RBFN	Financial data
Nourani et al. [68]	SOM–Wavelet Transform–FFNN	Satellite rainfall runoff data
Otok et al. [90]	Ensemble ARIMA–FFNN	Monthly rainfall in Indonesia
Sermpinis et al. [45]	RBFN–PSO	Global financial data
Shi and Han [171]	SVR–ESN hybrid	China Yellow River runoff
Simon et al. [64]	Double SOM	Polish electrical load time series
Skabar [84]	Bayesian FFNN	Australian Financial Index
Song [57]	Jordan RNN	Natural phenomena and sunspots
Valero et al. [63]	SOM, FFNN	Load demand in Spain electrical system
van Hinsbergen et al. [86]	Bayesian ANN	Urban travel time
Yadav and Srinivasan [65]	SOM–AR	Electricity demand in Britain and Wales
Yeh [93]	FFNN–ISSO	Natural phenomena and simulated data
Yin et al. [46]	RBFN	Tidal level at Canada's west coast
Zhang [88]	Hybrid ARIMA–FFNN	Natural phenomena and financial data
Zhao et al. [54]	Elman RNN–Kalman filter	By-product gas flow in the steel industry
Zimmermann et al. [96]	ECNN	Demand of products and raw materials

Feedforward-type ANN architectures (FFNNs, RBFNs, SOMs, SVRs, etc.) are by far the most popular among all ANN architectures employed for time series prediction tasks because of their relative simplicity, universal functional approximation properties, and stability. ANN training with alternative machine learning evolutionary algorithms (PSO, GA, ABC, etc.) and combined with ensemble modeling offers an attractive framework for producing accurate time series forecasts with associated uncertainty measures. Recurrent neural networks (RNNs) are hard to implement, but they are worth taking a look at, especially when we want to model long past time series behavior or when a time series behaves more like a chaotic dynamical system and less like a nonlinear autoregressive signal. RNN's standard training algorithm (namely, error backpropagation through time) requires intensive computing resources and has to be handled carefully in order to achieve convergence and stability. On the other hand, the echo state network (ESN) approach to time series RNN modeling offers a faster way to identify stable dynamical systems since fast and economical linear regression aimed at selecting appropriate nonlinear neural activations is at the core of ESN training.

Especially in the early days (late 1980s and early 1990s), properly fitting a suitable ANN architecture to a given time series dataset in order to produce accurate forecasts was more of an art than a science. The building process of a time series ANN model relied heavily on trial and error and was very sensitive to the practitioner's previous knowledge and experience with the data at hand. These limitations, together with seemingly conflicting empirical evidence regarding the forecasting power of ANNs, gave rise to doubts and skepticism about ANN's overall ability to predict future time series values. In our opinion, the works surveyed in Section 4 define well-structured time series ANN modeling strategies that successfully address the aforementioned issues; however, work still needs to be done. Time series ANN modeling is not as well-established as traditional time series analysis due to the following:

1. ANN modeling is still a fast-evolving field of study;
2. Further work still needs to be done in order to employ ANNs as useful tools for understanding and interpreting relationships among time series variables involved in the forecasting task at hand (opening the black box);
3. Although ensemble modeling and methods similar to the double SOM technique discussed in Section 4.4 provide solutions for quantifying the uncertainty of time series forecasts generated by ANN models, we think that work still needs to be done in order to construct statistically valid prediction intervals associated with time series point forecasts from ANN models.

On the other hand, traditional statistical linear regression models are simple to understand, easy to implement and interpret, and are always at the forefront of the time series modeling literature. Unfortunately, linear modeling offers only an incomplete framework since nonlinear features in temporal data play an important role in many time series forecasting tasks. Parametric nonlinear modeling is a difficult and cumbersome activity since many arbitrary initial assumptions have to be made about the true form of the unknown underlying data-generating process. Linear models are often used indiscriminately by many practitioners, even if the predictions turn out to be unsatisfactory, which is often the case given time series nonlinear characteristics for many real-world problems. People's predisposition and willingness to ignore the limitations of traditional linear models is also an obstacle to the adoption of ANN techniques applied to time series forecasting tasks. Linear models, when used appropriately, are very effective tools. In fact, combining nonlinear methods based on ANNs with traditional linear models is a powerful and effective strategy. ESNs represent a prime example: linearly trained weights allow the ESN to select nonlinear neural activations from its reservoir. SOM models potentially offer a solution to the black-box problem associated with neural network models since their local approximation properties can be combined with linear time series modeling techniques, allowing users to study and interpret existing relationships among the response variable and some of its time-lagged values. An approach of our own to the problem of building statistically valid prediction intervals for time series point predictions generated by ANN models is outlined next: The basic idea is that, if a time series model has good generalization properties, then its forecasts will be close to actual future observations, and therefore the linear correlation coefficient between forecasts and true future observations (once they become available) will be close to one. Under these circumstances, it makes sense to build a simple linear regression model (called an auxiliary linear model) using validation data (i.e., the most recent observations in the training set) as the response variable Y_t and corresponding predictions from a fully trained ANN model (called the main ANN model) as the independent variable X_t. Under favorable circumstances, the auxiliary linear model, after being built, would have a statistically insignificant intercept coefficient β_0 close to zero and a statistically significant slope coefficient β_1 close to one. The residuals from the auxiliary linear model would contain valuable information about the distribution of prediction errors associated with point forecasts generated by the main ANN model. Finally, we would employ our auxiliary linear model to compute standard errors associated with point forecasts generated by the main ANN model. These standard errors would be the basis for building prediction bands with a user-defined confidence level. In an upcoming paper, we will discuss our idea in more detail, putting to the test the associated hypotheses outlined here.

The recent big data phenomenon is now motivating researchers to take a closer look at machine learning techniques, specifically ANNs, which are well suited to huge time series datasets. Terabytes of satellite imaging data pour in constantly and incessantly. Such huge volumes of data would be impossible to analyze by traditional means. Machine learning techniques, including ANNs, become an essential tool in these situations since ANNs are good at identifying recurring patterns occurring in large volumes of data. The joint use of ANN and linear models applied to very large datasets with temporal structure could be a good opportunity for unifying traditional statistics and machine learning. Efforts should be made to standardize notation and techniques from both disciplines, so machine learning can be regarded by scientists and practitioners as an integral and important part of statistics.

Author Contributions: Conceptualization, A.E.M.-Z., J.E.M.-D., D.A.-C., and J.A.G.-D.-d.-L.; methodology, A.E.M.-Z., J.E.M.-D., D.A.-C., and J.A.G.-D.-d.-L.; software, A.E.M.-Z., J.E.M.-D., D.A.-C., and J.A.G.-D.-d.-L.; validation, A.E.M.-Z., J.E.M.-D., D.A.-C., and J.A.G.-D.-d.-L.; formal analysis, A.E.M.-Z., J.E.M.-D., D.A.-C., and J.A.G.-D.-d.-L.; investigation, A.E.M.-Z., J.E.M.-D., D.A.-C., and J.A.G.-D.-d.-L.; resources, A.E.M.-Z., J.E.M.-D., D.A.-C., and J.A.G.-D.-d.-L.; data curation, A.E.M.-Z., J.E.M.-D., D.A.-C., and J.A.G.-D.-d.-L.; writing—original draft preparation, A.E.M.-Z., J.E.M.-D., D.A.-C., and J.A.G.-D.-d.-L.; writing—review and editing, A.E.M.-Z., J.E.M.-D., D.A.-C., and J.A.G.-D.-d.-L.; visualization, A.E.M.-Z., J.E.M.-D., D.A.-C., and J.A.G.-D.-d.-L.; supervision, A.E.M.-Z., J.E.M.-D., D.A.-C., and J.A.G.-D.-d.-L.; project administration, A.E.M.-Z., J.E.M.-D., D.A.-C., and J.A.G.-D.-d.-L.; funding acquisition, J.E.M.-D. All authors have read and agreed to the published version of the manuscript.

Funding: This work was supported by the Universidad Autónoma de Aguascalientes through grant PII23-1. The corresponding author (J.E.M.-D.) was funded by the National Council of Science and Technology of Mexico (CONACYT) through grant A1-S-45928.

Institutional Review Board Statement: Not applicable.

Informed Consent Statement: Not applicable.

Data Availability Statement: Data sharing not applicable.

Acknowledgments: The authors wish to thank the anonymous reviewers for their comments and criticisms. All of their comments were taken into account in the revised version of the paper, resulting in a substantial improvement with respect to the original submission.

Conflicts of Interest: The authors declare no conflicts of interest.

Abbreviations

The following abbreviations are used in this manuscript:

ABC	Artificial bee colony
ANN	Artificial Neural Network
ARCH	Autoregressive conditional heteroskedasticity
ARIMA	Autoregressive integrated moving average
BP	Backpropagation
BPTT	Backpropagation through time
CV	Cross-validation
FFNN	Feedforward neural networks
GA	Genetic algorithm
MLP	Multilayer perceptron
NARX	Nonlinear autoregressive with exogenous inputs
PEM	Prediction error measure
PCA	Principal component analysis
PSO	Particle swarm optimization
RBFN	Radial basis function network
RNN	Recurrent neural network
SOM	Self-organizing map
SVM	Support vector machines

References

1. Alba-Cuéllar, D.; Muñoz-Zavala, A.E. A Comparison between SARIMA Models and Feed Forward Neural Network Ensemble Models for Time Series Data. *Res. Comput. Sci.* **2015**, *92*, 9–22. [CrossRef]
2. Panigrahi, R.; Patne, N.R.; Pemmada, S.; Manchalwar, A.D. Prediction of Electric Energy Consumption for Demand Response using Deep Learning. In Proceedings of the 2022 International Conference on Intelligent Controller and Computing for Smart Power (ICICCSP), Hyderabad, India, 21–23 July 2022; IEEE: New York, NY, USA, 2022; pp. 1–6.
3. Wang, Y.; Chen, J.; Chen, X.; Zeng, X.; Kong, Y.; Sun, S.; Guo, Y.; Liu, Y. Short-Term Load Forecasting for Industrial Customers Based on TCN-LightGBM. *IEEE Trans. Power Syst.* **2021**, *36*, 1984–1997. [CrossRef]
4. Tudose, A.M.; Picioroaga, I.I.; Sidea, D.O.; Bulac, C.; Boicea, V.A. Short-Term Load Forecasting Using Convolutional Neural Networks in COVID-19 Context: The Romanian Case Study. *Energies* **2021**, *14*, 4046. [CrossRef]
5. Panigrahi, R.; Patne, N.; Surya Vardhan, B.; Khedkar, M. Short-term load analysis and forecasting using stochastic approach considering pandemic effects. *Electr. Eng.* **2023**, in press. [CrossRef]
6. Alba-Cuéllar, D.; Muñoz-Zavala, A.E.; Hernández-Aguirre, A.; Ponce-De-Leon-Senti, E.E.; Díaz-Díaz, E. Time Series Forecasting with PSO-Optimized Neural Networks. In Proceedings of the 2014 13th Mexican International Conference on Artificial Intelligence (MICAI), Tuxtla Gutierrez, Mexico, 16–22 November 2014; IEEE: New York, NY, USA, 2014; pp. 102–111.
7. Box, G.E.; Jenkins, G.M. *Time Series Analysis: Forecasting and Control*; Holden Day: New York, NY, USA, 1970.
8. Tong, H. Nonlinear time series analysis since 1990: Some personal reflections. *Acta Math. Appl. Sin.* **2002**, *18*, 177–184. [CrossRef]
9. Tong, H. *Non-Linear Time Series: A Dynamical System Approach*; Oxford University Press: Oxford, UK, 1990.
10. Engle, R.F. Autoregressive conditional heteroscedasticity with estimates of the variance of United Kingdom inflation. *Econom. J. Econom. Soc.* **1982**, *50*, 987–1007. [CrossRef]
11. Granger, C.W.J.; Andersen, A.P. *An Introduction to Bilinear Time Series Models*; Vandenhoeck and Ruprecht: Göttingen, Germany, 1978.
12. Murphy, K.P. *Machine Learning: A Probabilistic Perspective*; MIT Press: Cambridge, MA, USA, 2012.
13. Drucker, H.; Burges, C.J.; Kaufman, L.; Smola, A.; Vapnik, V. Support vector regression machines. *Adv. Neural Inf. Process. Syst.* **1997**, *9*, 155–161.
14. Härdle, W. *Nonparametric and Semiparametric Models*; Springer: Berlin/Heidelberg, Germany, 2004.
15. McCulloch, W.S.; Pitts, W. A logical calculus of the ideas immanent in nervous activity. *Bull. Math. Biophys.* **1943**, *5*, 115–133. [CrossRef]
16. Rosenblatt, F. *The Perceptron—A Perceiving and Recognizing Automaton*; Technical Report 85-460-1; Cornell Aeronautical Laboratory: Buffalo, NY, USA, 1957.
17. Lapedes, A.; Farber, R. *Nonlinear Signal Processing Using Neural Networks: Prediction and System Modeling*; Technical Report LA-UR-87-2662; Los Alamos National Laboratory: Los Alamos, NM, USA, 1987.
18. As'ad, F.; Farhat, C. A mechanics-informed deep learning framework for data-driven nonlinear viscoelasticity. *Comput. Methods Appl. Mech. Eng.* **2023**, *417*, 116463. [CrossRef]
19. Maciel, L.S.; Ballini, R. Neural networks applied to stock market forecasting: An empirical analysis. *Learn. Nonlinear Model.* **2010**, *8*, 3–22. [CrossRef]
20. Cybenko, G. Approximation by superpositions of a sigmoidal function. *Math. Control Signals Syst.* **1989**, *2*, 303–314. [CrossRef]

21. Shumway, R.H.; Stoffer, D.S. *Time Series Analysis and Its Applications (with R Examples)*, 3rd ed.; Springer Science+Business Media, LLC: Cham, Switzerland, 2011.
22. Jones, E.R. *An Introduction to Neural Networks: A White Paper*; Visual Numerics Inc.: Houston, TX, USA, 2004.
23. Touretzky, D.; Laskowski, K. *Neural Networks for Time Series Prediction*; Lecture Notes for Class 15-486/782: Artificial Neural Networks; Carnegie Mellon University: Pittsburgh, PA, USA, 2006.
24. Whittle, P. *Hypothesis Testing in Time Series Analysis*; Hafner Publishing Company: New York, NY, USA, 1951.
25. Box, G.E. Science and statistics. *J. Am. Stat. Assoc.* **1976**, *71*, 791–799. [CrossRef]
26. Nisbet, B. Tutorial E—Feature Selection in KNIME. In *Handbook of Statistical Analysis and Data Mining Applications*, 2nd ed.; Nisbet, R., Miner, G., Yale, K., Eds.; Academic Press: Boston, MA, USA, 2018; pp. 377–391.
27. Bullinaria, J.A. Neural Computation. 2014. Available online: https://www.cs.bham.ac.uk/~jxb/inc.html (accessed on 1 December 2023).
28. Beale, R.; Jackson, T. *Neural Computing—An Introduction*; Institute of Physics Publishing: Bristol, UK, 1990.
29. Bishop, C.M. *Neural Networks for Pattern Recognition*; Oxford University Press: Oxford, UK, 1995.
30. Callan, R. *Essence of Neural Networks*; Prentice Hall PTR: Hoboken, NJ, USA, 1998.
31. Fausett, L. *Fundamentals of Neural Networks: Architectures, Algorithms, and Applications*; Prentice Hall: Hoboken, NJ, USA, 1994.
32. Gurney, K. *An Introduction to Neural Networks*; Routledge: London, UK, 1997.
33. Ham, F.M.; Kostanic, I. *Principles of Neurocomputing for Science and Engineering*; McGraw-Hill Higher Education: New York, NY, USA, 2000.
34. Haykin, S.S. *Neural Networks and Learning Machines*; Pearson Education Upper Saddle River: Hoboken, NJ, USA, 2009; Volume 3.
35. Hertz, J. *Introduction to the Theory of Neural Computation*; Basic Books: New York, NY, USA, 1991; Volume 1.
36. Mazaheri, P.; Rahnamayan, S.; Bidgoli, A.A. *Designing Artificial Neural Network Using Particle Swarm Optimization: A Survey*; IntechOpen: Rijeka, Croatia, 2022.
37. Arlot, S.; Celisse, A. A survey of cross-validation procedures for model selection. *Stat. Surv.* **2010**, *4*, 40–79. [CrossRef]
38. Hjorth, J.U. *Computer Intensive Statistical Methods: Validation, Model Selection, and Bootstrap*; Chapman and Hall: Boca Raton, FL, USA, 1994; pp. 65–73.
39. Makridakis, S.; Winkler, R.L. Averages of forecasts: Some empirical results. *Manag. Sci.* **1983**, *29*, 987–996. [CrossRef]
40. Barrow, D.K.; Crone, S.F. Crogging (cross-validation aggregation) for forecasting—A novel algorithm of neural network ensembles on time series subsamples. In Proceedings of the 2013 International Joint Conference on Neural Networks (IJCNN), Dallas, TX, USA, 4–9 August 2013; IEEE: New York, NY, USA, 2013; pp. 1–8.
41. Lahmiri, S. Intelligent Ensemble Systems for Modeling NASDAQ Microstructure: A Comparative Study. In *Artificial Neural Networks in Pattern Recognition*; Springer: Cham, Switzerland, 2014; pp. 240–251.
42. Broomhead, D.S.; Lowe, D. *Radial Basis Functions, Multi-Variable Functional Interpolation and Adaptive Networks*; Technical Report, DTIC Document; Controller HMSO: London, UK, 1988.
43. Hartman, E.J.; Keeler, J.D.; Kowalski, J.M. Layered neural networks with Gaussian hidden units as universal approximations. *Neural Comput.* **1990**, *2*, 210–215. [CrossRef]
44. Chang, W.Y. Wind energy conversion system power forecasting using radial basis function neural network. *Appl. Mech. Mater.* **2013**, *284*, 1067–1071. [CrossRef]
45. Sermpinis, G.; Theofilatos, K.; Karathanasopoulos, A.; Georgopoulos, E.F.; Dunis, C. Forecasting foreign exchange rates with adaptive neural networks using radial-basis functions and Particle Swarm Optimization. *Eur. J. Oper. Res.* **2013**, *225*, 528–540. [CrossRef]
46. Yin, J.c.; Zou, Z.j.; Xu, F. Sequential learning radial basis function network for real-time tidal level predictions. *Ocean Eng.* **2013**, *57*, 49–55. [CrossRef]
47. Niu, H.; Wang, J. Financial time series prediction by a random data-time effective RBF neural network. *Soft Comput.* **2014**, *18*, 497–508. [CrossRef]
48. Mai, W.; Chung, C.; Wu, T.; Huang, H. Electric load forecasting for large office building based on radial basis function neural network. In Proceedings of the 2014 IEEE PES General Meeting—Conference & Exposition, National Harbor, MD, USA, 27–31 July 2014; IEEE: New York, NY, USA, 2014; pp. 1–5.
49. Zhu, J.Z.; Cao, J.X.; Zhu, Y. Traffic volume forecasting based on radial basis function neural network with the consideration of traffic flows at the adjacent intersections. *Transp. Res. Part C Emerg. Technol.* **2014**, *47 Pt A*, 139–154. [CrossRef]
50. Elman, J.L. Finding structure in time. *Cogn. Sci.* **1990**, *14*, 179–211. [CrossRef]
51. Sprott, J.C. *Chaos and Time-Series Analysis*; Oxford University Press: Oxford, UK, 2003; Volume 69.
52. Ardalani-Farsa, M.; Zolfaghari, S. Chaotic time series prediction with residual analysis method using hybrid Elman–NARX neural networks. *Neurocomputing* **2010**, *73*, 2540–2553. [CrossRef]
53. Chandra, R.; Zhang, M. Cooperative coevolution of Elman recurrent neural networks for chaotic time series prediction. *Neurocomputing* **2012**, *86*, 116–123. [CrossRef]
54. Zhao, J.; Zhu, X.; Wang, W.; Liu, Y. Extended Kalman filter-based Elman networks for industrial time series prediction with GPU acceleration. *Neurocomputing* **2013**, *118*, 215–224. [CrossRef]

55. Jordan, M.I. Attractor Dynamics and parallelism in a connectionist sequential machine. In Proceedings of the Eight Annual Conference of the Cognitive Science Society, Amherst, MA, USA, 15–17 August 1986; Lawrence Erlbaum Associates: Hillsdale, NJ, USA, 1986.
56. Tabuse, M.; Kinouchi, M.; Hagiwara, M. Recurrent neural network using mixture of experts for time series processing. In Proceedings of the 1997 IEEE International Conference on Systems, Man, and Cybernetics—Computational Cybernetics and Simulation, Orlando, FL, USA, 12–15 October 1997; IEEE: New York, NY, USA, 1997; Volume 1, pp. 536–541.
57. Song, Q. Robust initialization of a Jordan network with recurrent constrained learning. *Neural Netw. IEEE Trans.* **2011**, *22*, 2460–2473. [CrossRef]
58. Song, Q. Robust Jordan network for nonlinear time series prediction. In Proceedings of the 2011 International Joint Conference on Neural Networks (IJCNN), San Jose, CA, USA, 31 July–5 August 2011; IEEE: New York, NY, USA, 2011; pp. 2542–2549.
59. Boussaada, Z.; Curea, O.; Remaci, A.; Camblong, H.; Mrabet Bellaaj, N. A Nonlinear Autoregressive Exogenous (NARX) Neural Network Model for the Prediction of the Daily Direct Solar Radiation. *Energies* **2018**, *11*, 620. [CrossRef]
60. Kohonen, T. *Self-Organizing Maps*; Springer Series in Information Sciences; Springer: Berlin/Heidelberg, Germany, 1995; Volume 30.
61. Barreto, G.A. Time series prediction with the self-organizing map: A review. In *Perspectives of Neural-Symbolic Integration*; Springer: Berlin/Heidelberg, Germany, 2007; pp. 135–158.
62. Burguillo, J.C. Using self-organizing maps with complex network topologies and coalitions for time series prediction. *Soft Comput.* **2014**, *18*, 695–705. [CrossRef]
63. Valero, S.; Aparicio, J.; Senabre, C.; Ortiz, M.; Sancho, J.; Gabaldon, A. Comparative analysis of Self Organizing Maps vs. multilayer perceptron neural networks for short-term load forecasting. In Proceedings of the Modern Electric Power Systems (MEPS), 2010 Proceedings of the International Symposium, Wroclaw, Poland, 20–22 September 2010; IEEE: New York, NY, USA, 2010; pp. 1–5.
64. Simon, G.; Lendasse, A.; Cottrell, M.; Fort, J.C.; Verleysen, M. Double SOM for long-term time series prediction. In Proceedings of the Conference WSOM 2003, Kitakyushu, Japan, 11–14 September 2003; pp. 35–40.
65. Yadav, V.; Srinivasan, D. Autocorrelation based weighing strategy for short-term load forecasting with the self-organizing map. In Proceedings of the 2010 the 2nd International Conference on Computer and Automation Engineering (ICCAE), Singapore, 26–28 February 2010; IEEE: New York, NY, USA, 2010; Volume 1, pp. 186–192.
66. Dablemont, S.; Simon, G.; Lendasse, A.; Ruttiens, A.; Blayo, F.; Verleysen, M. Time series forecasting with SOM and local non-linear models—Application to the DAX30 index prediction. In Proceedings of the Workshop on Self-Organizing Maps, Kitakyushu, Japan, 11–14 September 2003.
67. Cherif, A.; Cardot, H.; Boné, R. Recurrent Neural Networks as Local Models for Time Series Prediction. In *Neural Information Processing*; Springer: Berlin/Heidelberg, Germany, 2009; pp. 786–793.
68. Nourani, V.; Baghanam, A.H.; Adamowski, J.; Gebremichael, M. Using self-organizing maps and wavelet transforms for space–time pre-processing of satellite precipitation and runoff data in neural network based rainfall–runoff modeling. *J. Hydrol.* **2013**, *476*, 228–243. [CrossRef]
69. Bengio, Y.; Simard, P.; Frasconi, P. Learning long-term dependencies with gradient descent is difficult. *IEEE Trans. Neural Netw.* **1994**, *5*, 157–166. [CrossRef]
70. Pascanu, R.; Mikolov, T.; Bengio, Y. On the difficulty of training Recurrent Neural Networks. In Proceedings of the 30th International Conference on Machine Learning, Atlanta, GA, USA, 16–21 June 2013; IEEE: New York, NY, USA, 2013.
71. Hu, D.; Wu, R.; Chen, D.; Dou, H. An improved training algorithm of neural networks for time series forecasting. In *MICAI 2007: Advances in Artificial Intelligence*; Springer: Berlin/Heidelberg, Germany, 2007; pp. 550–558.
72. Nunnari, G. An improved back propagation algorithm to predict episodes of poor air quality. *Soft Comput.* **2006**, *10*, 132–139. [CrossRef]
73. Ioffe, S.; Szegedy, C. Batch normalization: Accelerating deep network training by reducing internal covariate shift. In Proceedings of the 32nd International Conference on International Conference on Machine Learning, ICML-2015, JMLR, Lille, France, 6–11 July 2015; pp. 448–456.
74. Yang, G.; Pennington, J.; Rao, V.; Sohl-Dickstein, J.; Schoenholz, S.S. *A Mean Field Theory of Batch Normalization*; Cornell Uiversity: Ithaca, NY, USA, 2019.
75. Werbos, P. Backpropagation through time: What it does and how to do it. *Proc. IEEE* **1990**, *78*, 1550–1560. [CrossRef]
76. Hochreiter, S.; Schmidhuber, J. Long Short-Term Memory. *Neural Comput.* **1997**, *9*, 1735–1780. [CrossRef]
77. Gers, F.A.; Schmidhuber, J.; Cummins, F. Learning to Forget: Continual Prediction with LSTM. *Neural Comput.* **2000**, *12*, 2451–2471. [CrossRef] [PubMed]
78. Calin, O. *Deep Learning Architectures: A Mathematical Approach*; Springer: Cham, Switzerland, 2020.
79. Roy, T.; kumar Shome, S. Optimization of RNN-LSTM Model Using NSGA-II Algorithm for IOT-based Fire Detection Framework. *IETE J. Res.* **2023**, in press. [CrossRef]
80. Jha, G.K.; Thulasiraman, P.; Thulasiram, R.K. PSO based neural network for time series forecasting. In Proceedings of the 2009 International Joint Conference on Neural Networks, IJCNN 2009, Atlanta, GA, USA, 14–19 June 2009; IEEE: New York, NY, USA, 2009; pp. 1422–1427.

81. Adhikari, R.; Agrawal, R.; Kant, L. PSO based Neural Networks vs. traditional statistical models for seasonal time series forecasting. In Proceedings of the 2013 3rd IEEE International Advance Computing Conference (IACC), Ghaziabad, India, 22–23 February 2013; IEEE: New York, NY, USA, 2013; pp. 719–725.
82. Awan, S.M.; Aslam, M.; Khan, Z.A.; Saeed, H. An efficient model based on artificial bee colony optimization algorithm with Neural Networks for electric load forecasting. *Neural Comput. Appl.* **2014**, *25*, 1967–1978. [CrossRef]
83. Giovanis, E. Feed-Forward Neural Networks Regressions with Genetic Algorithms: Applications in Econometrics and Finance. *SSRN* **2010**, *in press*. [CrossRef]
84. Skabar, A.A. Direction-of-change financial time series forecasting using neural networks: A Bayesian approach. In *Advances in Electrical Engineering and Computational Science*; Springer: Dordrecht, The Netherlands, 2009; pp. 515–524.
85. Blonbou, R. Very short-term wind power forecasting with neural networks and adaptive Bayesian learning. *Renew. Energy* **2011**, *36*, 1118–1124. [CrossRef]
86. Van Hinsbergen, C.; Hegyi, A.; van Lint, J.; van Zuylen, H. Bayesian neural networks for the prediction of stochastic travel times in urban networks. *IET Intell. Transp. Syst.* **2011**, *5*, 259–265. [CrossRef]
87. Kocadağlı, O.; Aşıkgil, B. Nonlinear time series forecasting with Bayesian neural networks. *Expert Syst. Appl.* **2014**, *41*, 6596–6610. [CrossRef]
88. Zhang, G.P. Time series forecasting using a hybrid ARIMA and neural network model. *Neurocomputing* **2003**, *50*, 159–175. [CrossRef]
89. Guo, X.; Deng, F. Short-term prediction of intelligent traffic flow based on BP neural network and ARIMA model. In Proceedings of the 2010 International Conference on E-Product E-Service and E-Entertainment (ICEEE), Henan, China, 7–9 November 2010; IEEE: New York, NY, USA, 2010; pp. 1–4.
90. Otok, B.W.; Lusia, D.A.; Faulina, R.; Kuswanto, H. Ensemble method based on ARIMA-FFNN for climate forecasting. In Proceedings of the 2012 International Conference on Statistics in Science, Business, and Engineering (ICSSBE), Langkawi, Malaysia, 10–12 September 2012; IEEE: New York, NY, USA, 2012; pp. 1–4.
91. Viviani, E.; Di Persio, L.; Ehrhardt, M. Energy Markets Forecasting. From Inferential Statistics to Machine Learning: The German Case. *Energies* **2021**, *14*, 364. [CrossRef]
92. Neto, P.S.d.M.; Petry, G.G.; Aranildo, R.L.J.; Ferreira, T.A.E. Combining artificial neural network and particle swarm system for time series forecasting. In Proceedings of the 2009 International Joint Conference on Neural Networks, IJCNN 2009, Atlanta, GA, USA, 14–19 June 2009; IEEE: New York, NY, USA, 2009; pp. 2230–2237.
93. Yeh, W.C. New Parameter-Free Simplified Swarm Optimization for Artificial Neural Network Training and its Application in the Prediction of Time Series. *IEEE Trans. Neural Netw. Learn. Syst.* **2013**, *24*, 661–665.
94. Crone, S.F.; Guajardo, J.; Weber, R. A study on the ability of support vector regression and neural networks to forecast basic time series patterns. In *Artificial Intelligence in Theory and Practice*; Springer: Boston, MA, USA, 2006; pp. 149–158.
95. Moody, J. Forecasting the economy with neural nets: A survey of challenges and solutions. In *Neural Networks: Tricks of the Trade*, 2nd ed.; Montavon, G., Orr, G.B., Müller, K.R., Eds.; Lecture Notes in Computer Science; Springer: Berlin/Heidelberg, Germany, 2012; Volume 7700, pp. 343–367.
96. Zimmermann, H.G.; Tietz, C.; Grothmann, R. Forecasting with recurrent neural networks: 12 tricks. In *Neural Networks: Tricks of the Trade*; Springer: Berlin/Heidelberg, Germany, 2012; pp. 687–707.
97. Lukoševičius, M. A practical guide to applying echo state networks. In *Neural Networks: Tricks of the Trade*; Springer: Berlin/Heidelberg, Germany, 2012; pp. 659–686.
98. Holland, J.H. *Adaptation in Natural and Artificial Systems*; University of Michigan Press: Ann Arbor, MI, USA, 1975.
99. Angeline, P.J. Evolutionary optimization versus particle swarm optimization: Philosophy and performance differences. In *Evolutionary Programming VII*; Springer: Berlin/Heidelberg, Germany, 1998; pp. 601–610.
100. Freitas, D.; Lopes, L.G.; Morgado-Dias, F. Particle Swarm Optimisation: A Historical Review Up to the Current Developments. *Entropy* **2020**, *22*, 362. [CrossRef] [PubMed]
101. Kennedy, J.; Eberhart, R. Particle swarm optimization. In Proceedings of the IEEE International Conference on Neural Networks, Perth, WA, Australia, 27 November–1 December 1995; IEEE: New York, NY, USA, 1995; Volume 4, pp. 1942–1948.
102. Eberhart, R.; Shi, Y. Evolving Artificial Neural Networks. In Proceedings of the International Conference on Neural Networks and Brain, PRC, Anchorage, AK, USA, 4–9 May 1998; Volume 1, pp. PL5–PL13.
103. Eberhart, R.; Shi, Y. Particle swarm optimization: Developments, applications and resources. In Proceedings of the 2001 Congress on Evolutionary Computation, Seoul, Republic of Korea, 27–30 May 2001; IEEE: New York, NY, USA, 2001; Volume 1, pp. 81–86.
104. Yu, J.; Wang, S.; Xi, L. Evolving artificial neural networks using an improved PSO and DPSO. *Neurocomputing* **2008**, *71*, 1054–1060. [CrossRef]
105. Munoz-Zavala, A.E. A Comparison Study of PSO Neighborhoods. In *EVOLVE—A Bridge between Probability, Set Oriented Numerics, and Evolutionary Computation II*; Springer: Berlin/Heidelberg, Germany, 2013; pp. 251–265.
106. Eberhart, R.; Dobbins, R.; Simpson, P. *Computational Intelligence PC Tools*; Academic Press Professional: Cambridge, MA, USA, 1996.
107. Clerc, M.; Kennedy, J. The particle swarm: Explosion, stability, and convergence in a multidimensional complex space. *IEEE Trans. Evol. Comput.* **2002**, *6*, 58–73. [CrossRef]

108. Slama, S.; Errachdi, A.; Benrejeb, M. *Tuning Artificial Neural Network Controller Using Particle Swarm Optimization Technique for Nonlinear System*; IntechOpen: Rijeka, Croatia, 2021.
109. Ahmadzadeh, E.; Lee, J.; Moon, I. Optimized Neural Network Weights and Biases Using Particle Swarm Optimization Algorithm for Prediction Applications. *J. Korea Multimed. Soc.* **2017**, *20*, 1406–1420.
110. Hagan, M.T.; Menhaj, M.B. Training feedforward networks with the Marquardt algorithm. *Neural Netw. IEEE Trans.* **1994**, *5*, 989–993. [CrossRef] [PubMed]
111. Riedmiller, M.; Braun, H. A direct adaptive method for faster backpropagation learning: The RPROP algorithm. In Proceedings of the IEEE International Conference on Neural Networks, San Francisco, CA, USA, 28 March–1 April 1993; IEEE: New York, NY, USA, 1993; pp. 586–591.
112. Møller, M.F. A scaled conjugate gradient algorithm for fast supervised learning. *Neural Netw.* **1993**, *6*, 525–533. [CrossRef]
113. Battiti, R. One step secant conjugate gradient. *Neural Comput.* **1992**, *4*, 141–166. [CrossRef]
114. Leung, F.H.F.; Lam, H.K.; Ling, S.H.; Tam, P.K.S. Tuning of the structure and parameters of a neural network using an improved genetic algorithm. *IEEE Trans. Neural Netw.* **2003**, *14*, 79–88. [CrossRef]
115. Sitte, R.; Sitte, J. Neural networks approach to the random walk dilemma of financial time series. *Appl. Intell.* **2002**, *16*, 163–171. [CrossRef]
116. de Araujo, R.; Madeiro, F.; de Sousa, R.P.; Pessoa, L.F.; Ferreira, T. An evolutionary morphological approach for financial time series forecasting. In Proceedings of the 2006 IEEE Congress on Evolutionary Computation, CEC 2006, Vancouver, BC, Canada, 16–21 July 2006; IEEE: New York, NY, USA, 2006; pp. 2467–2474.
117. Yeh, W.C.; Chang, W.W.; Chung, Y.Y. A new hybrid approach for mining breast cancer pattern using discrete particle swarm optimization and statistical method. *Expert Syst. Appl.* **2009**, *36*, 8204–8211. [CrossRef]
118. Goldberg, D.E. *Genetic Algorithms in Search, Optimization, and Machine Learning*; Addison-Wesley: Boston, MA, USA, 1989.
119. Zhao, L.; Yang, Y. PSO-based single multiplicative neuron model for time series prediction. *Expert Syst. Appl.* **2009**, *36*, 2805–2812. [CrossRef]
120. Mackey, M.C.; Glass, L. Oscillation and chaos in physiological control systems. *Science* **1977**, *197*, 287–289. [CrossRef] [PubMed]
121. Hyndman, R. Time Series Data Library. 2014. Available online: https://robjhyndman.com/tsdl/ (accessed on 1 December 2023).
122. Keirn, Z. EEG Pattern Analysis. 1988. Available online: https://github.com/meagmohit/EEG-Datasets (accessed on 1 December 2023).
123. Gershenfeld, N.; Weigend, A. The Santa Fe Time Series Competition Data. 1994. Available online: http://techlab.bu.edu/resources/data_view/the_santa_fe_time_series_competition_data/index.html (accessed on 1 December 2023).
124. Gudise, V.; Venayagamoorthy, G. Comparison of particle swarm optimization and backpropagation as training algorithms for neural networks. In Proceedings of the 2003 IEEE Swarm Intelligence Symposium. SIS'03 (Cat. No. 03EX706), Indianapolis, IN, USA, 26 April 2003; IEEE: New York, NY, USA, 2003; pp. 110–117.
125. Liu, C.; Ding, W.; Li, Z.; Yang, C. Prediction of High-Speed Grinding Temperature of Titanium Matrix Composites Using BP Neural Network Based on PSO Algorithm. *Int. J. Adv. Manuf. Technol.* **2016**, *89*, 2277–2285. [CrossRef]
126. Ince, T.; Kiranyaz, S.; Gabbouj, M. A Generic and Robust System for Automated Patient-Specific Classification of ECG Signals. *IEEE Trans. Biomed. Eng.* **2009**, *56*, 1415–1426. [CrossRef]
127. Hamed, H.N.A.; Shamsuddin, S.M.; Salim, N. Particle Swarm Optimization For Neural Network Learning Enhancement. *J. Teknol.* **2008**, *49*, 13–26.
128. Olayode, I.O.; Tartibu, L.K.; Okwu, M.O.; Ukaegbu, U.F. Development of a Hybrid Artificial Neural Network-Particle Swarm Optimization Model for the Modelling of Traffic Flow of Vehicles at Signalized Road Intersections. *Appl. Sci.* **2021**, *11*, 8387. [CrossRef]
129. Van den Bergh, F.; Engelbrecht, A. Cooperative learning in neural networks using particle swarm optimizers. *S. Afr. Comput. J.* **2000**, *2000*, 84–90.
130. van den Bergh, F.; Engelbrecht, A. Training product unit networks using cooperative particle swarm optimisers. In Proceedings of the International Joint Conference on Neural Networks, IJCNN'01, Washington, DC, USA, 15–19 July 2001; IEEE: New York, NY, USA, 2001; Volume 1, pp. 126–131.
131. Munoz-Zavala, A.; Hernandez-Aguirre, A.; Villa Diharce, E. Constrained optimization via particle evolutionary swarm optimization algorithm (PESO). In Proceedings of the 7th Annual Conference on Genetic and Evolutionary Computation, GECCO'05, Washington, DC, USA, 25–99 June 2005; ACM: New York, NY, USA, 2005; pp. 209–216.
132. Munoz-Zavala, A.; Hernandez-Aguirre, A.; Villa Diharce, E.; Botello Rionda, S. Constrained optimization with an improved particle swarm optimization algorithm. *Int. J. Intell. Comput. Cybern.* **2008**, *1*, 425–453. [CrossRef]
133. Kennedy, J. Methods of agreement: Inference among the EleMentals. In Proceedings of the 1998 IEEE International Symposium on Intelligent Control (ISIC) Held Jointly with IEEE International Symposium on Computational Intelligence in Robotics and Automation (CIRA) Intell, Gaithersburg, MD, USA, 17 September 1998; IEEE: New York, NY, USA, 1998; pp. 883–887.
134. Ozcan, E.; Mohan, C. Analysis of a Simple Particle Swarm Optimization System. *Intell. Eng. Syst. Artif. Neural Netw.* **1998**, *8*, 253–258.
135. Van den Bergh, F.; Engelbrecht, A.P. A Convergence Proof for the Particle Swarm Optimiser. *Fundam. Inform.* **2010**, *105*, 341–374. [CrossRef]

136. Kan, W.; Jihong, S. The Convergence Basis of Particle Swarm Optimization. In Proceedings of the 2012 International Conference on Industrial Control and Electronics Engineering, Xi'an, China, 23–25 August 2012; IEEE: New York, NY, USA, 2012; pp. 63–66.
137. Qian, W.; Li, M. Convergence analysis of standard particle swarm optimization algorithm and its improvement. *Soft Comput.* **2018**, *22*, 4047–4070. [CrossRef]
138. Xu, G.; Yu, G. On convergence analysis of particle swarm optimization algorithm. *J. Comput. Appl. Math.* **2018**, *333*, 65–73. [CrossRef]
139. Huang, H.; Qiu, J.; Riedl, K. On the Global Convergence of Particle Swarm Optimization Methods. *Appl. Math. Optim.* **2023**, *88*, 30. [CrossRef]
140. Zhang, G.P.; Qi, M. Neural network forecasting for seasonal and trend time series. *Eur. J. Oper. Res.* **2005**, *160*, 501–514. [CrossRef]
141. Vapnik, V.N. *The Nature of Statistical Learning Theory*; Springer-Verlag New York, Inc.: New York, NY, USA, 1995.
142. US Census Bureau. X-13ARIMA-SEATS Seasonal Adjustment Program. 2016. Available online: https://www.census.gov/srd/www/x13as/ (accessed on 22 October 2016).
143. Kiani, K.M. On business cycle fluctuations in USA macroeconomic time series. *Econ. Model.* **2016**, *53*, 179–186. [CrossRef]
144. Moody, J. Prediction risk and neural network architecture selection. In *From Statistics to Neural Networks: Theory and Pattern Recognition Applications*; Cherkassky, V., Friedman, J.H., Wechsler, H., Eds.; Springer: Berlin/Heidelberg, Germany, 1994; pp. 147–165.
145. Pi, H.; Peterson, C. Finding the embedding dimension and variable dependencies in time series. *Neural Comput.* **1994**, *6*, 509–520. [CrossRef]
146. Yang, H.; Moody, J. *Input Variable Selection Based on Joint Mutual Information*; Technical Report; Department of Computer Science, Oregon Graduate Institute: Eugene, OR, USA, 1998.
147. Mozer, M.C.; Smolensky, P. Skeletonization: A technique for trimming the fat from a network via relevance assessment. In *Advances in Neural Information Processing Systems*; ACM: New York, NY, USA, 1989; pp. 107–115.
148. Ash, T. Dynamic node creation in backpropagation networks. *Connect. Sci.* **1989**, *1*, 365–375. [CrossRef]
149. LeCun, Y.; Denker, J.S.; Solla, S.A.; Howard, R.E.; Jackel, L.D. Optimal brain damage. *Adv. Neural Inf. Process. Syst.* **1989**, *2*, 598–605.
150. Hassibi, B.; Stork, D.G. Second order derivatives for network pruning: Optimal brain surgeon. *Adv. Neural Inf. Process. Syst.* **1993**, *5*, 164.
151. Levin, A. Fast pruning using principal components. *Adv. Neural Inf. Process. Syst.* **1994**, *6*, 35–42.
152. Moody, J.E.; Rögnvaldsson, T. Smoothing Regularizers for Projective Basis Function Networks. *Adv. Neural Inf. Process. Syst.* **1996**, *9*, 585–591.
153. Wu, L.; Moody, J. A smoothing regularizer for feedforward and recurrent neural networks. *Neural Comput.* **1996**, *8*, 461–489. [CrossRef]
154. Liao, Y.; Moody, J. A neural network visualization and sensitivity analysis toolkit. In Proceedings of the International Conference on Neural Information Processing (ICONIP'96), Hong Kong, China, 24–27 September 1996; Amari, S.-I., Xu, L., Chan, L., King, I., Leung, K.-S., Eds.; Springer Verlag Singapore Pte. Ltd.: Singapore, 1996; pp. 1069–1074.
155. Schäfer, A.M.; Zimmermann, H.G. Recurrent neural networks are universal approximators. In *Artificial Neural Networks–ICANN 2006*; Springer: Berlin/Heidelberg, Germany, 2006; pp. 632–640.
156. Rumelhart, D.E.; Hinton, G.E.; Williams, R.J. *Learning Internal Representations by Error Propagation*; Technical Report, DTIC Document; Institute for Cognitive Science University of California:San Diego, CA, USA, 1985.
157. Zimmermann, H.G.; Neuneier, R. Neural network architectures for the modeling of dynamical systems. In *A Field Guide to Dynamical Recurrent Networks*; Wiley-IEEE Press: Hoboken, NJ, USA, 2001; pp. 311–350.
158. Werbos, P. Beyond Regression: New Tools for Prediction and Analysis in the Behavioral Sciences. Ph.D. Thesis, Harvard University, Cambridge, MA, USA, 1974.
159. Zimmermann, H.G.; Neuneier, R.; Grothmann, R. Modeling dynamical systems by error correction neural networks. In *Modelling and Forecasting Financial Data*; Springer: Boston, MA, USA, 2002; pp. 237–263.
160. Zimmermann, H.G.; Grothmann, R.; Schäfer, A.M.; Tietz, C.; Georg, H. Modeling Large Dynamical Systems with Dynamical Consistent Neural Networks. In *New Directions in Statistical Signal Processing*; MIT Press: Cambridge, MA, USA, 2007; p. 203.
161. McNeil, A.J.; Frey, R.; Embrechts, P. *Quantitative Risk Management: Concepts, Techniques, and Tools*; Princeton University Press: Princeton, NJ, USA, 2010.
162. Jaeger, H. *The "Echo State" Approach to Analysing and Training Recurrent Neural Networks—With an Erratum Note*; GMD Technical Report 148; German National Research Center for Information Technology: Bonn, Germany, 2001; p. 13.
163. Jaeger, H. Echo state network. *Scholarpedia* **2007**, *2*, 2330. [CrossRef]
164. Jaeger, H.; Haas, H. Harnessing nonlinearity: Predicting chaotic systems and saving energy in wireless communication. *Science* **2004**, *304*, 78–80. [CrossRef] [PubMed]
165. Jaeger, H.; Lukoševičius, M.; Popovici, D.; Siewert, U. Optimization and applications of echo state networks with leaky-integrator neurons. *Neural Netw.* **2007**, *20*, 335–352. [CrossRef]
166. Hyndman, R.; Athanasopoulos, G. *Forecasting: Principles and Practice*; OTexts: Melbourne, VIC, Australia, 2021; Volume 1.

167. Domingos, P. Occam's Two Razors: The Sharp and the Blunt. In Proceedings of the Fourth International Conference on Knowledge Discovery and Data Mining, New York, NY, USA, 27–31 August 1998; ACM: New York, NY, USA; AAAI Press: Washington, DC, USA, 1998; pp. 37–43.
168. Lin, H.W.; Tegmark, M. Why does deep and cheap learning work so well? *arXiv* **2016**, arXiv:1608.08225.
169. Busseti, E.; Osband, I.; Wong, S. *Deep Learning for Time Series Modeling*; Technical Report; Stanford University: Stanford, CA, USA, 2012.
170. Chatzis, S.P.; Demiris, Y. Echo state Gaussian process. *Neural Netw. IEEE Trans.* **2011**, *22*, 1435–1445. [CrossRef]
171. Shi, Z.; Han, M. Support vector echo-state machine for chaotic time-series prediction. *Neural Netw. IEEE Trans.* **2007**, *18*, 359–372. [CrossRef]

Disclaimer/Publisher's Note: The statements, opinions and data contained in all publications are solely those of the individual author(s) and contributor(s) and not of MDPI and/or the editor(s). MDPI and/or the editor(s) disclaim responsibility for any injury to people or property resulting from any ideas, methods, instructions or products referred to in the content.

MDPI AG
Grosspeteranlage 5
4052 Basel
Switzerland
Tel.: +41 61 683 77 34

Algorithms Editorial Office
E-mail: algorithms@mdpi.com
www.mdpi.com/journal/algorithms

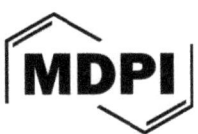

Disclaimer/Publisher's Note: The statements, opinions and data contained in all publications are solely those of the individual author(s) and contributor(s) and not of MDPI and/or the editor(s). MDPI and/or the editor(s) disclaim responsibility for any injury to people or property resulting from any ideas, methods, instructions or products referred to in the content.

www.ingramcontent.com/pod-product-compliance
Lightning Source LLC
LaVergne TN
LVHW070048120526
838202LV00101B/1834